W9-ACX-584

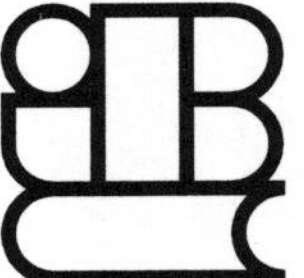

Qualitative Methods in Public Health

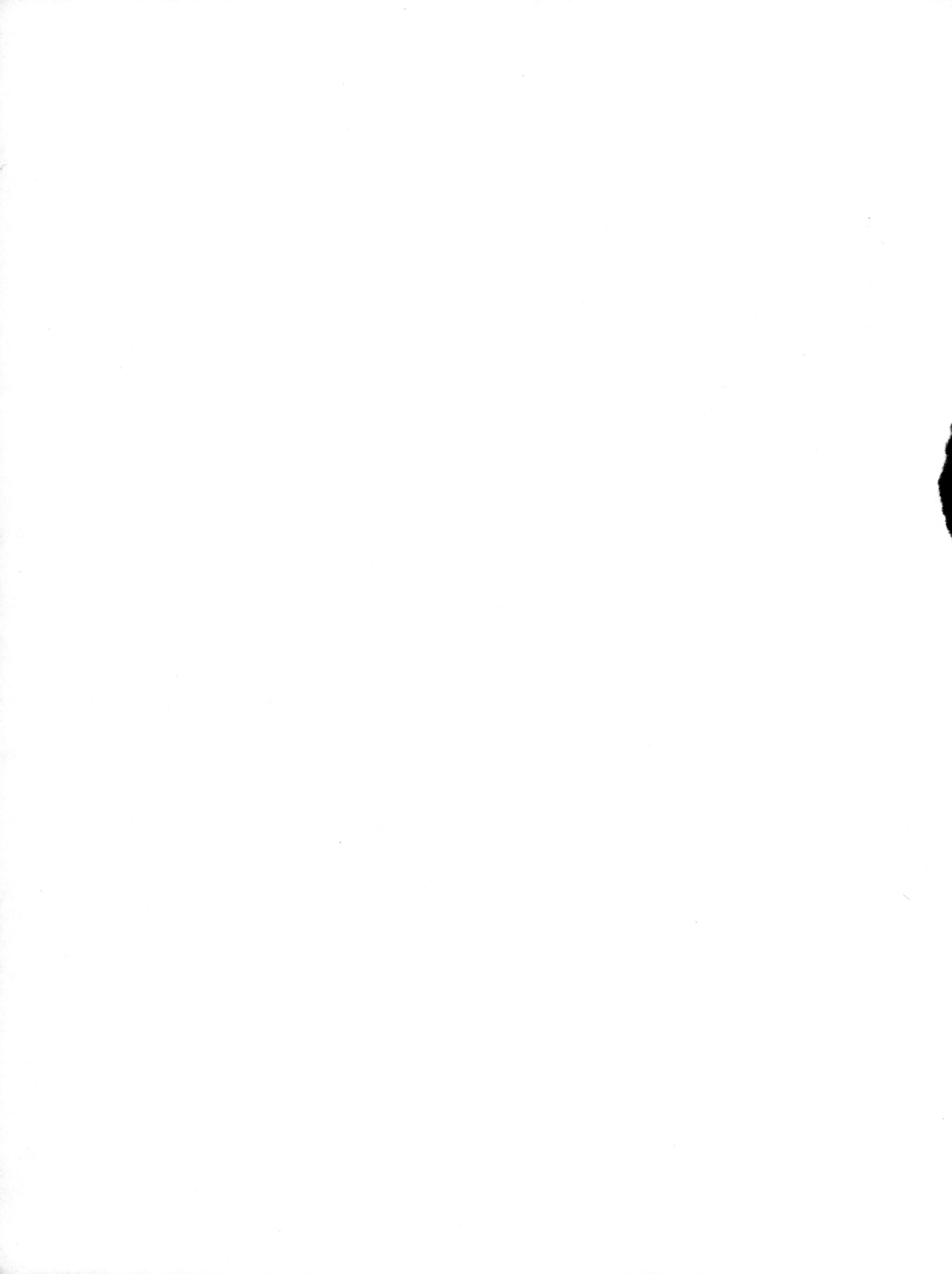

Qualitative Methods in Public Health

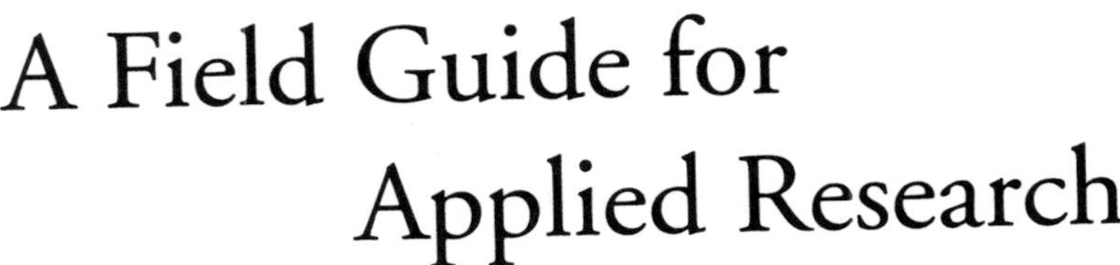

A Field Guide for Applied Research

Priscilla R. Ulin

Elizabeth T. Robinson

Elizabeth E. Tolley

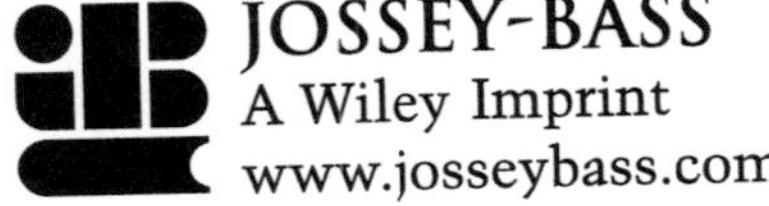

Published by Jossey-Bass
A Wiley Imprint
989 Market Street, San Francisco, CA 94103-1741 www.josseybass.com

Jossey-Bass books and products are available through most bookstores. To contact Jossey-Bass directly call our Customer Care Department within the U.S. at 800-956-7739, outside the U.S. at 317-572-3986 or fax 317-572-4002.

Jossey-Bass also publishes its books in a variety of electronic formats. Some content that appears in print may not be available in electronic books.

Library of Congress Cataloging-in-Publication Data

Ulin, Priscilla R.
Qualitative methods in public health: a field guide for applied research / Priscilla R. Ulin, Elizabeth T. Robinson, Elizabeth E. Tolley; foreword by Allan Steckler.—1st ed.
p.; cm.
Includes bibliographical references and index.
ISBN 0-7879-7634-2 (alk. paper)
1. Public health—Research—Methodology. 2. Qualitative research.
[DNLM: 1. Public Health. 2. Qualitative Research. 3. Research Design. WA 20.5 U39q 2004]
I. Robinson, Elizabeth T. II. Tolley, Elizabeth E. III. Title.
RA440.85.U43 2004
362.1'072—dc22 2004015978

Printed in the United States of America
FIRST EDITION
PB Printing 10 9 8 7 6 5 4 3 2 1

Contents

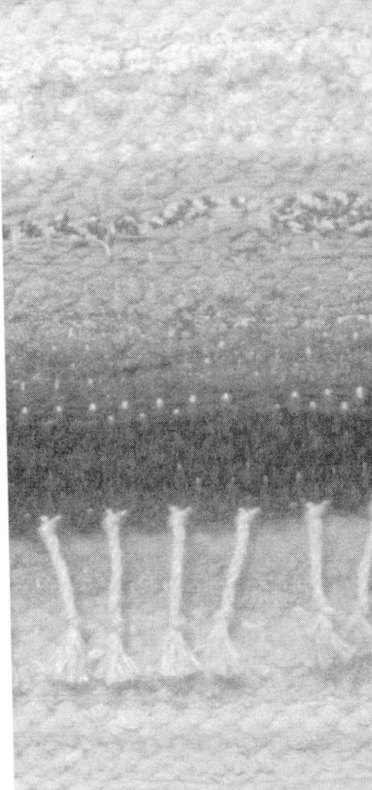

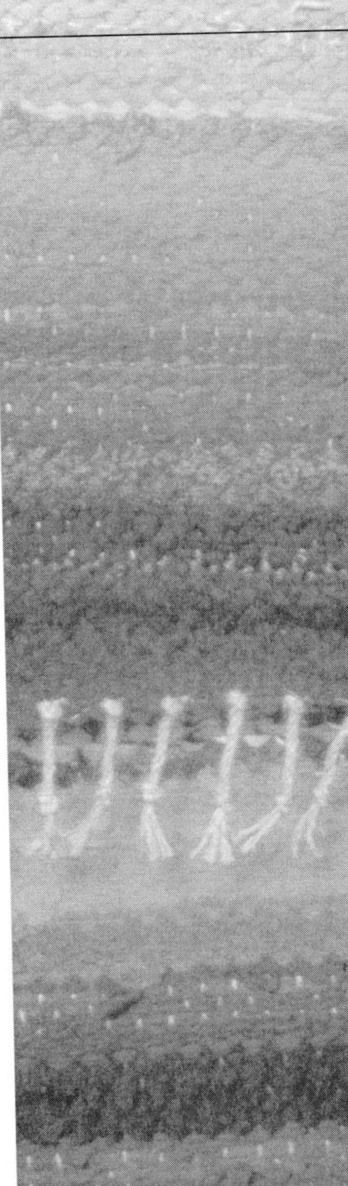

List of Boxes

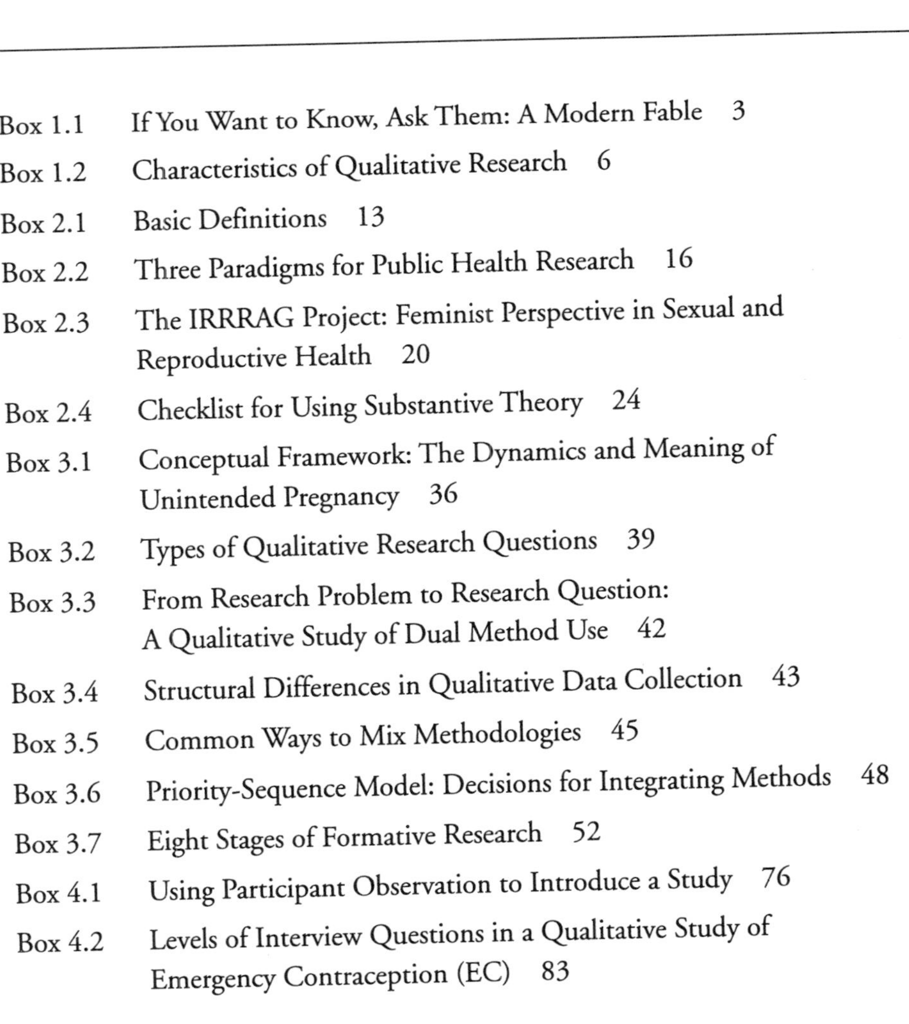

List of Field Perspectives

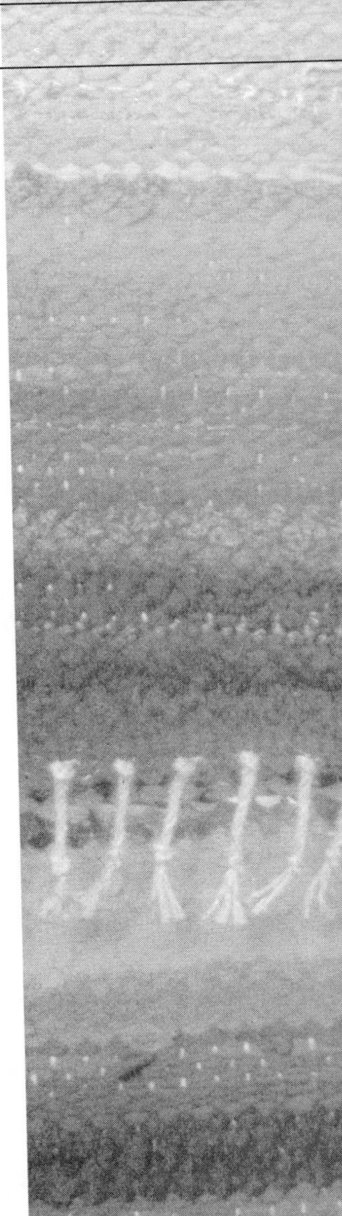

Foreword

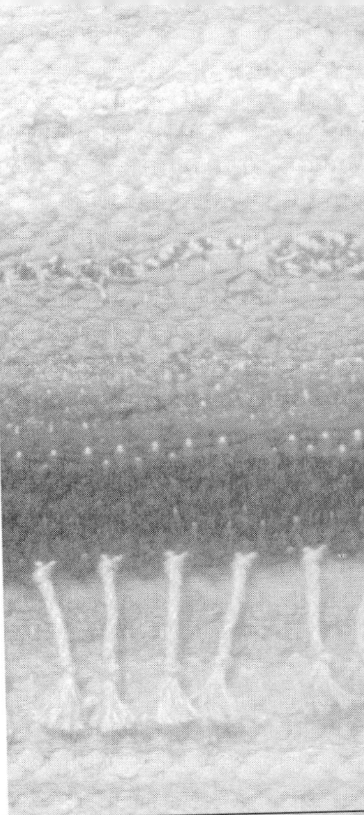

Allan Steckler, Dr.P.H.

University of North Carolina, Chapel Hill

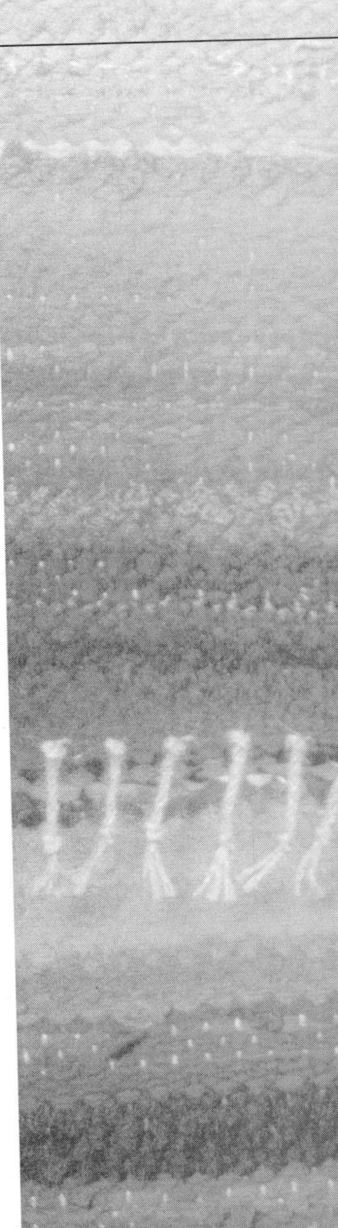

OVER THE LAST SEVERAL DECADES, there has been increasing recognition of complex forces that contribute to the public's health—factors that interact at individual, family, community, population, and policy levels. Social, economic, political, ethnic, environmental, and genetic factors all are associated with today's public health concerns. Public health problems are complex, not only because of their multicausality but also as a result of new and emerging domestic and international health problems. Consequently, public health practitioners and researchers recognize the need for multiple approaches to understanding problems and developing effective interventions that address contemporary public health issues.

Qualitative methods fill a gap in the public health toolbox; they help us understand underlying behaviors, attitudes, perceptions, and culture in a way that quantitative methods alone cannot. Qualitative methods are particularly suited to understanding the *how* and *why* questions. Similarly, qualitative results help us understand social, political, and economic factors associated with contemporary and emerging health problems. They also can be useful in understanding facilitators and barriers to the implementation of new public health programs. For all these reasons, qualitative methods are getting renewed attention and gaining new respect in public health.

Qualitative investigators apply anthropological research methods to study social, cultural, and health phenomena. Researchers using qualitative methods immerse themselves in a culture or group by observing its people and their interactions, often participating in activities, interviewing key people, taking life histories, constructing case studies, and analyzing existing documents or other cultural artifacts. The qualitative researcher's goal is to attain an insider's view of the group under study. For public health purposes, an insider's view tells us how people perceive and react to a given health problem and what interventions are most likely to be successful.

Qualitative methods are naturalistic in that they apply to real-world situations as they unfold naturally. They tend to be nonmanipulative, unobtrusive, and noncontrolling. Qualitative approaches often rely on personal contact over some period of time between the researcher and the group being studied. Building a partnership with study participants can lead to deeper insight into the context under study, adding richness and depth to the data. Thus, qualitative methods are inductive, that is, oriented toward discovery and process, have high validity, are less concerned with generalizability, and are more concerned with deeper understanding of the research problem in its unique context.

Qualitative data consist of narratives produced from open-ended interviews with key informants, individuals, and groups, as well as the researcher's field notes and other documents. Qualitative research usually produces a large amount of such textual data. Fortunately, we now have available a number of computer programs that assist in the analysis of qualitative data. Learning how to use such programs is an important skill for those who conduct applied public health qualitative research.

I have taught a qualitative research and evaluation methods course to graduate students in a school of public health for the past 12 years. During that time I used several different textbooks from disciplines other than public health, for example, anthropology and education. Although these books were excellent in their explanations of how to conduct qualitative research, they lacked public health application. For the past 3 years, however, I have been fortunate to have access to prepublication copies of *Qualitative Methods in Public Health: A Field Guide for Applied Research.* After an extensive search and review of a number of qualitative texts, my coteacher (Dr. Margaret Bentley) and I selected this book for several reasons. First, we found that the organization of the book follows very closely the units in our course, that is, overview, purposes, and rationale for qualitative methods; how to plan qualitative studies, how to collect qualitative data through field observations; individual and group interviews; how to use key informants; how to analyze qualitative data; and how to present qualitative study findings. This book gives a clear explanation of the purpose and reasons for each step in the research process, explains how to implement the step, and presents relevant examples and applications.

We also chose the book because of its clear links to public health practice and research. Our graduate students come from a number of disciplines, including health education, nutrition, maternal and child health, epidemiology, and health policy and administration. This textbook helps these students understand not only how to conduct good qualitative research but how to apply it in familiar settings. As the reader will discover, in comparison to other texts, *Qualitative Methods in Public Health* is relatively brief. Its conciseness is another strength of the book that we appreciate, because it allows us to supplement its use as a course text with relevant journal articles, while at the same time keeping the amount of assigned reading at a reasonable level. We also like the inclusion of Field Perspectives, examples that illustrate important methodological points. Such examples increase the "readability" of the text for students.

The students in our course are interested in both domestic and international public health problems. Some have previous international experience and clearly intend to pursue careers in global health, but others will work in the United States. Although the examples presented in the book often have international origins, they are applicable to both domestic and international settings. Seeing how qualitative methods can be conducted in different contexts is, for many students, an important benefit.

In addition to its value for researchers, this book is also an excellent resource for practitioners. It truly is a field guide, giving at each step of the qualitative research process clear explanations of why and how to conduct that step. It is a field guide also in the sense that examples throughout the text come from contemporary field experience. A practitioner with limited qualitative experience can read the book, or relevant parts of it, and begin to apply new techniques to everyday problem-solving.

In short, *Qualitative Methods in Public Health* makes a unique and important contribution to public health research and practice in both domestic and international settings. This book will be useful for anyone in public health embarking on a research project that would benefit from a qualitative approach.

March 2004

Erin T. McNeill, Ph.D.
1966–2003

Our book is dedicated to Dr. Erin T. McNeill, a friend and colleague whose vision helped us conceptualize and define the earlier edition, Qualitative Methods: A Field Guide for Applied Research in Sexual and Reproductive Health. *Erin saw the qualitative research enterprise as a tapestry—a fabric woven from threads of many textures and colors. The cover of the book is a tribute to her vision, reflecting the diverse lives and experiences of the people whose stories are told through qualitative research. Dedicated to the highest principles of social justice, Erin worked selflessly to expose human need, challenge stereotypes, and promote equity on all levels. She was a gifted teacher, a brilliant young theorist and researcher, and a devoted wife and loving mother. She left this world too soon.*

Preface

Shireen J. Jejeebhoy
Population Council, India

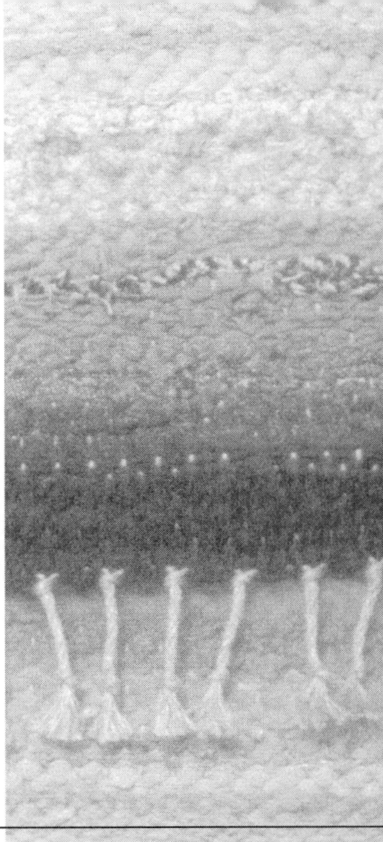

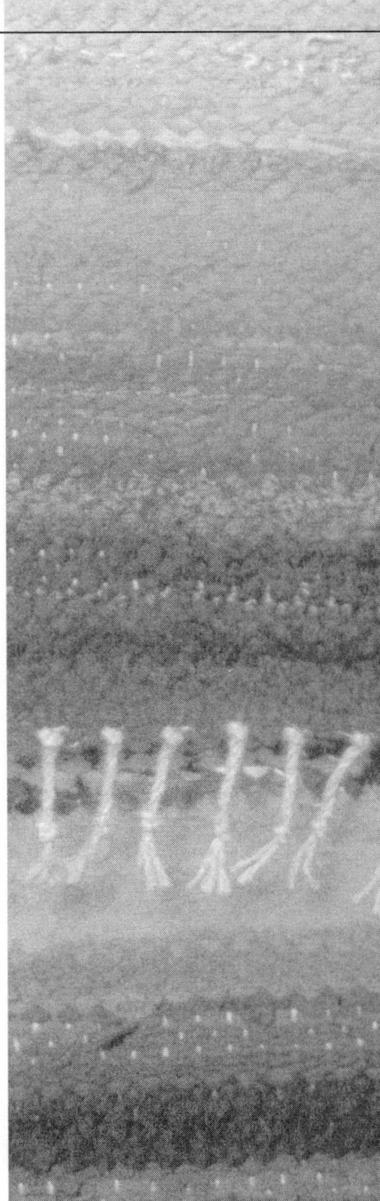

WHEN THE CENTRAL OBJECTIVES of an inquiry are to explore and explain behavior rather than to describe it, when the subject matter is unfamiliar and insufficiently researched, or when a suitable vocabulary with which to communicate with respondents is not available, researchers are well advised to address their research questions through the use of qualitative methods. Investigation into many social and behavioral aspects of public health fall into one or another of these categories and hence frequently call for qualitative designs. The potential contributions of this approach to research are many. Qualitative design can lead us to underlying behaviors, attitudes, and perceptions that determine health outcomes; it can help us explain social and programmatic impediments to informed choice or the use of services; it can shed light on the success of our interventions; and it can facilitate better understanding of the policy, social, and legal contexts in which health choices are made. Furthermore, qualitative design is flexible, encouraging discovery and further investigation of the unexpected. The value of combining qualitative and structured survey methods in a single design and allowing each to inform and reinforce the other cannot be sufficiently stressed.

Qualitative Methods in Public Health: A Field Guide for Applied Research fills an enormous need. Despite the merits of qualitative research, the field has thus far lacked comprehensive guidelines for planning and conducting qualitative research in health and behavior, including but not limited to sexual and reproductive health. The contexts in which health decisions are made, their antecedents and consequences, and the insights they provide us for program development are now within reach of public health researchers with access to this work. The volume presents practical strategies and methods for using qualitative research, along with the basic logic and rationale for qualitative research decisions. With its user-friendly but rigorous approach, this guide makes researchers aware of the complexities, advantages, and limitations of qualitative methods. Its eight chapters cover a wide range of topics and guide readers through every phase of research—from defining the language and logic of qualitative research to study design, data collection, analysis, interpretation, and even dissemination.

One strength of this book is that many of the examples are drawn from the field of sexual and reproductive health, allowing the reader to view aspects of decision making in research through the focused lens of one cross-cutting public health topic. *Qualitative Methods in Public Health* emphasizes the importance of addressing gender issues in research on sexual and reproductive health and describes in practical ways how to incorporate a gender focus. The guide provides useful examples where needed and contains insightful views by a range of experts who share their experiences and perspectives on qualitative research themes. It is systematically organized and attractively presented, enabling readers to access material that responds to their particular interests and research needs.

Although written largely in nonacademic language, the guide conveys the complexities of solid qualitative research and dispels any hopes that qualitative research is simple, quick, or easy to conduct. It is clear that the authors do not intend this guide to be an introductory research text. Rather, they intend it to be for those with formal training in the social sciences or those who are experienced in the practice of research and interested in expanding their repertoire to include qualitative methods. It complements *Social Science Methods for Research on Reproductive Health,* a guide that the World Health Organization's Special Programme of Research, Development and Research Training in Human Reproduction published in 1999 (Campbell et al. 1999).

The volume will undoubtedly make a mark. It appears at a time when the field of public health is asking new and difficult questions on factors underlying risk behaviors that require qualitative explanations. It provides researchers with the tools to make realistic decisions on complex research questions, highlights the value of building the capacity for qualitative research within research teams, and describes ways in which to promote dissemination and timely utilization of study findings.

The authors bring a range of strengths and experiences in international health and have produced a cogent and instructive, yet elegantly and clearly written, guide. *Qualitative Methods in Public Health* is essential reading for researchers interested in explaining many kinds of health behavior and understanding program effectiveness. I am confident that the volume will contribute to the generation of new and sound information on, and explanations of, critical areas related to population, health, and disease—including reproductive choice, sexual risk and protection, and gender relations. It merits wide dissemination.

Acknowledgments

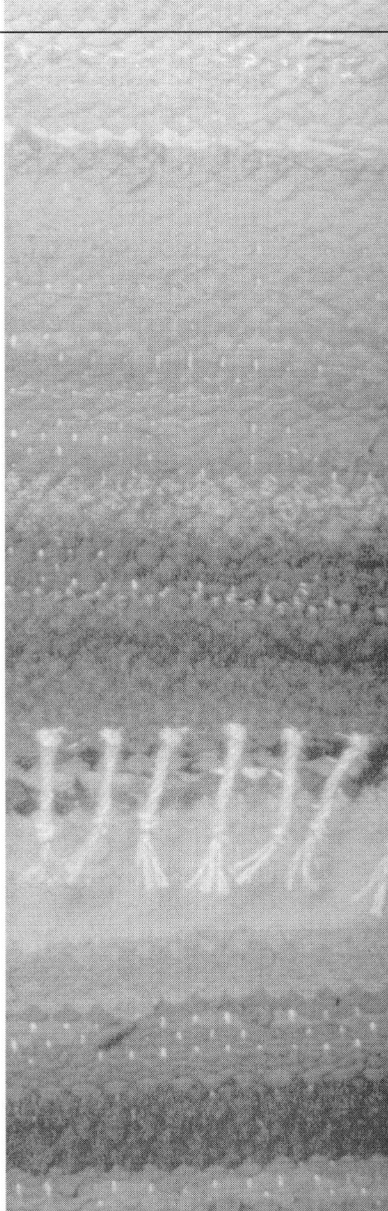

IT TAKES A VILLAGE to raise a child, and as we have experienced with this field guide, it takes a community of colleagues, friends, and scholars to capture new and old wisdom in a useful text. We thank each contributor for participation, large or small, in the process that has taken this effort from the initial spark to a printed book. Antonio Machado (1997) wrote, "Se hace el camino al andar" (paths are made by walking), and we have appreciated your presence, your questions, and the challenges your ideas have posed as this field guide has evolved to completion.

We would like to thank the many people at the U.S. Agency for International Development (USAID), CARE International, the Horizons Program, the MEASURE Project, and Mothercare, who shaped the content and form of this guide through their responses to the needs assessment Family Health International (FHI) conducted in preparation. USAID colleagues who offered advice include Dr. Felice Apter, Dr. Paul Delay, Dr. Duff Gillespie, Dr. Sarah Harbison, Dr. Laurie Krieger, Dr. Jeffrey Spieler, and Dr. Patricia Stephenson. USAID's Office of Population provided funding for the development and publication of an earlier version of this guide; we hope their confidence in our approach and the material support expressed in their decision is justified by the results. In particular, Dr. Harbison's commitment to develop a tool to help researchers apply qualitative methods to the study of reproductive health was pivotal in the development of this field guide.

Our panel of expert reviewers provided detailed critiques of the guide, improved the conceptual and technical mettle of the work, and challenged us to address the practical constraints and information needs of researchers new to qualitative methods. We thank Dr. Sarah Harbison (USAID), Drs. Valerie J. and Terence H. Hull (Australia National University, Canberra), Dr. Shireen J. Jejeebhoy (The Population Council,

India), Dr. John Knodel (University of Michigan, Ann Arbor), Dr. Kate MacQueen (Family Health International, Research Triangle Park, North Carolina); Dr. Susan Paulson (Miami University, Oxford, Ohio), Dr. Lawrence J. Severy (Family Health International), and Dr. Cynthia Woodsong (Family Health International). We deeply appreciate their insights, thoughtfulness, and candor. Our respect for their knowledge and experience is immeasurable.

Scientists at FHI who read and commented on early drafts challenged our assumptions, debated our conclusions, and helped us sharpen our perspective on the meanings of qualitative methods for applied research. Among these valued colleagues, Dr. Cynthia Woodsong stuck by us all the way—encouraging, critiquing, and sometimes adding her own articulate words to bring a message closer to the reader. In the end, it was Dr. Natasha Mack who rode with us over the finish line, helping us shape the final draft with judgment and precision.

We are no less grateful to the authors of the Field Perspectives. By sharing their rich experiences in qualitative research, these experts made sure that chapters in the book would match challenges in the field.

FHI staff without whose help we could not have compiled this guide include librarians Mr. William Barrows, who wrote a section on cataloguing information in qualitative research reports, and Ms. Carol Manion and Ms. Margaret Shiels, whose library and online reference skills have brought readers a wealth of valuable qualitative research literature. We thank Ms. Laura Johnson, too, for her early help organizing materials into electronic files and for advising us on software. Other staff too numerous to mention by name provided countless hours of gracious assistance in organizing materials, correcting our errors, typing and formatting, assembling text, corresponding with reviewers and contributors, and keeping on track. Ms. Karen Dickerson and Ms. Michele Lanham deserve our gratitude for the management of text revisions for this edition.

Mr. Andy Pasternack, Ms. Gigi Mark, and Ms. Sarah Miller, our ever-patient editors at Jossey-Bass, have our heartfelt thanks for being the best editors we have ever had.

Finally, we thank our families for supporting our work—Alan, Noah, and Zoë Dehmer; Mark, Elise, and Kyle Healy; and Richard, Don, and Marjorie Ulin and their families. They hold a special place in our hearts for listening to our stories, making do with our absences, and sharing in our excitement as we put it all into words.

Priscilla R. Ulin
Elizabeth T. Robinson
Elizabeth E. Tolley

Qualitative Methods in Public Health

text n. 1. original words of author [especially as opposed to paraphrase of or commentary on them . . . from Latin *textus,* tissue, literary style (in medieval Latin = Gospel); from Latin *textere* text—weave]

textile a & n 1. a. of weaving . . . woven, suitable for weaving, (textile fabrics, materials). 2. n. textile material; any cloth . . .

textual a. of or in the text . . .

texture a. & v. t. 1. arrangement of threads, etc. in textile fabric, characteristic feel due to this; arrangement of small constituent parts, perceived structure (of skin, rock, soil, organic tissue, literary work, etc.); representation of structure and detail of objects in art . . . 2. v.t. make by weaving; provide with texture [from Latin textura weaving] . . .

The words *text, textile,* and *texture* all share the same root; and their definitions have in common the notion of things interwoven—threads, ideas, or themes. The core material of qualitative research is the fabric of social life, and what emerges from qualitative research is very often text of one kind or another. Qualitative methods elicit narratives and discourse expressed as text, essentially stories. To tell a good story is to spin a fine yarn. The regular weaving and textual metaphors are not an accident in qualitative methods work. Social history can be interpreted as cloth with a warp and a weft made up of different threads, interlocking to produce a structure that is stronger and more permanent than its constituents. The pattern is often unique yet nevertheless recognizable. Counting the number and color of threads, or detailing the composition of the yarn alone, does not enable the observer to see the whole image that the final fabric produces in context.

The work of the qualitative researcher is to interpret the pattern or texture of that text—to discern the inherent pattern in the expressed ideas or images and actions. The art of qualitative research involves both weaving together the ideas and words of study participants and seeing or revealing to others the structure of the social fabric and its characteristics or "feel." Qualitative research is a means of looking at and better understanding life's rich tapestry to reach insights into the human heart and mind.

Source: Adapted from J. B. Sykes, ed., *The Concise Oxford Dictionary of Current English* (7th ed.; Oxford: Clarendon Press, 1982).

CHAPTER ONE

Invitation to Explore

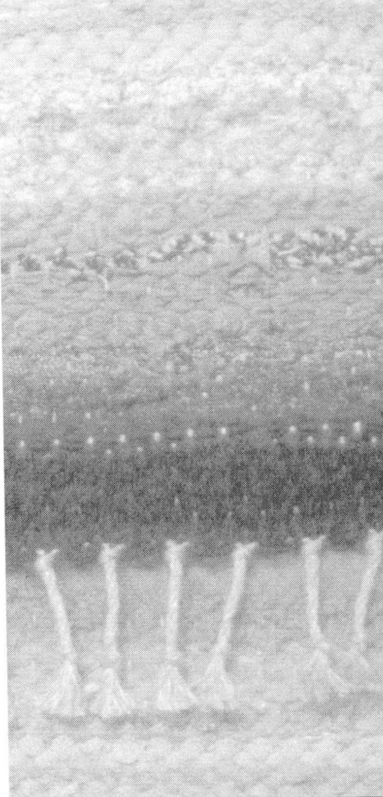

WHY DO SOME PROGRAMS succeed and others fail? Why are screening programs underused? Why does chronic disease go untreated? Why do countless couples know how to protect themselves from sexually transmitted infection but do not do so? How does a community mobilize itself to solve a persistent health problem? Questions like these may be all too familiar to readers of this field guide—public health practitioners, researchers, and program planners, many of whom have worked for years to protect health and prevent disease in highly vulnerable populations.

The field of public health is full of puzzling questions, complicated relationships, and slowly evolving events—phenomena leaving gaps in understanding that invite qualitative methods to fill.
(Rubin and Rubin 1995, p. 51)

Advances in the biomedical and population sciences have brought the means to better health within reach of people around the world. Yet evidence of escalating disease and inadequate health resources in many countries tell us that there is still much we do not know. How do women and men understand and actually use the technical information they receive to make critical decisions that affect their lives and their children's lives? By opening windows on cultural understandings of health and disease, methods of qualitative research can help us comprehend some of these old problems in new ways.

Our Purpose

The purpose of this book is to make the methods of qualitative science more accessible to researchers and practitioners challenged by problems that affect the public's health. The reader will observe that many of our illustrations are taken from the field of sexual and reproductive health–family planning, risk associated with sexually transmitted infection (STI) including HIV/AIDS, issues in adolescent pregnancy, and numerous instances of related decision making about health, sometimes in highly sensitive contexts. The first edition of this book, published under the title *Qualitative Methods: A Field Guide for Applied Research in Sexual and Reproductive Health* (Ulin and others 2002), was developed by staff at Family Health International, a nonprofit international public health organization, for developing country researchers in maternal and child health, health education, community medicine, nursing, and the applied social sciences. Our many years of experience with colleagues in these countries, working to understand the critical problems they face in AIDS prevention and reproductive health, showed clearly the need for a practical but comprehensive field guide for qualitative exploration. Since then, readers from other fields of public health and other parts of the world have told us that many of the principles and problems inherent in reproductive decisions and STI prevention also apply to their research and practice in other areas. Some have contributed examples from their own experience with qualitative methods, further expanding the applicability of this edition to a wide range of social and behavioral health problems.

We write not only for the qualitative researcher but for applied social scientists, epidemiologists, health providers, health educators, program managers, and others whose training and experience may be predominantly in quantitative methods. Our readers will be students as well as seasoned professionals looking for ways to probe more deeply the *whys* and *hows* of questions they may partially have answered in terms of *how much* and *how many.* They will want to know what qualitative methods can offer to improve their practice or strengthen their research findings. And many of our readers will be training others to ask the same kinds of questions, to listen, and to observe.

Numerous disciplines have contributed to the phenomenal growth of public health. Sociology, anthropology, psychology, economics, demography, medicine, and nursing, among others, have brought their unique perspectives and methods to a multidisciplinary understanding of health and wellness. Parallel advances in these disciplines have resulted in different ways of conceptualizing and addressing issues as diverse as health decision making, health promotion, child survival, compliance, substance abuse, adolescent sexuality, domestic violence, and gender relations. Similar progress in service delivery research and evaluation have given us a broader understanding of providers' knowledge and values, client-provider communication, and issues related to the accessibility and quality of health care for populations at risk.

Much of this work has focused on objective questions, such as numbers of births, patterns of contraceptive use, trends in disease prevalence, and numerous factors that predict health behavioral outcomes. Research designs traditionally have been quantitative, describing measurable phenomena, projecting trends, and sometimes discovering causal relationships. Psychological research in health behavior has developed primarily from a quantitative perspective, contributing useful rating scales and behavioral indicators, along with case study methods and tools for observation. Anthropologists and qualitative sociologists have approached some of the same problems from different perspectives, focusing on cultural norms and relationships that influence how people interact and act on everyday experiences (Bernard 1995; Knodel 1997). Their meth-

BOX 1.1

If You Want to Know, Ask Them: A Modern Fable

A country plagued with high rates of STI and low condom use invited a team of experts to introduce a new contraceptive option: the female condom. This new barrier device, they argued, was an effective alternative to the male condom and would at last give women the control they needed to protect themselves or their partners against infection.

Working with local counterparts, the team initiated a program to strengthen STI prevention and treatment services, inform people about the female condom, train providers in its use, stock the shelves of clinics and dispensaries, and recruit lay outreach workers to carry the message to women in the communities. Six months later, encouraging results showed that rates of infection had dropped; women and men were indeed seeking treatment for STI symptoms. Twelve months later, treatment rates were still up, but rates of new infection were not declining as expected.

The team was forced to conclude that introduction of the female condom was not a cost-effective strategy because it had little sustained impact on the incidence of STI. The team leader, however, began to suspect that there might be more to the story. She invited a social scientist with qualitative research skills to investigate further the failure of the female condom to lower STI rates. This researcher designed a follow-up study that used in-depth interviews, focus groups, and clinic observation to explore the meaning of the new device to different community groups. He and his trained interviewers soon learned that clinicians were not distributing the female condom because they feared being accused of lacing the condoms with HIV virus—a rumor that was circulating in the community. Data from providers about the popular belief that the female condom could carry HIV were reinforced by comments from women in the communities. Talking with women revealed that most women knew about the method but did not ask for it, believing that providers (who rarely suggested it) either did not have it or thought it was ineffective or even dangerous.

In both men's and women's focus groups, participants discussed what the female condom meant to them. Men were candid in their criticism of giving women control over pregnancy and therefore license to engage in extramarital affairs. They surprised the researchers with their anger at a program that "encouraged promiscuity" while claiming to promote reproductive health. Some even questioned the motives of women "who would want to collect a man's semen" in a condom. Against a backdrop of cultural beliefs in the power of witchcraft to bring harm to one's enemies, men's anxiety concerning illicit use of the female condom was a serious and understandable obstacle to the program.

Women felt caught between program messages urging them to try the female condom and partner resistance. Although most were attracted to the idea of independent protection, they also understood that control carried its own risks. By accepting the female condom, they possibly would trade the risk of infection for the risk of abandonment by partners who could accuse them of infidelity.

Listening to people tell how they made their decisions gave program developers the information they needed to understand and address specific social and cultural issues in female condom promotion. But even more important was the realization that the forces motivating sexual and reproductive decisions are complex and often more powerful than competing health promotion messages. We may not know why some programs succeed and others fail, but the simple lesson from this situation is that if you want to understand how and why people make the decisions they do, ask them.

ods rely primarily on techniques of observation, participation, guided discussion, in-depth interviewing, life histories, and secondary analysis of documentary data.

Yet there is much overlap among different disciplinary approaches. Quantitative researchers at times use qualitative methods to guide a sampling design or to develop a sensitive data collection tool. Anthropologists and qualitative sociologists turn to quantitative methods when they want to describe a population or measure some tendency they may have observed qualitatively. Quantitative research with representative samples can produce hard, factual, reliable outcome data that usually are generalizable to wider populations (Steckler and others 1992). But most quantitative studies lack contextual detail and reflect a limited range of responses (Carey 1993). On the other hand, qualitative methods elicit rich, contextual data, but their small samples and flexible design usually are not appropriate if the study objective is to describe larger populations with statistical accuracy (Patton 1990). As a result, researchers increasingly are exploring creative new ways to combine techniques, letting the strengths of one method compensate for the limitations of another to yield a more powerful methodology (Wolff and others 1991).

We have written this guide not to promote one methodology over another, but because many quantitatively trained health professionals, policymakers, and researchers are looking for ways to expand their methodological options with new tools for answering difficult questions.

In searching the literature on qualitative research, we found it divided between manuals that summarize specific techniques for designing and conducting health-related studies (Yoddumnern-Attig and others 1993; Hudelson 1996; Campbell and others 1999) and more comprehensive texts for general academic audiences (Denzin and Lincoln 2000; Patton 1990; Rossman and Rallis 1998). Missing from most manuals was a theoretical basis for qualitative decisions, and few texts included strategies to address practical health research issues and problems that arise in the field. Nor did we find clear guidelines for dealing with the large volume of transcripts that qualitative data collection on sensitive topics often generates. Another gap in the literature was the lack of direction for writing and disseminating qualitative results. Our intent, therefore, is to show first how qualitative methods can shed new light on perplexing questions and second to provide basic skills to design, conduct, and disseminate the research.

What Is Qualitative Research?

A challenge to the author of any book on qualitative research is to answer the commonsense question: What is it? Although there is no short, comprehensive definition, the unique organizing framework is a theoretical and methodological focus on complex relations between (1) personal and social meanings, (2) individual and cultural practices, and (3) the material environment or context. Similarly, there is no universal blueprint for doing qualitative research, but the availability of rigorous methods for qualitative inquiry can take us down many rewarding paths to understanding life in ways that consider the perspectives and experiences of people who live it. Note that although qualitative analysis can answer questions about how people make sense of the world, it also can address many objective dimensions of human action and interaction, relating these findings to the contexts in which they occur.

Many problems central to public health research and practice are deeply embedded in their cultural contexts. People in communities confront decisions and challenges that are conditioned by membership in multiple social groups—whether or not to use contraception, how to get through pregnancy and childbirth safely, where to go for help in times of illness, and how to give young people the skills and confidence they will need for healthy adulthood. Contradictions and competing priorities can make many seemingly commonplace decisions difficult: Spend money on prescription drugs or save for retirement? Protect oneself from sexually transmitted infection and risk losing the attention and economic support of a sexual partner or accept the risk of disease? Running through the fabric of economic, sexual, and reproductive lives is the pervasive influence of gender, a theme that resonates in the voices of the women and men in our research.

Qualitative researchers seek answers to their questions in the real world. They gather what they see, hear, and read from people and places and from events and activities. . . . their purpose is to learn about some aspect of the social world and to generate new understandings that can be used by that social world.

(Rossman and Rallis 1998, p. 5)

The fact that people differ in the ways they interpret—and consequently act on—ordinary situations has profound implications for health research. If it is true that what people define as real is real in its consequences (Thomas and Thomas 1929), then applied behavioral research in public health must have the capacity to uncover multiple perspectives and understand their implications for health decision making. Qualitative researchers have taken seriously this charge, with the result that we now have at our disposal powerful techniques for "hearing data" (Rubin and Rubin 1995, p. 12), listening to what people are saying about their own lives in their own words.

Qualitative researchers know that there are always at least two key players: the participant who contributes the information and the researcher who, as learner and co-interpreter, guides the process toward the understanding that both seek to articulate. Together they form a partnership for exploring different social understandings of reality. Creating a qualitative research partnership requires a high level of skill. It also carries with it profound ethical obligations, because the relationship is based on trust and mutual understanding of a common goal.

Application of Research to Action

We have chosen to focus on applied research because it informs action and enhances decision making on practical issues, unlike basic research, which is conducted to generate theory and produces knowledge for its own end. Although applied research can add immeasurably to our understanding of human behavior, its outcomes are "judged by their effectiveness in helping policymakers, practitioners, and the participants themselves make decisions and act to improve the human condition" (Rossman and Rallis 1998, p. 6). Most well-designed qualitative studies have elements of both the basic and the applied, because rigorous applied research has a theoretical base, and scholars ground their theory in concrete findings. Unfortunately, however, too many examples of hastily constructed qualitative research attempt to apply faulty findings to policy or program issues.

BOX 1.2

Characteristics of Qualitative Research

- Asks why, how, and under what circumstance things occur
- Seeks depth of understanding
- Views social phenomena holistically
- Explores and discovers
- Provides insight into the meanings of decisions and actions
- Uses interpretive and other open-ended methods
- Is iterative rather than fixed
- Is emergent rather than prestructured
- Involves respondents as active participants rather than subjects
- Defines the investigator as an instrument in the research process

Such studies often have an inadequate theoretical base or use data collection techniques that are inappropriate to the purpose of the research. These misguided efforts do not constitute science and seldom contribute significantly to solutions to problems.

At least three important developments are fueling the demand for qualitative expertise in the international health arena:

- Advances in cross-cultural understanding of health and health-related behavior
- Global health patterns
- Increased awareness of issues in human rights

Discussion of these items follows.

ADVANCES IN CROSS-CULTURAL UNDERSTANDING OF HEALTH AND HEALTH-RELATED BEHAVIOR

Sophisticated quantitative methods have produced an extensive base of knowledge for understanding such phenomena as population growth, disease patterns, and many aspects of human behavior that are determinants of health and sickness. But each new finding leads to more questions and new research problems that often require a different approach to data collection and analysis. For example, knowing the contraceptive prevalence rate in a population leads us to ask why fertility is still high in some sectors. Or with the wide availability of primary health care services, we must ask why so many potentially serious diseases continue to go undetected in their early stages. Qualitative methods are adding a new dimension to the ongoing search for answers to these and other complex questions.

Designs for quantitative surveys increasingly are incorporating qualitative techniques in an effort to improve the validity of interview tools through better understanding of the language and perspectives of study populations. Hearing participants' customary language for sexual issues helps the survey researcher compose standardized items in familiar words or prestructure response categories from actual experience. Program planners too are finding that participation of local people in collecting qualitative data and analyzing local problems leads to more relevant programs and a greater sense of community ownership. In Zambia, for example, CARE International used a participatory approach to design a peer outreach program, the Partnership for Adolescent and Sexual Reproductive Health Project, to reduce sexual health risk among periurban adolescents. The active participation of young people and others in in-depth interviewing was instrumental in the design of the project and its successful implementation (Shah 1999).

GLOBAL HEALTH PATTERNS

Demographic and health statistics speak to the urgent need for solutions to public health problems everywhere. Growing health disparities between rich and poor countries highlight different research needs. In the United States, tobacco use, poor diet and physical inactivity, and alcohol consumption together account for roughly one-third of total deaths (Mokdad and others 2004). In the poorest areas of the world, preventable and treatable diseases, such as diarrhea, measles, and malaria, take a heavy toll on human life. In Africa alone more than 2.3 million people die from vaccine-preventable diseases annually (Carr 2004). Complications of pregnancy, childbirth, and unsafe abortion claim the lives of over five hundred thousand women every year, 99 percent of them in developing countries (World Health Organization 1996). In sixteen sub-Saharan African countries, more than 10 percent of fifteen- to forty-nine-year-olds are infected with HIV; and in the hardest-hit countries, the toll exceeds one-third of the population (UNAIDS 2000b). Moreover, many health experts are only just beginning to acknowledge the full impact of social problems like gender-based violence, the feminization of poverty, economic crises, persistent regional conflict and refugee resettlement—all played out in a climate of increasing globalization and overburdened resources. This book illustrates the principles of qualitative research in the context of global health, with reference to social and behavioral determinants of many preventable health problems. Qualitative research is not a solution but rather a route to better understanding of the human condition, with the hope of contributing to more rational decision making for improved health program effectiveness and impact. Given the magnitude of the problems we face, we must use all the tools at our disposal and use them well.

INCREASED AWARENESS OF ISSUES IN HUMAN RIGHTS

International discussion of population and health has brought attention to the need for a new global consensus on population and development, human rights, and gender. There is growing recognition that if we hope to address pressing needs for improved health and social development, we urgently need to understand better the complexities of human behavior. (Among the more widely publicized international gatherings were the International Conference on Population and Development in Cairo in 1994 and the Fourth World Conference on Women in Beijing in 1995.) The desire to probe interrelationships among, for example, health decisions, human rights, gender equity, equality, and empowerment calls for new ways to address old, intractable questions. Investigators from the fields of women's studies and applied disciplines in the social sciences continue to search for better understanding of key developmental processes such as gender socialization and role awareness, raising new questions that invite a more qualitative approach to research.

Concern for the status of women is a critical element in development policy, but human rights and the ethics of inclusion add another dimension. We are seeing a gradual shift of priorities toward new goals for community participation, human rights advocacy, and gender equity, broadly defined. This trend has strengthened research outcomes by influencing how research is conceptualized and conducted. Our research questions are more likely now to include attention to gender relations in reproductive health decision making and to status and power as significant factors in the study of health service delivery. Qualitative methods enable researchers to explore more fully the nature and consequences of gender identities and relations in reproductive health. As they become more aware of the powerful role of status in everyday life, researchers themselves are adopting participatory approaches to research that are consistent with qualitative work. This shift is creating new collaborative relationships with study participants and heightened awareness of the researcher's ethical responsibility in the data collection partnership.

Getting Started

This volume takes you step-by-step through the qualitative research process from its theoretical base to its application in public health problems, with particular emphasis on issues in sexual and reproductive health, and finally to dissemination of findings for program and policy change. Key elements in the process will be interaction and interpretation. By *interaction,* we mean broadly the art and science of asking, observing, listening, reflecting, probing—always with the purpose of engaging people in meaningful dialogue. We advocate qualitative techniques, independent of or in association with quantitative methodology, as a way of discovering how people act and interact in the familiar contexts of their lives. Our purpose is to share what we have learned with other researchers who are similarly committed to systematic policy and program development for healthier and more empowered populations.

The chapters that follow build the qualitative process—understanding, designing, implementing, and using methods to answer questions and solve problems that challenge workers in public health. Chapter Two, The Language and Logic of Qualitative Research, begins with a brief overview of the theoretical basis for qualitative research, emphasizing the practical application of theory to research design and analysis. To help the reader locate qualitative research in the theoretical universe, we review three important paradigms, or theoretical frameworks, that have guided methodological decisions in social and behavioral health research. We emphasize the complementarity of these frameworks and the added value of linking them in well-coordinated designs to solve complex problems. Chapter Two also reviews key qualitative concepts, explaining what they mean and how they are interrelated. We conclude Chapter Two with a discussion of standards for judging the scientific rigor of qualitative research. We maintain that different assumptions and purposes make the criteria for evaluating quality in quantitative and qualitative studies analogous but not interchangeable.

Chapter Three, Designing the Study, reviews the basic steps in research design, from defining the area of inquiry and the purpose and problem of the research to analyzing, writing, and disseminating the findings. We also discuss conceptual and initial frameworks that link concepts and relationships to qualitative data collection strategies. We then review aspects of informed consent that are particularly relevant to qualitative studies, including the ethical responsibility of the researcher in an open-ended interview or discussion. To underscore the point that combining qualitative and quantitative methods can increase the power of the design and result in a more comprehensive understanding of the topic of study, we present a practical strategy for mixed-method design.

Chapter Four, Collecting Qualitative Data: The Science and the Art, describes the principal methods of data collection. We identify three fundamental methods—observation, in-depth interviewing, and focus group discussion. Observation is further divided into nonreactive (including documentary research) and participant observation. Techniques of in-depth interviewing and focus group discussion are presented in detail, along with participatory research methods and other selected structured qualitative approaches: freelisting and pile sorts, photo narrative, storytelling, network analysis, and body mapping. We recommend a semistructured approach to data collection and discuss the construction and use of topic guides.

In Chapter Five, Logistics in the Field, we focus on implementation. This chapter contains practical recommendations for introducing a study; building a research team; working with stakeholders and policymakers; selecting and training data collectors; developing field materials; and recording, transcribing, and translating data.

Chapter Six, Qualitative Data Analysis, is a comprehensive overview in which the reader learns how to process and interpret text using manual methods as well as a coding technique appropriate for conducting computer searches and synthesizing findings. Included in this discussion are some guidelines for analysis of data in mixed-method studies. We then detail the concept of rigor in qualitative studies, showing how qualitative concepts analogous to validity and reliability can be used to judge the findings' trustworthiness. In this chapter we also emphasize the importance of selecting appropriate software for computer text analysis and summarize some of the distinguishing features of several programs in common use.

Chapter Seven, Putting It into Words: Reporting Qualitative Research Results, discusses the steps in writing up qualitative study findings. These steps incorporate ethical norms that govern how we present results, integrate thematic ideas into a meaningful narrative, determine our audiences, and select a presentation format that is both appropriate to the study methods and relevant to potential readers. The chapter offers practical advice on how to organize qualitative findings in written reports, report combined qualitative and quantitative results, and enhance the credibility and communicability of qualitative writing. We include criteria that external reviewers commonly use to evaluate manuscripts.

Chapter Eight, Disseminating Qualitative Research, outlines ways to effectively disseminate and promote the use of results. We suggest some possible outcome indicators for dissemination and use of study findings and challenge researchers to reconsider their roles in planning and implementing dissemination.

Finally, one of our objectives in writing this field guide is simply to share with readers the rewards and frustrations of doing qualitative research. Therefore, we offer numerous examples from our own research and from the practical experiences of others who already have embarked on this journey. Throughout the book you will find short field perspectives written by some of these colleagues. They speak to you from lessons they have learned in their own experiences with qualitative methods, offering stories, ideas, reflections, and advice to help you on your way.

CHAPTER TWO

The Language and Logic of Qualitative Research

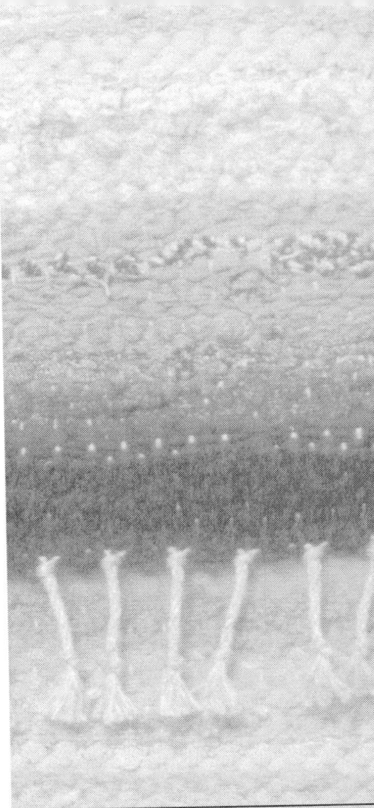

Theories help you locate where your problem lies and where to find likely solutions.

(Smith JB, personal communication with authors, unreferenced)

REPRODUCTIVE HEALTH researchers and practitioners daily confront a myriad of challenging questions. How will a new vaccine be received? What public health messages will young adolescents tempted to try street drugs or alcohol actually hear? How do people make fertility decisions? How can an HIV-negative woman have a safe relationship with an infected partner? It is useful to have an idea of how an innovation will be disseminated, how a group of people will react to a public health message, how couples decide how many children to have, or how a woman will negotiate the use of condoms with her infected partner.

We cannot know for certain how any individual will respond to any of these issues, but if we turn to the lessons learned from countless observations and studies of related human behavior, we begin to have some idea of a range of responses. Thus, we have the beginning of our research questions; and from the set of more general statements from many lessons learned, we develop conceptual and theoretical frameworks. These frameworks provide the logic and the language that guide our research. Through a common understanding of how the world works (or doesn't work), theory provides researchers and practitioners with reference points for understanding human behavior in a more general context.

The purpose of theory in the social sciences is to make sense of the world and to understand and anticipate how people will react to each other and to events. For most applied researchers in public health, the test of a good theory is how well it helps us define our research problems, design our studies, and produce useful results.

At a minimum, *theory* can be defined as a scientific but tentative statement of relationships among diverse phenomena. A quantitative research problem often begins with theory and examines hypothetical relationships within it—a deductive process. Qualitative research more often builds theory, moving from observations and open questions to more general conclusions—an inductive process. In actual practice most researchers use elements of both deductive and inductive logic. Both approaches collect and analyze data, draw tentative conclusions, test conclusions, and reinterpret earlier findings based on new evidence. Research across disciplines has at its core a common scientific logic. However, the process of applying the basic logic of scientific inquiry to tangible problems in public health differs depending on the problem and the researcher's theoretical perspective.

Frameworks for Research: Paradigms and Theories

Research frameworks range from broad to very specific theoretical approaches that often contain their own vocabulary and logical assumptions. Broad theoretical frameworks, also called paradigms, provide researchers with a unified set of concepts, principles, and rules for conducting research. More specific frameworks can be found in substantive theories supported by research findings. A *paradigm* is a worldview that presents a definition of the social world linked to related sources of information (data) and appropriate ways (methods) to tap these sources (Guba and Lincoln 1994).

Whether consciously or not, every researcher works from some theoretical orientation or paradigm. Perspectives can vary a great deal among researchers who see the world through different cultural, philosophical, or professional lenses. One researcher might seek evidence of the regularity of patterned behavior in trends, rates, and associations. Another might focus on how people understand or interpret what they experience. Both contribute valuable data to describe social behavior but from different paradigmatic perspectives. The questions they ask and the methods they use will be determined to a large extent by their separate paradigms. For example, researchers working from a demographic perspective generally operate within a different theoretical orientation or paradigm than do researchers with a social development perspective. Your view of the world—your basic philosophical grounding—influences the problems you study, the sources of data you consider appropriate, the methods you choose to gather your data, and the way you carry out your studies.

In applied research a paradigm can be an ally—a powerful strategic tool to guide you through the many practical decisions that arise in the design and implementation of your research. We recommend constant awareness of your theoretical position and its influences on the kinds of questions you ask. As you examine your own views of social life, your theoretical perspective is likely to become an increasingly deliberate choice, consistent with the problems you study.

Substantive Theory

Substantive theories are more concrete than the broad theoretical frameworks for research discussed earlier. Also called operational or working theories, they represent conclusions about the social world that emerge from specific findings of research studies. Applied

BOX 2.1

Basic Definitions

concepts or constructs The major components of a theory—its building blocks or key elements. The key concepts of the Stages of Change theory (Prochaska and others 1992), for example, describe individual behavior change in the following stages: precontemplation, contemplation, preparation for action, action, and maintenance of the new behavior.

paradigm An overarching but ever-changing framework that influences how we perceive and understand the world. Paradigmatic assumptions establish boundaries for scientific inquiry. A researcher who embraces a feminist paradigm, for example, might conceptualize sexual decision making through the lens of power differences between sexual partners. Similarly, a researcher studying the same phenomenon from an interpretivist perspective would want to know what sexual decisions mean to men and women in the larger contexts of their lives.

substantive theories These theories organize conclusions about the social world as they emerge from the specific findings of scientific studies. Theories of health behavior change, for example, and have been elaborated and refined from the results of numerous studies that document how people perceive health risk and make decisions to alter or not alter risky behavior.

theoretical or conceptual models Such models usually draw on more than one theory to help people understand a problem in a specific setting or context. For example, the Health Belief Model (Rosenstock and others 1994) incorporates a number of well-tested social-psychological theories to explain and predict health behaviors.

theory A "set of interrelated concepts, definitions and propositions that presents a systematic view of events or situations by specifying relations among variables in order to explain and predict the events or situations" (Glanz and others 2002, p. 21). Theories specify the determinants of phenomena of interest (Bandura 1986).

variables Things that can change or differ, quantitatively or qualitatively. Common variables thought to account for differences in health behaviors include intention, ability or skill, norms, environmental constraints, anticipated outcomes, self-standards, emotion, and self-efficacy (Fishbein 1997/1991).

Source: Adapted from Glanz and others 2002, pp. 21–27.

research in public health commonly uses substantive theory to define and explain specific behavior in relation to program development and policy. In fact, applied researchers often maximize their ability to explain a phenomenon by combining elements of more than one theory to construct a model. Appendix One contains examples of several substantive theories that may be of use in social and behavioral health research.

Putting Theory to Work

In Chapter One we endorsed the practice of mixing methods in applied research. In this chapter we will show how choosing research methods is contingent on both practical and theoretical considerations. Methodological decisions are practical strategies tailored to specific problems, but they also reflect the researcher's theoretical orientation to a problem (see Box 2.2). The qualitative methodology of in-depth interviewing, for example, is a natural outgrowth of an interpretivist paradigm that casts young mothers as experts whose interpretation of their experience can help researchers learn about early childbearing.

If a key theoretical assumption of your work is that individuals have the power to make independent health decisions, then you may decide to use structured, quantitative methods to categorize individual traits and behaviors. On the other hand, if you believe that control of health decisions is variable and dependent on one's position in social relationships and networks, then it would be advisable to include qualitative methods. We present overviews of three of the most common and important theoretical paradigms used in public health research: positivism (a largely quantitative approach), interpretivism, and feminism (both qualitative approaches). Because qualitative research is a rapidly growing field accompanied by theoretical debate, we will also discuss briefly some of the controversies surrounding the use of methods from these frameworks. In light of trends in the wider field of qualitative research, we advocate a pragmatic approach that recognizes theoretical distinctions but is able to incorporate relevant elements from all three in carefully designed studies.

Finally, because assumptions regarding the quality of research are grounded in one's theoretical orientation, we introduce criteria for judging the rigor of qualitative studies, emphasizing that qualitative and quantitative criteria of excellence are equally important but inherently different.

QUANTITATIVE OR QUALITATIVE?

What is social reality, and how do we explain it? The question has stirred debate and polarized social science research between quantitative and qualitative methods. The issue centers on "the capacity of the data, as collected by one method or the other, to describe, understand, and explain social phenomena" (Pedersen 1992, p. 43). Theoretical purists argue that because each methodology reflects a different understanding of research, human behavior, and the nature of social life, the two are incompatible (Greenhalgh 1997). The purist position would require the researcher to choose one or the other approach on the principle that mixing methods violates the assumptions on which either framework is constructed (Patton 1990; Carey 1993). The debate revolves around such fundamental questions as, "what is health and disease, who decides what are important research questions, and whose 'truth' is the 'real truth'?" (Meetoo and Temple 2003, p. 6).

One viewpoint proposes that all [social scientific] data can in principle be measured or classified; therefore, when we confront non-quantified data, our task is to refine them through analysis so that they are subject to quantification or categorization.
(Selltiz and others 1976, p. 460)

Our position, on the other hand, like that of many quantitative and qualitative researchers today, chooses pragmatism over "one-sided paradigm allegiance" (Patton 1990, p. 38). Our purpose in presenting more than one theoretical framework is to help readers understand similarities and differences, strengths and limitations, and the contribution that each can make to applied health research. The methods that emerge from these frameworks "offer a distinct set of strengths and limitations that are markedly different but potentially complementary when combined in a mixed-method research design" (Wolff and others 1991, p. 2). Throughout this guide, therefore, we will advocate methodological appropriateness—using theory and related methods to make reasoned decisions "appropriate to the purpose of the study, the questions being investigated, and the resources available" (Patton 1990, p. 39).

THREE THEORETICAL PARADIGMS FOR PUBLIC HEALTH RESEARCH

In this section we describe three important theoretical frameworks, or paradigms, and apply them to common problems in sexual and reproductive health. Together they have generated much of the substantive theory, or knowledge, in social and behavioral health today: research based on positivist principles, research that uses an interpretivist approach, and research shaped by a feminist perspective. Given the assumptions of each of these broad theoretical orientations, the positivist perspective is generally, but not exclusively, associated with quantitative methods, whereas interpretivist and feminist orientations typically lead to the use of qualitative research strategies.

Box 2.2 (see p. 16) summarizes the logic and language of the three paradigms and outlines major points with a selection of examples from the methodological toolboxes of each theoretical framework. Interested readers are referred to more comprehensive sources such as the *Handbook of Qualitative Research* (Denzin and Lincoln 2000).

Quantitative Research from a Positivist Perspective Much of what is known today about population and reproductive health can be attributed to research that has developed from quantitative principles in the natural sciences. Quantitative methods have become the norm for describing the state of the world's population—demographic models that project trends in fertility, morbidity, and mortality; epidemiological surveillance techniques to describe patterns of disease, including the proliferation of sexually transmitted infection (STI) and the spread of the HIV/AIDS epidemic; and standardized household surveys that provide statistical data on knowledge, attitudes, and practices related to health behavior.

A basic assumption of this paradigm is that the goal of science is to develop the most objective methods possible to get the closest approximation of reality. Researchers who work from this perspective explain in quantitative terms how variables interact, shape events, and cause outcomes. They often develop and test these explanations in experimental studies. Multivariate analysis and techniques for statistical prediction are among the classic contributions of this type of research. This framework has evolved largely from a nineteenth-century philosophical approach called positivism, which maintains that reliable knowledge is based on direct observation or manipulation of natural phenomena through empirical, often experimental, means.

Quantitative studies in social science use highly standardized tools with precisely worded questions. Working with representative samples, the interviewer might ask the following questions: How many pregnancies have you had and at what intervals? What contraceptive methods have you used? Who has influenced your decision? Which of the following has led you to discontinue the method you had begun? In data analysis the answers to open-ended questions are typically classified according to

BOX 2.2

Three Paradigms for Public Health Research

	Positivist	Interpretivist	Feminist
Basic assumptions	The social world is composed of observable facts. Reality is objective, independent of the researcher.	The social world is constructed of symbolic meaning observable in human acts, interactions, and language. Reality is subjective and multiple as seen from different perspectives.	The social world is governed by power relations that influence acts and perceptions. Reality is negotiated and differs according to status and power.
Sources of evidence	Facts are revealed through standard scientific processes and are context-free.	Meanings are derived from perceptions, experiences, and actions in relation to social contexts.	Power, control, and contextual factors can be heard in personal accounts that reflect different versions of reality.
Methods	Prestructured data collection, controlled measurement, clinical trials are the norm. Examples: surveys, clinical trials, rating scales, structured observation.	Semistructured, open questions, and observation enable participants to express thoughts and actions in natural ways. Examples: in-depth interviews, focus group discussions, participant observations, case histories.	Participatory forms of observation and guided conversation enable both marginal and dominant groups to voice opinions and tell their stories. Examples: participatory action techniques, reflexive listening, challenges to political and personal barriers to entrenched positions.
Research intention	Quantitative studies seek explanation, verification, and prediction of human behavior through causal or associative relationships.	Qualitative studies seek discovery, understanding, and insight into the circumstances of human behavior.	Feminist studies seek insight into the influence of gender on human behavior, including differentials in power and control, in an agenda for social change.
Level of participation	Research subjects answer specific, predetermined questions in a structured response format.	Research participants are active partners in data collection and respond to semistructured questions spontaneously and naturally.	Research participants have relative freedom to direct the data collection process and define follow-up.
Impact on study participants	Impact is neutral. Research subjects may gain new information or insight from the results.	Participants are aware of their engagement in the research process; may gain insight into their own perspectives and behaviors, as well as the research topic.	Participation is empowering. Results may lead to a participant-defined action agenda and empowerment to initiate or participate in policy change.

prestructured categories that represent the researcher's theoretical understanding of the problem.

Control of extraneous and competing variables, as this framework defines them, is important in quantitative design. The framework applies rules for incorporating factors from the social environment based on assumptions that are different from other frameworks. Using experimental and quasi-experimental designs, quantitative researchers attempt to distribute evenly the effect of contextual variables through randomization. Their rationale is that context contains hidden determinants, which may affect measurement of causal or associative relationships and bias the outcomes of the study. Control is thus fundamental to quantitative research assumptions because it provides a means to isolate extraneous variables and focus more clearly on the relationships that were highlighted in the research problem.

Controlling effects also helps researchers to identify and explain in quantitative terms the influence of factors in the study environment on key relationships. For example, if your research problem were to identify factors that predict fertility trends in Peru, you would measure the variable relationships among selected possible determinants of fertility and the relative strengths with which each of these factors can predict the number of births per Peruvian woman. You would control for sociodemographic and other variables that might explain the observed relationships. You would obtain accurate measurements, but because it is impossible to identify, measure, and control every variable that could influence whether a woman will give birth, you would always have unanswered or partially answered questions. A versatile investigator might at this point turn to qualitative techniques to explore some of the quantitative findings in greater depth.

In quantitative studies accuracy, reliability, and relative freedom from bias are critical criteria for judging the quality of findings. The inherent difficulty of ensuring accuracy in any social or behavioral inquiry has led quantitative researchers to stress neutrality, uniformity, objectivity, and replicability. Such goals are consistent with the positivist goal to study phenomena objectively and to express findings in terms of measurable outcomes and relationships. A quantitative strategy emphasizes structure: consistent operational definitions throughout the study, precisely worded questions, and statistical analysis. However, this structure limits the scope of the research by requiring the formulation of research problems and questions in measurable terms.

Over the years demographers, epidemiologists, biostatisticians, and other quantitative scientists have met many methodological challenges. Their painstaking efforts to answer difficult questions have resulted in an impressive knowledge base in population studies and public health. But still missing is a deeper understanding of the circumstances that help to explain why and how people make the decisions they do. Even when working in a quantitative framework, therefore, researchers often seek other ways of understanding human behavior, specifically in the methods of qualitative research (Pedersen 1992), based on different principles and theoretical assumptions.

Qualitative Research from an Interpretivist Perspective The theoretical framework for most qualitative research emerges from an interpretivist perspective, a paradigm that sees the world as constructed, interpreted, and experienced by people in their interactions with each other and with wider social systems (Ulin 1992). Research focuses not only on objectively verifiable facts but also on the many subjective meanings that people attach to them. Identifying, sorting, and analyzing those meanings in relation to objective behavior—decisions, actions, practices—are the methodological substance of the interpretivist framework.

Three key components of this framework are subjective perceptions and understandings, which arise from experience; objective actions or behaviors; and context. Qualitative researchers explore phenomena in the light of related social, cultural, political, and physical environments of the people they are studying–the holistic approach characteristic of the interpretivist perspective. Qualitative analysis also allows the researcher to link findings from the three components to explore the multiple relations among them. For example, a woman usually does not define contraception simply as a means to prevent pregnancy. She interprets its significance in the light of personal and cultural experience and from what other people say and believe about it, including health workers, her partner, her friends, or influential family members. If, as several studies have found, a woman—or the people she listens to—believes that contraceptive pills will "accumulate in her stomach and cause cancer," then that belief may be a key factor in her decision to accept or reject the method.

On another level the social and material contexts in which a woman acts also affect her decisions and behavior. If a woman cannot afford contraceptive pills and the economic environment offers very limited opportunity to generate income, or if isolated living conditions or restrictive social norms make it impossible for her to get to a health clinic for her monthly prescription, these contextual factors will influence both her perceptions and her behaviors.

Approaching this problem from an interpretivist perspective, you would take seriously the woman's subjective understanding of oral contraception and link it to her actions and their potential impacts. Using flexible, in-depth techniques, you would compare your findings with the perspectives and actions of other women, looking for different as well as similar constructions that could explain patterns of behavior. You might also examine the wider context of women's experiences with oral contraception in that culture; for example, barriers to information and service, partner communication concerning family planning, extended family norms, and the influence of fertility on the changing status of women in their extended families.

The kinds of research questions that arise in an interpretivist framework are mainly those that address why, how, and under what circumstances rather than what and how many. Why do people who were abused as children tend to be overrepresented among abusive adults? Under what circumstances will parents accept a school's responsibility for sex education? How do economically dependent women protect themselves from HIV transmission when their partners are at risk? Why has the intrauterine device (IUD) been widely accepted in some countries and rejected in others? Each of these questions leads deeper into questions of subjective meaning–the meaning that life events and experiences have on health decisions and health behavior. The same questions can be addressed from a quantitative perspective but in terms of discrete indicators with measurable dimensions. Qualitative methods of participant observation, in-depth interviews, and focus group discussions would elicit data on subjective understandings.

The methods associated with this perspective tend to be those that enable participants to speak freely and understand the investigator's quest for insight into a phenomenon that the participant has experienced (Barnett and Stein 1998). As subsequent chapters will show, interpretivist methodology seeks information in as natural a context as possible, where the researcher can observe activities and events as they occur and encourage people to respond from their own perspectives and experiences and in their own words. In the IUD example, the results might be a deeper understanding of motivations, decisions, and circumstances associated with IUD use. They would not answer more descriptive questions concerning extent, patterns, and prediction of use or measurable indicators of knowledge and attitudes concerning the method—issues that a quantitative framework would better address. The reader should note, however, that a combined methodological strategy in this example would make it possible to use the strengths of each approach while compensating for each one's limitations.

Working on the assumption that "research participants construct [their own] accounts of reality" as they experience it, Meetoo and Temple (2003) used an interpretivist framework to investigate self-care among people with diabetes. Their design included methods that would enable them to see how participants built their different accounts: semistructured interviews, structured fixed-response interviews, and diaries. The seemingly inconsistent results, especially comparing face-to-face interview data with the more private diary entries, demonstrated to the researchers the importance of circumstances, or context, in determining different dimensions of self-help.

Qualitative Research from a Feminist Perspective Like interpretivist scholars, feminist theorists believe that how people interpret their experience is not only a valid but an essential focus of research. But until feminist theory was articulated in the 1960s, neither the positivist nor the interpretivist perspectives had fully taken into account the profound influence of power relations, especially—but not uniquely—in the area of women's health (Ulin 1992). Although critical theorists such as Antonio Gramschi and Michel Foucault have greatly advanced studies of the social dynamics of power, grounded in the work of Karl Marx and other critical scholars, feminist scholars have brought this current of thought into the field of gender relations, an issue of consummate importance in many fields of public health.[1]

Feminist work sets the stage for other research, other actions, and policy that transcend and transform.
(Olesen 2000, p. 215)

Feminist research has grown from a commitment to gender equity and increasing equality between men and women, and it continues to advance these aims, but the feminist perspective addresses power relationships of many kinds, not just those between men and women. A feminist perspective on health is not simply about women;

BOX 2.3

The IRRRAG Project: Feminist Perspective in Sexual and Reproductive Health

The International Reproductive Rights Research Action Group (IRRRAG) was founded in 1992 by Rosalind Petchesky on the premise that "until we know more about the local contexts and ways of thinking in which women in their everyday lives negotiate reproductive health and sexual matters, we cannot assume that reproductive and sexual rights are a goal that they seek and therefore one that has universal applicability" (Petchesky and Judd 1998, p. 1).

One IRRRAG project—part research and part movement for social justice—is an example of how feminist theory has been effectively applied to qualitative research in sexual and reproductive health. Using primarily qualitative methods, IRRRAG researchers talked with women in Egypt, Malaysia, Nigeria, Mexico, Brazil, the Philippines, and the United States about how they conceptualize and act on their sexual and reproductive rights. Feminist and participatory research models guided the project, which focused on two key questions:

1. How do women across diverse countries, cultures, and generations arrive at and negotiate a sense of entitlement with regard to their reproductive and sexual health and well-being?
2. Under what life circumstances and by what terms and strategies do women begin to take charge of their reproductive and sexual bodies? (Petchesky and Judd 1998, p. 8).

The project was "centrally concerned with issues of moral and political [power] and women's formulation and pursuit of claims to decision-making authority" (Petchesky and Judd 1998, p. 8). Thus, an agenda for action, or social change, was built into the research with the intention to "uncover and enhance the conditions for women [that will enable them to] challenge existing power relations" (Petchesky and Judd 1998, p. 8).

A distinguishing element in the project was the commitment to feminist research principles and practices, including the use of democratic consensus building within the international research team. Together the team built a conceptual framework that highlighted understanding women's beliefs about sexual and reproductive rights and interpreting those insights. The study explored how women formulate and express their ideas about rights and entitlement and how, through both accommodation and resistance, they attempt to negotiate their rights in the contexts of their daily lives.

The IRRRAG researchers discovered that many women do not feel a sense of entitlement to basic human rights on their own behalf until they become mothers. Only when they needed to protect the rights of their children did the women in the study believe they were entitled to any rights at all. The conceptual framework for the study helped to explain this finding as follows: the women's lives were sharply limited by their gender-defined status and roles, that is, by social and cultural expectations for the appropriate behavior (and rights) of women at different ages. As wives and mothers, women in the study were expected to assert and defend their rights to safeguard their children and the well-being of their families. It was less acceptable, however, for a woman to demand her own rights to personal growth, leisure, or sexual pleasure, because these are outside the usual boundaries of women's traditional reproductive and productive family roles.

The IRRRAG study illustrates how a feminist theoretical perspective can be the basis for a research design, incorporating substantive theoretical constructs such as rights, entitlement, accommodation, and resistance. It also demonstrates the practical relevance of theory, because a woman's sense of entitlement can be directly related to sexual and reproductive decisions that shape her life. The finding that women in the IRRRAG study countries often do not believe they are entitled to reproductive rights until they are mothers is critical information for women's advocates. It helps to explain why, despite intensive informational and educational campaigns, many women still cannot accept family planning until they have borne a child.

it is about power and the recognition that long-standing differences in access to power have a profound effect on the health of populations. This perspective is rapidly restructuring how we design our research, adding concepts and tools to answer numerous important questions we have not before had the means to ask.

Feminist research frameworks are concerned with the gender and power dimensions of social phenomena that shape people's lives. An important premise of feminist theory is that social life and behavior are constrained in various ways by what is considered acceptable behavior based on gender. Feminist research focuses on the political dimension inherent in understanding these constraints from the standpoints of people in different power and gender positions. The power relationships that maintain boundaries on people's lives often cast women in subordinate positions relative to men, but they apply equally to other forms of power imbalance, for example, those defined by race, economic status, and access to scarce resources.

Recent substantive theories of subordination and domination, constructed within a feminist paradigm, have been instrumental in improving the quality of family planning and reproductive health care delivery (Bruce 1990). Health practitioners and researchers are familiar with the power differential that all too often silences the voices of clients in health care settings. Communications workshops for health providers, as well as efforts to empower women to participate more actively in their health care, have been an outgrowth of studies that identify gender gaps in client-provider relationships. Male involvement in reproductive health decisions is frequently addressed from a gender perspective. For example: How do couples negotiate sexual decisions? How do men learn about fertility, and why do they remain on the margins of many reproductive health programs?

Feminist theorists point out that women's voices have not been heard in the process of developing and delivering health care to women. Similarly, when we leave men out of sexual and reproductive health programs or research, we are not hearing what they experience and what they think about a host of issues, including sexual relationships, family planning, and protection against infection. As a result our policy and program perspectives may be too narrow and may neglect questions that are important to men.

The influence of feminist thought and methodology can be found in much of the social and behavioral health literature today, often bridging qualitative and quantitative methods while keeping lived experience central to the investigation (Barnett and Stein 1998; Tolman and Szalacha 1999). For example, in development studies, household survey results have highlighted gender differences in relation to other social characteristics such as age, ethnicity, and class. These differences can be further explored with methods that enable people to speak out on issues that are meaningful to them (Caro 1995). Researchers who work from the feminist paradigm tend to select qualitative methods that empower participants who have not previously had a voice in significant debates, including population and health delivery issues that affect women's lives. By alerting us to the potential for bias when researchers do not listen to the voices of certain groups of people, feminist researchers are helping us reformulate how we design and conduct our studies.

Putting It All Together

QUALITATIVE CONCEPTS AND THEIR RELATIONSHIPS

Theoretical components of qualitative health research include concepts and principles that have evolved—and continue to evolve—under the influence of interpretivist and feminist paradigms. A basic premise of qualitative logic is that because people interpret things, events, and interactions in different ways, they arrive at different understandings, responses, or actions. Public health messages, for example, mean different things to different people because they interpret them differently. To a qualitative researcher, the meanings that people take from an AIDS prevention message may be attributed to differences in social context, with its profound influence on human thought and behavior. Qualitative researchers are always probing contradictions and inconsistencies in the human condition, because it is at this level that we begin to understand the dynamics of human behavior.

Understanding how qualitative research explores these dynamics means becoming familiar with the language that expresses basic qualitative concepts and principles. We have grouped some of the most important concepts to show their relationships:

- *Qualitative research is systematic discovery.* Its purpose is to generate knowledge of social events and processes by understanding what they mean to people, exploring and documenting how people interact with each other and how they interpret and interact with the world around them. It also seeks to elucidate patterns of shared understanding and variability in those patterns.
- *Qualitative researchers value natural settings where the researcher can better understand people's lived experiences.* The natural context of people's lives is a critical component of qualitative design, because it influences the perspectives, experiences, and actions of participants in the study. It is the interpersonal and sociocultural fabric that shapes meanings and actions.
- *Researchers express qualitative data in participants' words, in images, and sometimes in numbers.* Language, verbal and nonverbal, has symbolic meaning—an expression may mean one thing to the study participant and a different thing to the interviewer. Qualitative researchers listen carefully to language as participants tell about their experiences without the constraints of externally imposed structure. When we refer to raw data as narrative, we mean participants relating their ideas and experiences in ways that can offer insight into important research concepts and questions.
- *The qualitative research process is flexible, emergent, and iterative.* The study design is never fixed; there is constant interplay between design and discovery. Findings emerge continuously. The investigator is always in touch with the research process, observing how participants respond to the topic and examining data for fresh insights that might lead to altering a technique, modifying questions, or changing direction to pursue new leads. Analysis does not wait until all the data are collected; it begins in the field.

- *Reflexivity—the researcher's critical self-awareness—is a vital process in which you question and observe yourself* at the same time you listen to and observe the participant. With its emphasis on egalitarian relationships, feminist methodology has contributed greatly to this point. In contrast to the detachment required in many quantitative studies, your presence is a vital component of the qualitative research process in two ways. First, you are in a partnership with the participant—working together to explore themes and find answers. Second, as you listen to your participant-partner, interpret, and respond, you are a key research instrument yourself, not only absorbing information but also influencing how it is elicited. Self-examination, documented with other observations in the field notes, is part of the iterative process of interpretation and revision that moves the data collection toward its goal.

Theoretical Models in Practice

Applied qualitative researchers often use substantive theory from the field of health behavior.[2] These behavioral frameworks offer a rich array of concepts and theoretical relationships that can help define qualitative research problems more clearly and guide the research design. If your research is principally concerned with behavior change, we recommend reviewing several frameworks and models and selecting concepts that fit your theoretical perspective on the research problem. Many studies, both qualitative and quantitative, have included concepts from behavioral frameworks that do the following:

- Describe cultural models of health and illness to understand "individual and group-level knowledge and beliefs about health threats, transmission dynamics, and behavioral norms"
- Identify the social contexts in which beliefs and values are manifested in actions
- Identify the conditions that promote or prevent change in risk behaviors
- Determine the conditions necessary for maintaining individual behavior change (Trotter 1997, pp. 259–260)

If you are designing a study for a community health intervention to promote screening for breast cancer, you might look for a framework that enables you to identify perceptions of risk in the target population, as well as reasons that women might or might not accept the new program. One example of such a framework would be the health belief model, which would help you design your research around theoretical constructs that have been tested in numerous studies of health behavior change (Rosenstock 1974). Or if your research problem focuses on the dynamic between empowerment and constraint, as in a study of women's contraceptive choices in a pronatalist society, the locus of control model might help conceptualize the distinction between women's belief that they control their own decisions and the contrasting belief that outside forces control what they do (Wallston and others 1978). Frequently, elements of two or more models are combined to construct a theoretical "picture" of the phenomenon under study. (These models are summarized in Appendix One.) Some qualitative researchers, on the other hand, refer to models and frameworks only in the analysis and interpretation of their data, comparing themes that emerge from their findings to concepts and relationships in a larger body of theory. Others use a grounded theory approach (Glaser and Strauss 1967), as described by Rance in a field perspective at the end of this chapter. Rather than build the study on preexisting theory, an investigator "discovers" theory in many context-rich observations, always searching for new insights, comparing interpretations of emerging data, and allowing a theoretical framework to evolve.

Setting Standards for Qualitative Research

At the heart of the debate on research standards is the much-used but often misunderstood concept of subjectivity. To a quantitative scientist, data are facts that must be isolated as much as possible from the researcher's personal, or subjective, values; subjectivity can mean distortion. Although the notion of a perfectly objective social science is a widely acknowledged myth, the accuracy of quantitative data often depends on the separation of fact from subjective judgment. In theoretical frameworks that guide and emerge from qualitative research, on the other hand, subjectivity is an important element in the research process. We believe that we perceive the world only partially and therefore, as researchers, must describe as many aspects of reality as we can and be open to many ways of interpreting the social world. Our access to these multiple worldviews is through the subjective experiences and understandings of study participants. The qualitative researcher's use of self as a reflexive

BOX 2.4

Checklist for Using Substantive Theory

When applying a theory or model, consider the following:

- What dimensions of the problem does the theory or model concern?
- Is it specific to the unit of study (for example, individual behavior, group influences, environmental issues)?
- How does the theory or model explain this portion of your research problem?
- What information does the theory or model suggest that you gather?
- How accurately does the theory or model coincide with your understanding of the problem?
- What aspects of the problem does the theory or model fail to consider?
- In your judgment how helpful is the theory or model in working with the problem and determining how best to study it?
- What are its limitations?

Source: Adapted from van Ryn and Heaney 1992.

(self-aware) partner in collecting and interpreting information further strengthens the position that subjectivity, applied appropriately and systematically, is a positive element in qualitative science.

JUDGING QUALITY: THE SEARCH FOR TRUSTWORTHY DATA

Qualitative and quantitative criteria of excellence are equally important but inherently different (Devers 1999). All of us who design research or use research findings are concerned with quality, but the criteria of evaluation differ in qualitative and quantitative research practice: they are analogous but not interchangeable. Each has its own appropriate and no less rigorous standards. The most widely adopted criteria have been those developed from the positivist framework, which uses validity, reliability, objectivity, precision, and generalizability to judge the rigor of quantitative studies intended to describe, predict, and verify empirical relationships in relatively controlled settings.

On the other hand, qualitative research that aims to explore, discover, and understand cannot use the same criteria to judge research quality and outcomes. We will synthesize the work of several qualitative scientists who have articulated standards or criteria for judging qualitative data (Lincoln and Guba 1985; Miles and Huberman 1994; Kirk and Miller 1986). Lincoln and Guba suggest that the fundamental criterion for qualitative reports is trustworthiness. How, they ask, can a researcher be certain that "the findings of an inquiry are worth paying attention to, worth taking account of?" (Lincoln and Guba 1985, p. 398). In answer, practitioners and consumers of qualitative science ask a new set of questions: How can we know that the data are credible, dependable, confirmable, and transferable? We introduce these concepts because evaluating the trustworthiness of qualitative data is directly related to the fundamental logic of qualitative theory. In Chapter Six we discuss standards of quality in greater detail in relation to data analysis.

Credibility In quantitative science *validity* is the extent to which a measurement taps the concept it intends to measure. The outcome is accepted as true within reasonable limits. Credibility, also called truth value, is the corresponding criterion for qualitative research. Validity assumes correct operational measures for the concepts being studied and, in experimental studies, a potential cause-effect relationship (Yin 1994); credibility focuses on confidence in the truth of the findings, including an accurate understanding of the context:

- Do the findings show a logical relationship to each other, that is, are they consistent in terms of the explanations they support?
- Are the findings grounded in, and substantiated by, the narrative data, that is, are the narrative data sufficiently rich to support the specific findings? Do the findings indicate a need for more data?
- Does the original study population consider reports to be accurate? (Miles and Huberman 1994)

Dependability An important test of quantitative reliability is the extent to which findings can be replicated. The goal is not only to obtain the same results in a study (which, given intervening time and change, may not be possible) but to be able to replicate the processes used to obtain these results, even though they may be very different in different cultural contexts (King and others 1994). For qualitative researchers inquiring into unique constellations of multiple phenomena and meanings, this goal would be meaningless. In other words, the same method is not likely to produce the same results unless the answers are prestructured to conform to definitions imposed by the research design. For qualitative researchers the methodological parallel to reliability is whether the results are dependable, whether the research process is consistent and carried out with careful attention to the rules and conventions of qualitative methodology. We ask ourselves:

- Are the research questions clear and logically connected to the research purpose and design?
- Are there parallels across data sources?
- Do multiple field-workers have comparable data collection protocols?

Given the contextual nature of qualitative research, we do not expect to produce exactly the same answers. On the other hand, we do anticipate that if the data are dependable, we will find logically consistent patterns of response that remain reasonably stable over time.

Confirmability Objectivity is a traditional standard of quality in quantitative data. The term generally implies maintaining distance between the observer and the observed and minimizing any possible influence of the researcher's values on the process of inquiry. Either strategy would be counterproductive in most qualitative studies. From a qualitative perspective, the analogous goal is to confirm, by audits and other methods that we will discuss in Chapters Five and Six, that the data reflect as accurately as possible the participants' perspectives and experiences. Confirmability thus means a way of knowing that, even as a coparticipant in the inquiry, the researcher has maintained the distinction between personal values and those of the study participants. Applying the concept of reflexivity, qualitative researchers have an obligation to observe and document their own roles in the research process, including assumptions, biases, or reactions that might influence the collection and interpretation of data. Applying reflexivity contributes to the confirmability of the results.

Transferability Also called extensibility, *transferability* is the qualitative analogue to the concept of generalizability. Generalizability of the findings to a wider population is a goal of most quantitative studies. Indeed, if every unit in the study sample has an equal chance of being selected, and the sample is large enough to minimize the probability of error, then this goal can be met within certain specified margins. It is a statistically representative sample. Although generalizability by this definition is not relevant to the goals or the methodology of most interpretive work, it is nevertheless important to know "whether the conclusions of a study . . . [are] transferable to other contexts" (Miles and Huberman 1994, p. 279). The importance of context in qualitative studies leads some researchers to doubt that results from one context should be transferred to another, while it may lead others to apply conclusions from their data too casually. Our position is on middle ground: lessons learned from qualitative studies can be applied to other contexts if samples have been carefully selected to represent viewpoints and experiences that reflect key issues in the research problem. Our goal is to produce data that are conceptually, not statistically, representative of people in a specific context. Because context is a key influence in any qualitative research, the researcher must account for contextual factors when transferring data from one situation to another. Repeating the study in another population, with similar conclusions, lends credibility to the results and further specifies the circumstances under which the findings will occur. Thus, well-documented knowledge might be extended to similar populations, but "the burden of proof lies less with the original investigator than with the person seeking to make an application elsewhere. The original inquirer cannot know the sites to which transferability might be sought, but appliers can" (Lincoln and Guba 1985, p. 404).

Credibility, dependability, confirmability, and transferability are the standards for evaluating the rigor of qualitative studies that are consistent with the worldview, information sources, and methods of the interpretivist paradigm. In subsequent chapters we will return to these criteria of quality with further discussion of specific techniques for ensuring the rigor of qualitative studies.

Conclusion

As researchers we each have a fundamental curiosity about our subject of inquiry. But in designing and implementing the research, we must move beyond ordinary curiosity to a disciplined use of the rules and conventions of our theoretical perspective or paradigm. A great deal has been written from the quantitative point of view that will continue to guide much of our work in public health. For this book we have set our theoretical compass largely, though not entirely, by the interpretivist and feminist paradigms. We believe that, alone or in combination with appropriate quantitative methods, these two theoretical positions can generate qualitative research that addresses many complex issues in public health research and practice. In this chapter we have urged readers to examine their own theoretical perspectives, to ask themselves what perspective their work reflects, where their ideas come from, and whether it might be useful to look at a problem through a different lens. It is important to incorporate self-reflection in the research process, to know how one's own worldview influences the questions under investigation. If you understand and use your theoretical perspective as a guide, you will discover new ways to a better understanding of human thought and behavior.

Qualitative research is grounded in a philosophical position, which is broadly "interpretivist" in the sense that it is concerned about how the social world is interpreted, understood, experienced, or produced.

(Mason 1996, p. 4)

NOTES

1. *Gender* is "the roles that men and women play and the relations that arise out of these roles. They are socially constructed, not physically determined" (Pan American Health Organization 1997, p. 28).
2. Appendix One presents summaries of several working behavior change models that have contributed conceptually to both qualitative and quantitative research in public health.

Field Perspective

Modes of Inquiry: Positioning the Self

David Bell, M.A., Ed.D.

Clark University

I began my career as a counseling psychologist in my native South Africa, trained to answer questions through standardized tests and psychological instruments. My training was grounded in the empirical, quantitative paradigm. As a doctoral student at the University of Massachusetts, however, I began to realize that my experience working in South Africa's rural communities, townships, and former homelands had shaped my views in different ways. My work in community advocacy and empowerment among the oppressed, the poor, and until recently the disenfranchised was challenging my traditional notions of research. Answers to my research questions were coming more from my interpretation of people, their behavior, and the words they used to express the realities of their lives and less from instruments, numbers, and statistical formulas. At first I felt confused and insecure. Would others see my work as relevant and legitimate if I adopted a more qualitative and interpretivist approach to research?

The uncertainty I felt as a researcher in relation to the people I was supposed to study began to influence the questions I was asking and the methods I was choosing to answer them. Instead of asking questions that emerged from standardized measures and instruments and relating everything to existing theory, I began exploring everyday life from the perspectives of the people I was studying. I was becoming aware that I could look at research problems differently: I had the power to choose the appropriate methodology for the research question, and I was able to incorporate my personal beliefs and research style at the same time. Research was no longer a clinical and academic act; it was human interaction on a very personal level.

But defining and justifying the critical distinctions between these different approaches was far more difficult than simply selecting new methods and feeling comfortable about the questions. Given the many ways that research can be conducted, how would I justify one methodological choice above another? How could I know what would work best for a particular research problem and provide the most appropriate and relevant information?

As I wrestled with these questions, I turned to a typology that included two useful continua. The first, a subjectivity-objectivity continuum, helped me articulate two related questions: Can the act of research (and the actions of the researcher) be impersonal and objective? Or is research a more human act that, by its very nature, is subjective and personal? An affirmative answer to the first question would justify the quantitative studies I had been conducting. It did, however, raise the uneasy question of whether and how objective research affects the very people that the research findings were designed to assist. Was it helping or harming?

The second question, whether research is subjective, also struck a familiar chord with my experience in the former homelands and townships where I had been working. I questioned whether outsiders had any right to use the lives of people in these communities as laboratories for their research. Could my own research lie somewhere between the two poles of the continuum? Could such a midpoint still be respected? Was I one type of researcher in one context and a different type of researcher in another? I saw that the primary stakeholders in the research we were doing were the participants themselves. It was my responsibility as a researcher not only to collect reliable data but also to enable participants to speak for themselves. I had to be a partner and a listener in the human act of research.

The second continuum that helped me organize my thoughts was a radical change–status quo continuum. This continuum challenged me to think about the social and political implications of my role as a researcher. These are the questions it raised: Does my research focus on the underlying unity and cohesiveness of the world (finding information and evidence to explain the status quo)? Or am I really seeking evidence of fundamental and deep-seated structural conflicts and inequities, thereby arguing for radical change? As I considered the purpose of my work in rural South African communities, I concluded that my research would have to do both. On the one hand, participants described many aspects of community life that were strong and good. Although resources were in short supply, people were finding creative ways to help each other and their neighbors. I wanted our research results to reinforce that spirit of self-help and cooperation.

On the other hand, the oppressive consequences of apartheid on people's lives were continuing into the postapartheid era, and in fact, many women continued to feel oppressed by gender inequities in their own households. How could we document what was happening during this critical transition? We put aside our standardized tools and asked the people, "What does it mean to be oppressed? Describe oppression for us in as many ways as you can." The result was that both women and men began to look more introspectively at their potential for equal participation in their newly won independence. We then asked, "What would need to change in your community to make life more rewarding for everyone? And how can that happen?" Now we were approaching the radical change end of the continuum. People were learning to ask their own questions, analyze the answers, and use the results to plan for change.

Inherent in all of the questions listed here is the power relationship that exists in almost any form of social inquiry or research. Research can be either empowering or disempowering for both researcher and participants. Placing the power to ask and interpret research questions solely in the hands of the researcher takes the power of understanding problems away from those who are the focus of the research. The phenomenon of power and empowerment is therefore central to the selection of a research methodology. Research that is empowering enables people in their communities to contribute to the process and interpret the findings. Empowerment research goes a step farther in that it develops the skills and competence of people in communities to formulate their own questions and conduct their own research. Research findings, therefore, should contribute directly to improving participants' quality of life.

Examining your intention to empower, or to disregard power, is a critical step for all social researchers. How you position yourself on these continua will ultimately influence the kinds of research you conduct.

Note: *Based on theoretical models developed in the field of education (Burrell and Morgan 1979; Rossman and Rallis 1998).*

Field Perspective

Interrogating Data: A Grounded Theory Approach

Susanna Rance, Ph.D.

La Paz

Nowadays I go by the motto "Stick close to your data." I read and reread my field notes and transcripts to see what they tell me. This approach owes much to the grounded theory method—theory "that is inductively derived from the study of the phenomenon it represents" (Glaser and Strauss 1967).*

In practice, grounded theory typically implies the essential features of qualitative research, including observing from a cultural perspective, building flexibility and iteration into the data collection process, and being reflexive—or examining the influence of one's own attributes and assumptions on the research process. Although I do not follow all the steps that Glaser and Strauss prescribed, I hang on to certain principles that have served me in successive medical ethnographies in Bolivia. First, start with an open mind and leave your research agenda as flexible as possible. Next, rather than taking preexisting theory as a given and bringing it down onto your data, interrogate the data and allow fresh theory to develop systematically from your questions.

Drawing on the grounded theory approach, I have found the following questions to be useful:

- Which particularly vivid expressions, or in vivo codes (Strauss 1987), show me how my research participants represent their own realities?
- How do I order and group these expressions into my own sociologically constructed codes?
- What do I learn in confronting the "messy" record of my own interventions in the field?
- What problems and questions come to mind as I reflect on my research experience?
- What new theories do these questions suggest, and how can I test their validity in contrasting circumstances and settings?
- Which research methodologies seem most appropriate for exploring these issues further?

As an example I cite my analysis of interview transcripts from a 1994 study on abortion in periurban migrant settlements. Time and again I found that the same speaker, in the course of an extended interview, would express contradictory views on the subject. One woman who swore abortion was a sin that she would never commit later described her attempts to "lose" a pregnancy "naturally" through a series of self-inflicted procedures. A physician who first condemned abortion as a crime went on to describe it as a social problem whose frequency could be understood in terms of poverty, lack of sex education, and inadequate communication within the family.

From my rereading of these transcripts emerged the question: How could I understand these contradictions? I was unwilling to settle on any one group of expressions as indicative of a speaker's homogenized position. I came to abandon the notion of attitudes that had shaped my former research proposal. In commencing a new study on abortion, I started to search for theories and methods that would enable me to deal constructively with difference. Discourse analysis offered me a coherent approach, with its focus on text as a topic for analysis in its own right rather than as an informative resource (Potter and Wetherell 1987). Variability in accounts, instead of being a problem, was embraced as inevitable, fascinating, and illustrative of the different voices a speaker might assume at particular moments, within specific interactions.

Having found my method, I went on to design a study on medical discourses on abortion in Bolivian hospital settings. I followed the methodological recommendations of Cicourel (1973) and concentrated on a small number of research subjects observed in a wide variety of interactions. Through following just one willing doctor in each hospital, I was able to register their changing voices concerning abortion. I then fed my interpretation of the rationale giving rise to these variations to the entire medical team for their critical comments.

Analysis of these data led me in turn to a further series of questions. What kind of research subjects "did abortion," and who "interrupted a pregnancy"? How did (legally allowed) therapeutic interruption of pregnancy come to be registered in medical histories and hospital statistics as treatment of incomplete abortion? How did medical students and professionals confront the conflict between the condemnation of abortion in their embryology classes and the reality of its practice on gynecology wards?

These questions led me into a further year of fieldwork in the medical school. There I presented students and teachers with real-life hospital stories about abortion, narrated by a series of different speakers. I analyzed their responses and our discussions within the framework of different approaches to medical education. My research in the end has come to center on the uneasy relations between sociology and medicine.

The grounded theory approach has remained a constant in my research through years of queries, doubts, and changes. Each time I become intrigued by a new theory, I try to remember to stick close to my data and ask: Is this what the texts are really saying? Does the theory still hold? Back to the trying and testing and always, new questions.

**Although Glaser and Strauss were not the first to advocate an approach in which substantive theory is "discovered" from data, they named the process and described it in terms of both theory and method.*

CHAPTER THREE

Designing the Study

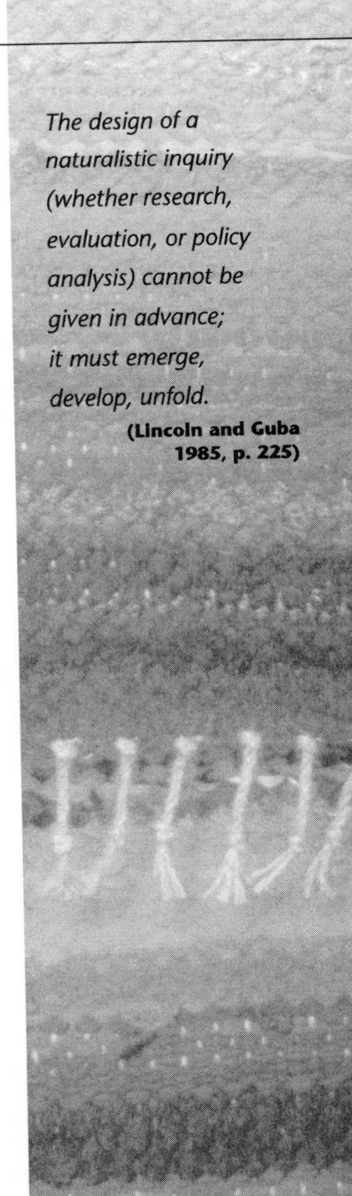

The design of a naturalistic inquiry (whether research, evaluation, or policy analysis) cannot be given in advance; it must emerge, develop, unfold.

(Lincoln and Guba 1985, p. 225)

A WELL-ARTICULATED DESIGN is the basis for all research proposals. It presents the rationale for conducting the study in the first place, and it builds a persuasive argument for the methodology you choose for accomplishing your objectives. Design decisions at this stage will demonstrate the value and rigor of your proposed research. They will also show clearly the relationship between your research problem and the conceptual or theoretical framework that will guide your design (see Chapter Two).

As experienced investigators know, the process of designing research is rarely linear. The steps are interdependent and overlapping, each one challenging the researcher to think ahead to subsequent steps. Qualitative researchers rethink and modify elements of the design even as the data are emerging. However, for the purpose of this discussion, we present important design questions in the following sequence:

- What is the general area of inquiry?
- What is the purpose of the research?
- How is the research problem defined?
- What is the larger conceptual framework?
- What questions will address the research problem?
- What methods will best address the research questions?
- Who should participate?
- What ethical standards will assure the protection of study participants?
- How should the data be collected?

- How will data collectors be trained and monitored?
- How will the data be analyzed?
- How will the results be disseminated?

Written answers to these questions should provide your initial design strategy with sufficient detail by which others can judge the relevance and rigor of your proposed research. Such documentation often becomes the basis for proposals submitted to donors for funding. (See Appendix Three for an example of a study design.) Donors looking for evidence that the design is appropriate to the study's purpose often have their own criteria for judging quality and relevance (see Appendix Nine).

Establishing an Area of Inquiry

Most applied researchers are drawn to an area of inquiry out of personal interest or experience, a desire to help solve a problem, or perhaps in response to a request from a stakeholder or donor. The choice is rooted in values and expectations that the inquiry will in some way benefit society. In public health, areas of inquiry might be the need for dental care in a community health service, the introduction of a new method of cancer screening, the prevalence of HIV in a low-risk population, or perhaps the high incidence of health-related absenteeism in a textile mill. It also is not unusual to develop a cluster of different studies in one problem area, employing combinations of qualitative and quantitative methods, all of which focus on a single broad domain.

Stating the Research Problem and Purpose

As you narrow your focus to a more manageable field, you begin to define the broad area in terms of specific issues that will form the core of the study. If the area of inquiry is quality of prenatal care, the research problem might be to explore women's perceptions of the care they receive at a clinic, the nature and consequences of client-provider interaction, or women's decisions whether or not to seek prenatal care. If the inquiry focuses on occupational hazards in the workplace, the purpose might include exploring the context in which accidents occur and the immediate responses of coworkers in the vicinity. To some extent these and related questions can be addressed by quantitative methods, but exploring circumstances and subjective responses places the problem in an interpretivist framework. Stated in this way, they suggest that the design will enable the researcher to understand and interpret the situation from participants' varied points of view.

A research problem may also come from earlier studies, perhaps a query as to why or under what circumstances a finding has occurred. For example, a household survey carried out in Haiti at the height of the AIDS epidemic revealed that women reported significantly lower risk behavior than men but greater fear of acquiring HIV (Adrien and Cayemittes 1991). Subsequent qualitative research addressed the gap between risk status and fear of AIDS, exploring in greater depth women's perceptions of their own vulnerability (Ulin and others 1995). Or an initial research problem may be generated by a donor organization interested in a particular issue, such as how to allocate limited resources in a country to reduce unwanted pregnancy or expand access to treatment for drug-resistant tuberculosis.

Literature review helps to make a case for the importance of the problem, to build it into a conceptual framework, and to avoid duplication of effort. When you state the problem and purpose of your research, you usually are describing a gap in scientific knowledge, a puzzle to put together, or a mystery to solve. Referring to previous research adds clarity to the problem by placing it in a larger empirical context. It is useful to know the extent to which quantitative research has examined the problem and to identify questions that other qualitative studies may have left unanswered. Are earlier studies consistent or inconsistent? Qualitative researchers welcome divergent findings, because they suggest multiple and sometimes contradictory dimensions of a problem and spur further investigation.

In applied research we usually extend the statement of purpose to potential use of the results, for example, to help improve access to, and quality of, prenatal care or to help lower the rate of sexually transmitted infection (STI) in a population. Even at this early stage of design, it is important to think ahead to the results or the kinds of information that you will want to report and to the potential recipients who will use it. Therefore, an important resource for research questions may be policymakers and program managers who need to know how to make programs more accessible, health care more effective, or services more acceptable. In designing a qualitative study of contraceptive use in Mali, we asked local family planning managers to share some of their concerns. Their interest in the involvement of husbands in family planning decisions led to a modification of the research problem, with results that ultimately played an important role in the analysis and dissemination.

Let us be done with the arguments of [qualitative versus quantitative methods] . . . and get on with the business of attacking our problems with the widest array of conceptual and methodological tools that we possess and they demand.

(Trow 1957, p. 35)

Remember that a single researcher might view a problem from different perspectives at different times, depending on the information needed. From a quantitative perspective, the researcher might wish to describe the scope of a problem or test a hypothesis concerning its occurrence. Using a qualitative perspective, one might shift focus to understanding why the same problem occurs or how it is perceived. From a feminist perspective, the researcher might introduce the concept of power as a determinant of an individual's or group's position on an issue. In most areas of inquiry in social and behavioral health, more than one perspective is useful for understanding a problem to the fullest extent possible.

When the purpose of a study is to form or guide practical decisions about a program or intervention, it becomes formative research. Many public health studies fall in this category, whether or not they are labeled as such. Recognition that your research idea has a formative purpose will affect how you then conceptualize the variables and relationships in the design. We will discuss formative research in more detail later in this chapter.

Conceptualizing the Problem in a Larger Framework

One way to keep your design centered on the research problem is to take the time to develop a conceptual framework. A *conceptual framework* is a set of related ideas behind the research design. It may be a simple list of concepts and their possible associations or a more elaborate schematic diagram of key influences, presumed relationships, and possible outcomes of the research problem (see Box 3.1). Motivated by a compelling problem or some critical gap in knowledge, most researchers begin a study with at least a tentative notion of what factors may be important and how they might fit together in a logical scheme. Literature review can identify findings from previous research that will suggest ways of conceptualizing the current problem.

BOX 3.1

Conceptual Framework: The Dynamics and Meaning of Unintended Pregnancy

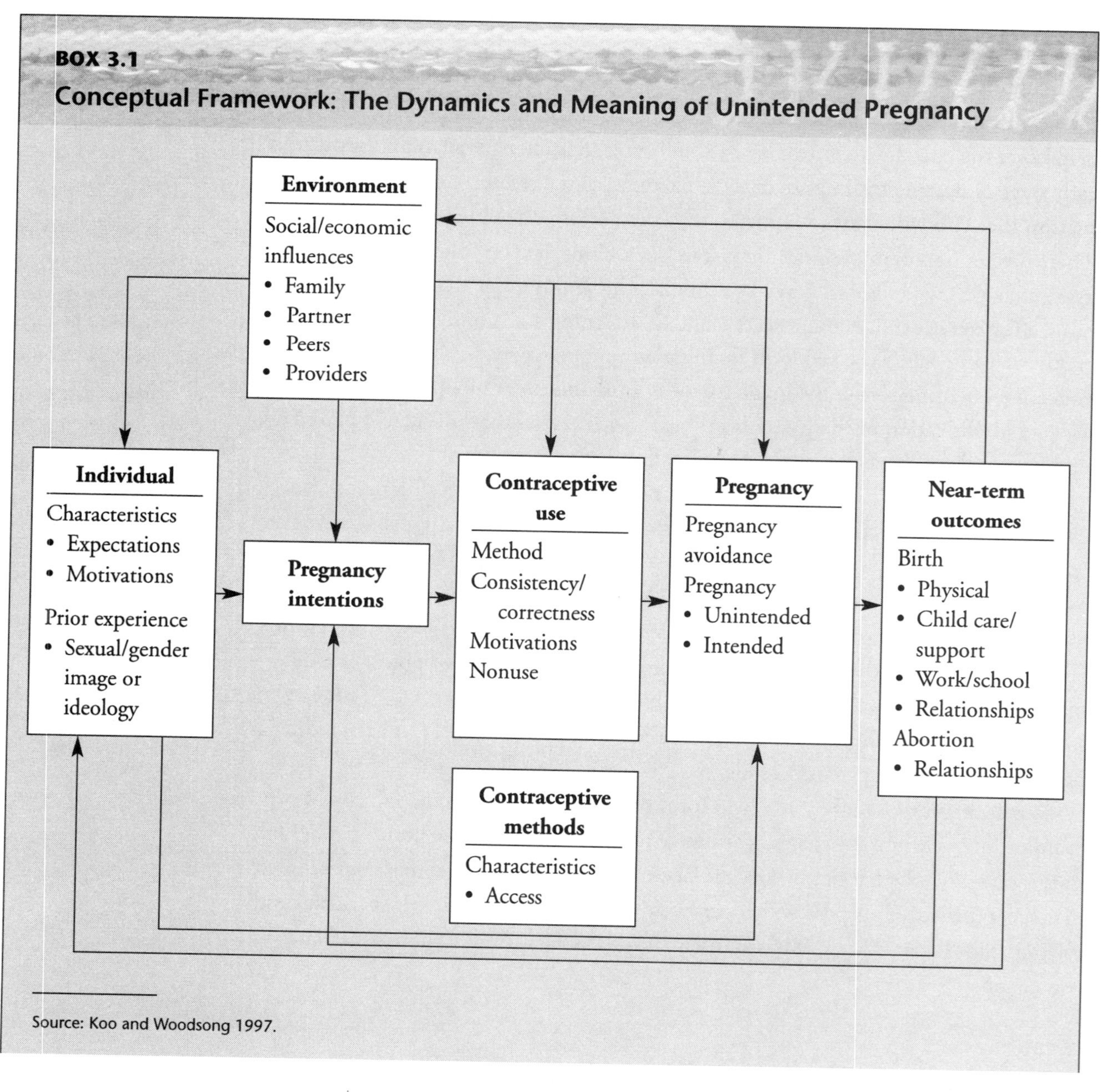

Source: Koo and Woodsong 1997.

Most qualitative researchers start with a set of thoughtfully defined concepts and tentative associations as they design the research and begin to work with study participants. As the study progresses, concepts and their relationships become clearer, articulated in the participants' voices. In many cases researchers discover the framework's elements during the study rather than anticipating them at the design stage. Thus, some studies conclude with a schematic diagram that shows graphically how concepts interrelate.

A conceptual framework does more than help outline research questions. It also provides a context in which others will be able to understand the research. Evidence-based findings contribute to theoretical generalizations, which in turn can be useful to other investigators developing new research. Whether a simple list of concepts or a more elaborate schematic diagram, your framework will be the springboard from which you will both launch your investigation and communicate what you are studying.

For example, one study (Koo and Woodsong 1997) drew on both qualitative and quantitative methods to investigate the dynamics and meaning of unintended pregnancy in a sample of women and their sexual partners. The researchers' purpose was to develop and test measures of pregnancy intendedness, focusing on contextual influences on decision making. To conceptualize the dynamics of unplanned pregnancy, they constructed the model in Box 3.1.

This model contains several clusters of variables:

- Environment: influences in the social, economic, and interpersonal environment that affect contraceptive choice
- Individual factors: characteristics, motivations, experiences, and gender images of women, their partners, and significant older family members
- Pregnancy intentions: couples' conscious or unconscious attitudes that influence contraceptive behavior
- Contraceptive use: the "gate" by which sexually active couples enter or avoid pregnancy—method choice, consistency and correctness of use, or nonuse
- Contraceptive methods: method characteristics and access
- Pregnancy: the occurrence of a pregnancy, classified as (1) successful avoidance and (2) pregnancy intended or unintended
- Near-term outcomes: whether the pregnancy results in birth or abortion; and if a birth, whether the woman receives assistance with child care and support, whether she can return to work, and what effect the birth has on family and social relationships

The conceptual framework enabled the researchers to consider many different facets of the problem and possible relationships among them in order to identify appropriate qualitative and quantitative research strategies. The framework also proved useful in presenting the proposal to a funding agency in that funders could visualize quickly core concepts and interrelationships to be studied. Preliminary hypotheses, developed from the conceptual framework, further clarified goals and expectations of the research. However, from a qualitative perspective, the reviewers understood that the hypotheses were illustrations only and that working hypotheses would be developed from the results of focus group discussions in the first round of data collection.

As this example demonstrates, a conceptual framework is a tentative mapping of the research domain. The example also illustrates the iterative process of qualitative design. The researchers used their framework as a guide, continually examining assumptions and methods in the light of new evidence. As new constructs and new relationships emerged, the structure of the framework changed. For example, research questions related to pregnancy intentions suggested an open-ended, exploratory approach: How or by what process and under what circumstances do couples arrive at decisions to space pregnancies? But the researchers also recognized that questions concerning the parameters of contraceptive method choice—source of supply, frequency and consistency of use or nonuse—could be better answered in a survey design. From survey data they then compiled personal profiles of a subsample of participants' experiences with contraceptive methods. The profiles helped them construct a qualitative instrument that they used to explore the decisions, relationships, and meanings of these choices in qualitative interviews with the subsample. In this way the researchers analyzed qualitative and quantitative data separately for some components of the framework yet fully integrated them in others.

Asking Qualitative Research Questions

As this discussion demonstrates, a thoughtfully constructed conceptual framework can be a valuable compass to help keep your work oriented to the central research problem while ensuring flexibility and credible results.

A carefully defined research problem is an invitation to examine the issue with more specific research questions. There are different kinds of qualitative questions, as outlined in Box 3.2. The research problem will determine whether your design should focus on people's experiences, actions, and behaviors; on their opinions and values; on their feelings or emotional responses; or on what they know or believe to be true in certain situations. Most qualitative studies combine two or more of these elements. Note that some of the questions in Box 3.2 could be asked from either a qualitative or a quantitative perspective.

A quantitative interviewer might suggest several topics and ask respondents to rate their importance. Qualitative questions give participants more freedom to structure their answers as they wish. For example, a health department might want to know what its family planning program can do to reduce rates of unwanted pregnancy in the local adolescent population, suggesting a need for formative research. Stated this broadly, though, one could do little except speculate on a possible solution.

First, you would need to break the big question into specific, researchable questions:

- What are actual rates and trends in adolescent pregnancy?
- What services do local family planning clinics offer young people?
- At what age do adolescents become sexually active?
- What are contraceptive use rates among teenagers?

BOX 3.2

Types of Qualitative Research Questions

Type of Question	Purpose	Examples
Experience/behavior questions	Intended to elicit descriptions of experiences, behaviors, actions, activities; what a person has done, seen, heard, or thought.	If I were present when you talk to your adolescent son about AIDS, what would I hear? How did you introduce your partner to the idea of using a condom as well as the IUD?
Opinion/value questions	Aimed at how people interpret specific events or issues; answers reflect a decision-making process and may reveal goals, opinions, norms, intentions, desires, and values.	What do you think about a girl your age getting pregnant? In the reorganization of this health service, what programs do you think should have highest priority? In your opinion who should have the final say in decisions about how many children to have?
Feeling questions	Probes emotional responses to experiences. Typically spontaneous, often not the result of a decision, often nonrational. May emerge in responses to other kinds of questions.	How did you feel when you learned you were HIV positive? How do women react to situations where they fear physical violence?
Knowledge questions	Intended to discover what people consider factual information—what people think is true. Interviewer records but does not correct misinformation, except at the end of the interview.	Tell me about some different kinds of family planning you know. If a man and woman have just had unprotected sex, is there anything they can do to avoid a pregnancy? What are some ways that a person can get the AIDS virus?

Source: Adapted from Timyan 1991.

Much of this information can be obtained from records, surveys, and other quantitative sources. It is valuable information for describing the extent of the problem, constructing the context, and understanding the problem of unwanted pregnancy in this population.

As you continue to explore the problem, however, you probably will want to know where adolescents themselves stand on this question. An interpretivist perspective can guide you in articulating additional, specific questions:

- How have adolescents experienced reproductive health services?
- How have young people understood the information they have received about sex and sexual health?
- How do young couples negotiate sexual protection?
- What do early sexual relationships mean to adolescents in terms of costs and benefits?
- What has happened when adolescents have tried to reduce their risk of pregnancy or STIs?

Adopting a feminist perspective, on the other hand, you might decide to examine the meaning of negotiation in relation to the balance of power in the partner relationship and the ability of adolescents to participate in decisions affecting their health.

Questions like these call for a qualitative approach, because in different ways they ask why adolescent pregnancy in this community is so high. They expand and elaborate on the original research question—how to reduce adolescent pregnancy—by addressing some of the underlying dynamics of adolescent sexual experience. They also have the potential to elicit a range of information, including knowledge, experience, opinions, and feelings, as well as their social context—types of questions that are summarized in Box 3.2.

However specific such questions seem in the beginning, later data collection may uncover material that leads to new and more insightful questions, which in turn may suggest yet more ways to understand and articulate the nature of adolescent pregnancy. What do clinic personnel believe is their responsibility to young people who want contraceptive advice? To what extent do young women discuss pregnancy and disease prevention with their partners? Such is the iterative nature of qualitative research at the level of problem definition. Even after the data collection begins, you may find that you continue to refine and build on your research questions in the light of new insights.

A source of formative questions not to be overlooked is stakeholders in the project, individuals and groups who understand the context of the problem and whose own goals will be served by the results of the research. In the example from Mali cited earlier, the researchers had not been aware that service providers were worried that so many women were coming to the family planning clinic in secret. Asking practitioners "What information would help you provide better service?" can generate new questions that will lead to more relevant and useful conclusions.

Leaders of women's advocacy groups can also be a valuable source of collaboration if your research problem is consistent with their agenda for women. In our experience advocacy organizations often lack the resources to conduct research and are eager to share their own knowledge as insiders to develop mutually rewarding research questions.

When you take your research questions to the field, remember that in the iterative process of qualitative inquiry, your design work may not be finished. Qualitative research problems are often deeply stratified, composed of layers of meaning that have not been accessible to other methods in the past. Thus, it may take several iterations before the experienced researcher is satisfied with a set of research questions that will tap the problem's underlying dimensions. The natural evolution of a qualitative research question is a growth process in which a basic question (for example: Why are people not coming to this clinic?) can continue to generate new and more refined questions. On the other hand, the tendency of good research questions to grow and multiply must not imply design without form. Vigilance is needed to ensure that emerging research questions retain an internal consistency and clear relationship to the basic problem or purpose of the research.

Box 3.3 illustrates how an initial set of questions can emerge from a single broad research problem. Questions from the dual method contraceptive study in this example suggest that participants will come from at least three groups: sexually active women, sexually active men, and reproductive health care providers. Discussion of these topics may lead to additional questions that would explore further the implications of participants' comments. Understanding the problem—how to introduce dual method use—might be further enriched by using quantitative techniques as well.

Selecting Data Collection Methods

Once your research problem has become a set of questions, you are ready to put them to work. Using your conceptual framework as a guide, the challenge now is to match the research questions with the methods and techniques that can yield the richest information. Box 3.4 compares the characteristics, strengths, and weaknesses of four types of data collection, from the least structured, qualitative format to a more structured, typically quantitative design. Researchers sometimes combine these types to address different dimensions of a research problem. However, our focus here will be mainly on techniques for asking qualitative questions in an open-ended format. Later in this chapter we will return to these comparisons in the discussion of collecting data.

Because this guide cannot adequately cover all qualitative techniques, we focus on three major methodological strategies: observation, including study of existing documents; in-depth interview; and focus group discussion. We will discuss each in more detail in Chapter Four. Observing, interviewing, and managing group discussion, aided by careful note taking and transcription, are basic methods of qualitative science. Once you master the principles and skills of observation and interaction and learn to use documentary materials to understand human behavior, you will have a valuable set of tools that you can adapt to numerous research problems and circumstances, from formative

BOX 3.3

From Research Problem to Research Question: A Qualitative Study of Dual Method Use

Research Problem

To assess the feasibility of introducing dual-method use (DMU), the use of condoms with another contraceptive method, among couples at risk of pregnancy and sexually transmitted infection (STI)/HIV.

Research Questions

How and to what extent do women perceive themselves to be at risk of pregnancy and STI/HIV?

How do women view DMU?

- What experiences have women had with the simultaneous use of condoms and another method?
- What do they know about DMU?
- How do they describe negative and positive aspects of DMU?
- How do they perceive others' experiences with DMU?
- To what extent will women accept DMU?
- Under what circumstances do women believe DMU is an appropriate choice?
- If a woman believes DMU is appropriate and effective, why might she not use it?
- Whose decision does she believe it is to use two methods?

How do men view DMU?

- What do men believe is the purpose of using two methods?
- Under what circumstances do they believe couples should or should not rely on two methods?
- What do they see as the partner's role in promoting or discouraging DMU?

What are providers' opinions of DMU?

- How do providers describe their current practice regarding recommendation of DMU to couples?
- Under what circumstances do providers believe DMU is indicated and not indicated?
- What obstacles do providers identify in promoting DMU?
- How do they think providers can circumvent these obstacles?

inquiry to program evaluation. Be aware as you design your study that the methods you choose in the beginning may not be the only ones you will use. Even with the study under way, a qualitative researcher must have the flexibility to modify the design, pursue new leads, add new questions, or turn to other subgroups in the population for different perspectives. For example, pilot data from a focus group may reveal that people are reluctant to disclose their views on certain topics in front of others or that they are not accustomed to expressing opinions on controversial issues. You then may decide that individual interviews or one of the projective techniques discussed in Chapter Four will be a more comfortable and rewarding approach.

We urge readers to consult the Suggested Readings and Selected Internet Resources at the end of this volume to explore other possibilities for gathering qualitative data. We also encourage you to devise your own techniques, adapting strategic frameworks

BOX 3.4

Structural Differences in Qualitative Data Collection

Type of Interview	Characteristics	Strengths	Weaknesses
Informal conversational interview	Questions emerge from the immediate context and are asked in the natural course of things; there is no predetermination of question topics or wording.	Increases the salience and relevance of questions; interviews are built on and emerge from observations; interviews can be matched to individuals and circumstances.	Different information collected from different people with different questions; less systematic and comprehensive; certain questions do not arise naturally; data organization and analysis can be quite difficult.
Interview guide approach	Topics and issues to be covered are specified in advance in outline form; interviewer decides sequence and wording of questions in the course of the interview.	The outline increases the comprehensiveness of the data and makes data collection somewhat systematic for each respondent; logical gaps in data can be anticipated and closed; interviews remain fairly conversational and situational.	Important and salient topics may be inadvertently omitted; interviewer flexibility in sequencing and wording questions can result in substantially different responses from different perspectives, thus reducing the comparability of responses.
Standardized open-ended interview	The exact wording and sequence of questions are determined in advance; respondents are asked the same basic questions in the same order; questions are worded in a completely open-ended format.	Respondents answer the same questions, thus increasing comparability of responses; data are complete for each person on the topics addressed in the interview; reduces interviewer effects and bias when several interviewers are used; permits evaluation users to see and review the instrumentation used in the evaluation; facilitates organization and analysis of the data.	Little flexibility in relating the interview to particular individuals and circumstances; standardized wording of questions may constrain and limit naturalness and relevance of questions and answers.
Closed, fixed response interview	Questions and response categories are determined in advance; responses are fixed; respondent chooses from among these fixed responses.	Data analysis is simple; responses can be directly compared and easily aggregated; many questions can be asked in a short time.	Respondents must fit their experiences and feelings into the researcher's categories; may be perceived as impersonal, irrelevant, and mechanistic; can distort what respondents really mean or experience by so completely limiting their response choices.

Source: Adapted from Patton 1990, pp. 280–289.

such as those presented in Chapter Two to new research problems and contexts. Many of the innovative techniques reported in qualitative literature today have come from the creative improvisation of researchers seeking better ways to help participants express their perspectives on and experiences with often sensitive topics. These field-driven techniques have included information-generating strategies such as asking young people to photograph significant moments in their lives and training HIV-positive women to interview each other. In both examples the interpretations of the study participants enhance analysis.

INDIVIDUAL INTERVIEWS OR FOCUS GROUPS?

Whether to interview participants individually or in groups is a common design question not always easy to answer. In-depth individual interviews establish a one-to-one relationship between interviewer and respondent, whereas participants in group interviews relate to each other as well as to the interviewer. In an in-depth interview, information comes from the thoughtful reflection of one person aided by exchange with the interviewer—one person's point of view. In focus groups information comes from interaction among members of the group—several points of view.

Highly sensitive topics, such as injection drug use, sexual behavior, or domestic violence, may argue for an individual interview format with maximum privacy and intimacy. However, if study participants are already accustomed to informal exchange on the topic among themselves—for example, discussion of disease prevention among commercial sex workers—then the investigator might choose a focus group. Ask the question: Sensitive to whom? Questions that would cause embarrassment in a group of middle-class women might be easy for women whose livelihood depends on sexual services at enormous risk to their own health and well-being. In our study of family planning decision making in Mali, many of the participants were covert users of contraception, often in defiance of the pronatalist wishes of husbands and elders (Castle and others 1999). Individual interviews were the only option for encouraging these women to share their experiences while protecting their secret. Researchers encounter similar constraints in studies of injection drug users or of women who have broken the law by seeking abortion. In such cases the problem of disclosure can often be resolved in individual interviews with assurance of privacy and confidentiality.

When the research problem focuses on cultural norms, attitudes, or reactions of a group to some aspect of their environment, group discussion can be a rewarding technique. What expectations determine family health decisions in a rural Bolivian community? What factors are likely to encourage parents' support of a new program for adolescent health or invite young people's participation? How can vulnerable women negotiate protection against STIs and HIV/AIDS? Questions such as these focus on group norms rather than individual behavior. In each example a group of people committed to the issue will probably enjoy an opportunity to express their opinions, hear other people's views, challenge one another, and participate in studying a topic of compelling interest. By stimulating interest in a common problem and listening to others' views, participation can also motivate people to initiate change. As they wrestle with questions posed by the moderator (and sometimes by others in the group), participants' comments and debate among themselves will shed light on their community's wider perspectives, revealing clues to the context, or the social environment, in which individuals make decisions that affect their lives. Spontaneous exchange among participants also will show nuances in the language of ideas—the terms people use and the verbal frameworks they commonly construct for understanding their worlds.

Mixing Methods

Because no single research method can tap all dimensions of a complex research problem, it is often valuable to combine two or more methods, drawing conclusions from a synthesis of the results. Multiple method use, also called triangulation, unquestionably results in a broader perspective on the problem and often more persuasive findings for policymakers. Similar results from two or more methods could increase the credibility of the findings, whereas dissimilar results might raise new questions about alternative interpretations (see Box 3.5).

BOX 3.5

Common Ways to Mix Methodologies

If you understand the basic principles and techniques of qualitative and quantitative strategies, you will discover useful ways to combine them:

- A formative phase (for example, focus group discussions) that precedes a quantitative phase (for example, household survey) can provide information for generating hypotheses and designing the instrument, as well as identifying language meaningful to the study population.
- Quantitative data can also be used in a formative phase, providing useful background information for designing a qualitative study.
- Quantitative data on study participants (for example, sociodemographic data and sexual and reproductive histories) can help to interpret qualitative results or highlight important subgroup differences.
- A qualitative phase that occurs at the end of a quantitative study can help to interpret quantitative findings or evaluate an intervention.
- Qualitative and quantitative techniques can be used independently to examine a problem from different perspectives.
- Qualitative (open-ended) questions can be included in a quantitative instrument to collect limited data on issues that cannot be answered in the structured format.
- Qualitative exit interviews can be conducted with a sample of quantitative survey participants to check the external validity or comprehensiveness of the measures.

Note that different results from one method do not necessarily invalidate the results of another. Given that reality is defined in many ways and in many contexts, different data collection tools may reveal a variety of perspectives, different ways that people conceptualize and evaluate the same situation. Like a photographer attempting to capture a perfect likeness, the careful researcher considers the research problem from different angles, using quantitative or qualitative methods or integrating both in various combinations.

Increasingly, researchers are discovering the benefits of using more than one theoretical perspective to study a problem (Tashakkori and Teddlie 1998; Knodel 1997; Obermeyer 1997). Their research reports demonstrate that combining qualitative and quantitative strategies in a single study can result in a more powerful design than either used alone. For example, a study of condom acceptability in a population at risk of STI/HIV transmission might include a structured survey of knowledge, attitudes, and practices regarding condom use (a quantitative component), in addition to in-depth interviews with a subset of the survey population (a qualitative component) and observation in pharmacies that sell condoms (both quantitative and qualitative). Each technique would yield different but complementary results, and together they would give you a more complete picture than one approach alone.

In applied social and behavioral research, few problems do not have the potential for qualitative and quantitative inquiry. In a study that explored how cultural differences influence minority caretakers' responses to Alzheimer's disease and related dementias, Weitzman and Levkoff (2000) conducted qualitative interviews with forty caretakers, followed by 120 structured interviews using several standardized scales. The authors discovered that this combination highlighted the interplay between culture and care more clearly than could any single method alone. They concluded that rigor in research means "not being beholden to a particular research method, but rather letting the questions point to the methods even if it means combining methods" (p. 203).

Similarly, a study of the students' use of a school health service might include records of student attendance with age and grade, students' health complaints, the school nurse's observations, and treatment or referral (a quantitative component). In-depth interviews with students, parents, and school personnel (a qualitative component), and observation in the nurse's office (both quantitative and qualitative), would yield three sets of complementary results. Together they could offer a comprehensive understanding of student health care from multiple perspectives.

In a different application of mixed methods, a team of investigators sought to develop a valid and reliable instrument that could help monitor the prevalence and nature of domestic violence against women (Smith, Earp, and DeVellis 1995; Smith, Tessaro, and Earp 1995). Their first concern was to reconceptualize violence by exploring the meanings that battered women attach to the particular physical and psychological violence that they experienced. Data came from transcripts of focus groups in which women were encouraged to talk to each other about what battering meant to them. From these meanings the researchers developed a conceptual framework that replaced the traditional concept of violent acts as discrete events (number, frequency, and behavioral characteristics) with a continuous concept that captured battered women's sense of perpetual vulnerability. From the qualitative transcripts, the researchers then identified potential scale items that seemed to highlight women's continuous perception of susceptibility to danger, loss of power, and loss of control in relationships with male partners. These items became the basis for construction of the Women's Experiences with Battering (WEB) scale, a valid and concise measure for studying relations between battering and health or health behavior, estimates of prevalence, and evaluation of the impact of interventions on battered women's situations.

In either qualitative or quantitative study design, written material such as clinic reports, letters, newspapers, and advertising also can be combined with other sources of data. Documentary evidence offers valuable insight into the context of relationships, decisions, and actions, sometimes helping to explain or expand on data gathered with other methods. Chapter Four will discuss documentary methods in greater detail.

A PRACTICAL STRATEGY FOR MIXED-METHOD DESIGN

Much has been written in support of mixed methodology, but the reader is often left to manage the technical task of combining very different techniques in a coherent design. Once you have established the strategic relevance of two or more methods to the research questions, you will need to decide how to coordinate them. For this purpose we advocate the priority-sequence model (see Box 3.6), an approach that integrates the "complementary strengths of different methods through a division of labor . . . within the same overall project" (Morgan 1998, p. 366). The division of labor requires two basic decisions, one that assigns priority and one that determines sequence.

The four-cell model represents four basic designs in which "(a) the principal method is either qualitative or quantitative (priority) and (b) the complementary method occurs as a preliminary or a follow-up stage to the primary method (sequence)" (Morgan 1998, p. 367). In each cell of the model, the primary method is abbreviated in capital letters and the complementary method in lowercase letters; arrows indicate their sequence in the design. Thus, the model shows four types of design:

1. *A principally quantitative study that begins with a smaller qualitative study.* The qualitative component might be a formative phase of participant observation or focus group discussions, to develop the content of a survey questionnaire. A Demographic and Health Survey, for example, might use the results of exploratory work to ensure that the survey instrument covers important topics in language familiar to the respondents. In clinical trials a preliminary qualitative phase could provide valuable information on the trial population and the likely acceptability of the contraceptive method to be tested.

2. *A principally qualitative study that begins with a complementary quantitative study.* A preliminary survey, for example, might guide selection of study sites and help to define the sample. Qualitative research in public health frequently begins with a review of secondary data from national health, census, and other population surveys in order to relate the research problem to a larger demographic context. Quantitative findings from surveys may highlight important issues that raise questions to explore with qualitative methods.

BOX 3.6

Priority-Sequence Model: Decisions for Integrating Methods

Quantitative	Qualitative
1. Qualitative preliminary qual ➔ QUANT Smaller qualitative study helps guide the data collection in a principally quantitative study. • Can generate hypotheses, develop content for questionnaires and interventions, and so on. *Example:* Focus groups shape culturally sensitive versions of a new health promotion campaign.	2. Quantitative Preliminary quant ➔ QUAL Smaller quantitative study helps guide the data collection in a principally qualitative study. • Can guide purposive sampling, establish preliminary results to pursue in depth, and so on. *Example:* A survey of different units in a hospital locates sites for more extensive ethnographic data collection.
3. Qualitative follow-up QUANT ➔ qual Smaller qualitative study helps evaluate and interpret results from a principally quantitative study. • Can provide interpretations for poorly understood results, help explain outliers, and so on. *Example:* In-depth interviews explain why one clinic generates higher levels of patient satisfaction.	4. Quantitative follow-up QUAL ➔ quant Smaller quantitative study helps evaluate and interpret results from a principally qualitative study. • Can generalize results to different samples, test elements of emergent theories, and so on. *Example:* A statewide survey of a school-based health program pursues earlier results from a case study.

Source: Morgan 1998, p. 368.

3. *A principally quantitative study with a complementary qualitative study as a follow-up.* An important purpose of the qualitative phase in this design is to help interpret the results of the quantitative study. The qualitative component may or may not be part of the initial study design. For example, a national survey of AIDS knowledge, attitudes, and practices might turn up the finding that the majority of respondents understood the basics of prevention but chose not to protect themselves. The researchers could then explore this finding by inviting survey respondents to participate in focus groups to discuss what AIDS transmission and protection meant to them and to others in their community. Similarly, quantitative researchers sometimes build into their designs a plan for

analysis that includes a small qualitative study at the end, in which individuals from the study population discuss and help interpret selected findings.

4. *A principally qualitative study with a complementary quantitative study as a follow-up.* In this design the quantitative phase may be a valuable way to test the extent to which qualitative findings are generalizable in a larger population. Or one might want to look at qualitative data on attitudes toward STIs from a different perspective by using standardized rating scales in a subsample of the study population. For example, a qualitative study of STI risk among adolescents identified fear of infection, embarrassment, and age as important constructs in attitudes regarding protection. In a follow-up study, the researchers constructed scale items from the adolescent participants' comments; then, having validated the scales and confirmed their reliability, they applied scale analysis techniques to study quantitatively the dimensions, fear, and embarrassment in relation to age. Construction of the WEB scale, cited previously, is another example of this type of integration.

In some mixed-method studies, qualitative and quantitative components may be equally important. Different methods of data collection may occur simultaneously, guided by complementary objectives. In analysis the researcher might draw on both at the same time to address the central problem. Or analysis of data from one method might serve to illuminate data from the other. Both formative and evaluation research can benefit from the multiple perspectives of a mixed methodology.

Combining different qualitative techniques is also useful but only if the data collection and methods of analysis are carefully matched to the research questions. For example, a study of adolescent sexuality in Malawi combined in-depth interviews, participant observation, and focus group discussions. The purpose was to examine the social and information networks of adolescent girls: the ways they learn about sexuality, their perception of the risk of HIV infection, their experience with sex, and the skills they learn to avoid infection. The authors reported that "focus group discussion elicited more socially correct answers and produced good data on social norms but not very good data on deviations from those norms. By contrast, in-depth, one-on-one interviews were necessary to elicit good data on actual knowledge and experience." Using more than one qualitative research method "not only broadens the quality of information that can be obtained about sexuality and reproductive health issues in a community, it also opens the way to finding culturally acceptable ways of disseminating information inside your community with the support of and benefit to all its members" (Helitzer-Allen and others 1994, p. 81).

Formative Research

GETTING TO KNOW THE AUDIENCE

Formative research is the name given to any inquiry that takes place before a program or scientific investigation for the purpose of defining the selected population, creating appropriate programs or research procedures, and ensuring that the program or study to follow will be culturally relevant and acceptable. Your study's purpose will help you determine whether or not to take a formative approach to your study design. Formative studies draw on many methods of social and behavioral research, and often they combine quantitative and qualitative methods to achieve their end.

In program development a formative phase may be as simple as asking a few preliminary questions or as comprehensive as a multistage research investigation. Formative inquiry often is associated with rapid assessment methods in program development, in which a shortage of resources may require the investigator to collect as much useful information as possible as efficiently as possible. The conclusions reached by a rapid assessment are necessarily more limited than those from a more extensive formative investigation, but they may be all that is needed to launch a project. For example, a school health educator might begin a new AIDS awareness program by asking students what they know about HIV/AIDS and what they think would be important to include in classroom discussion. The same questions repeated at intervals during implementation of the program would help the health educator monitor the process (process evaluation) and might suggest modifications to keep the program on track.

Decisions on policy issues frequently are guided by formative research that helps busy policymakers anticipate and understand the implications of the policy in the population that will be affected. In a field perspective at the end of this chapter, Hatzell describes a situation in which Department of Health officials urgently needed guidance for research allocation decisions that would affect their HIV/AIDS prevention program. Turning to their public health research unit, they were able to get the information they needed. Based on findings from structured interviews with women and a qualitative analysis of open-ended questions, the ministry concluded that vulnerable women were likely to use the female condom and that funds therefore should be allocated for this purpose.

These examples of a rapid assessment approach to formative research stand in contrast to a more extensive formative study prior to development of an intervention for diabetes prevention in a Pacific Island population (Cortes and others 2001). Such formative inquiry may include combining qualitative and quantitative methods, integrating qualitative methods into clinical trials, assessing community needs, or preparing for any research or program that requires preliminary information. The purpose of the diabetes prevention study, for example, was to explore dietary patterns and perceptions of the disease, as well as local terminology. A quantitative survey of food intake, along with sociodemographic descriptive factors and anthropometric measurements, provided quantitative baseline information. Qualitative data collection focused on beliefs and perceptions relating to food, activity, illness, and body size. In addition to mixing qualitative and quantitative methods, this study employed a mix of qualitative techniques, including in-depth interviews, freelisting of foods and illnesses, pile sorts of foods, ranking of foods for fattiness, valuation of body size, and unstructured observation of eating behavior. Data analysis led to a set of guiding principles with recommendations for intervention that the researchers then incorporated into the diabetes prevention program. The researchers also identified effective media of communication for intervention and presented their conclusions as a model for the use of formative research to enhance prevention and treatment programs for diabetes.[1]

Community assessments are another use of formative research. In their introduction to the manual *Assessing Safe Motherhood in the Community: A Guide to Formative Research,* the authors point out that "a well-conducted Community Assessment will show where intervention is needed to enable mothers and newborns to thrive by preventing as many problems as possible; ensuring community recognition of problems; encouraging prompt and proper response to complications; and by providing for accessible, responsive, and competent care" (Nachbar and others 1998, p. 13).

Similarly, action-oriented community diagnosis, a tool developed by Eng and Blanchard (1991), enables researchers to identify group as well as individual needs and, by bringing community residents into the diagnostic process, motivate interested groups to find solutions based on the results of their own community assessment. This approach is particularly useful for linking individuals' health perceptions and needs to conscious behavioral change.

A different but common application of formative research is in the design of pharmaceutical and biomedical studies. For example, trials to evaluate the efficacy of a vaccine require large samples of individuals at risk. Whether individuals will volunteer for vaccine trials, whether they will remain in the study, and how they will respond to risk-reduction counseling are questions that can be addressed by social and behavioral scientists collaborating with biomedical researchers who will use the results to shape the trial (Francis and others 2003; Guest and others 2004).

Empirical evidence in estimates of the parameters of disease is equally important when it comes to developing programs to prevent, reduce, or eradicate the disease. Nichter (1990) has developed a model to guide epidemiologists and others through the formative transition from a population-based health problem to a culturally relevant intervention. This model, reproduced in Box 3.7, highlights the research questions that should precede program development and enable public health scientists to identify gaps in their understanding of the target population before embarking on a costly initiative. Formative questions can also be asked when a program seems to have failed, as in Box 1.1 (p. 3).

Whether paving the way for health intervention, informing policy, or creating a database for research design, formative research can produce valuable information for evidence-based decisions at all levels of practice.

Selecting a Sampling Strategy

In decisions about whom to interview, researchers are commonly guided by the paradigm, or theoretical framework, they have chosen for a study. From an interpretive perspective, the investigator views ordinary people as experts by virtue of the experiences and ideas they can share and their willingness to help explore the research problem. As always in the iterative process of qualitative research, selection criteria may change as the study progresses, allowing the researcher to follow new leads with information from new sources (Rubin and Rubin 1995).

BOX 3.7

Eight Stages of Formative Research

1. *To inform:* What are people thinking now, saying now, and doing now about the problem?
   - Range of ideas about the problem, sense of risk, concern.
   - Language used to talk about the problem in context; lay interpretation of public health or medical terminology introduced.
   - Self-care practices: long-standing and emergent.
   - Health care seeking: When, where, after how much delay, reasons why various services are and are not preferred?
   - Expectations from providers and programs: What do people expect? What do they receive? How do they evaluate quality of care?
   - Compliance with treatment or prevention guidelines: patients, practitioners, and health care system.
   - Interactive sets of factors contributing to the distribution of the health problem (health disparity) and differences in health care outcomes.
   - History of previous intervention attempts.
2. *To identify:* What are the important problems that need to be solved?
   - In the community (broadly defined, attentive to factions, action sets, power relations).
   - At local health centers and hospitals.
   - During health provider training and so on.
   - In the health care system at large, other institutions.
   - In the private sector, marketplace.
3. *To generate a list of options* for interventions in the community and clinic(s).
   - Options are generated through discussion with community members and health staff who are invited to reflect on problem areas and data collected during stage one.
4. *To foster critical assessment and problem solving:* What are the pluses and minuses of possible interventions?
   - This requires considerations of feasibility (money, time, reorganization).
   - Thoughts about how different stakeholders (doctors, nurses, and so on) will respond to each option.
   - What are constraints to change and opportunity costs?
   - What is the benefit for the people you want to reach?
   - Who is likely not to be reached?
   - Is it worth the effort?

Strength-weakness-analysis-target (SWAT) analysis of intervention options:

Options	Pluses +	Minuses -

This step requires consideration of the motivations and opportunities for change at this moment, resources, complementary and competing programs, and so on.

5. *To investigate how best to implement* promising interventions.
   - Details matter.
   - Who, when, where, how much?
   - Exploration of supportive collaborations.

6. *To monitor responses* to interventions in real time.
   - To facilitate midcourse correction.
   - Reflection, refinement.

7. *To evaluate:* What are intervention goals, and how do we know if we are reaching them?
   - Process as well as outcome evaluation.
   - Difference across intervention sites.
   - Impact of secular trends.

8. *To assess* how the intervention and its results are being presented to the public and the scientific community.
   - By participants, funding agencies, and the press.
   - What motivates such presentation?
   - Response to this presentation of knowledge.

Source: Model developed for the International Network of Clinical Epidemiology by Mark Nichter (1990); reproduced by permission of Mark Nichter.

GENERALIZATION VERSUS INSIGHT

A typical goal of quantitative research is to generalize findings to larger populations, achieving a high degree of reliability. To minimize sampling error, every case in a sampling frame must have an equal probability of selection. The purpose of most qualitative studies, on the other hand, is to produce information-rich data from a sample chosen for its ability to speak to the research issue (Patton 1990). Qualitative research emphasizes depth more than breadth, insight rather than generalization, illuminating the meaning of human behavior. Although qualitative researchers sometimes use numbers and frequencies to record observations, conceptual rather than numerical considerations determine sample selection. The challenge for the qualitative researcher, therefore, is to select participants who will be able to provide the most meaningful information on the topic. The extent to which results may be relevant to other populations will be enhanced by careful documentation of the conceptual links between research problem, sample selection process, and emerging data.

The validity, meaningfulness, and insights generated from qualitative inquiry have more to do with the information-richness of the cases selected and the observational/analytical capabilities of the researcher than with sample size.
(Patton 1990, p. 185)

SELECTION: THEORETICAL OR A PRIORI?

In qualitative design there are two basic approaches to selecting participants; each places more emphasis on the level of experience or insight of potential respondents than on their random selection. One of these approaches, called theoretical sampling, is particularly appropriate when the main purpose of data collection is to generate substantive theory (Strauss and Corbin 1990). Beginning with a small number of individuals or groups, the researcher asks, "Given what I am learning, what information do I need next and where—or in what groups—will I find it?" (Flick 1998, p. 65). In other words, theoretical sampling is continuous and gradual, guided by data collection, analysis, and interpretation as theory builds. It is especially consistent with the goals and techniques of grounded theory, presented in more detail in Chapter Two.

A priori sampling is the approach most familiar to applied researchers in public health. Based on your research problem and purpose, you define in advance of data collection the sample's characteristics and structure. If your purpose is to understand health attitudes and behaviors of adolescents in a community, you will select participants from this group as well as other individuals whose opinions on adolescent health or whose actual experiences with young people give them special insight into your area of inquiry. If different perspectives and behaviors are known to prevail in the population, then you would choose participants who differ in these respects. At this point you will also decide the numbers of participants in each category and the background characteristics that will help you interpret their responses.

Note that a priori selection does not preclude sampling additions and changes as the study progresses. The most important consideration in qualitative sampling is the data's richness, or explanatory value. In the adolescent health example, you might discover that young people with conservative religious views perceive sexual norms differently than do their peers with a different religious orientation. The next step could be to invite a sample of religious leaders in the community to help you explore religious influences on adolescent health decisions.

SAMPLE SIZE

When a goal of the study is to generalize findings from a sample to a larger population, as in many quantitative designs, the researcher can calculate a representative sample size from a formula. In qualitative studies optimum size is less clear. The investigator is guided by the degree to which incoming data adequately answer the research questions—an ambiguous rule at best. But if sample size depends on completeness of the data (Rubin and Rubin 1995), how do you know when data are complete? If the research problem is a simple one, it is possible that one individual could provide the whole answer. In public health, however, most research design is not that simple. Generally, you collect data from as many groups or individuals as necessary to answer the research questions. When little new information is coming from your observations, interviews, or focus group discussions, you can be reasonably confident that you have saturated that source of information to the point of redundancy (Glaser and Strauss 1967).

In most funded research, such indeterminate measures as saturation and redundancy are likely to be impractical for budgeting and the length of time researchers might take to reach that point unacceptable to donors. Qualitative researchers might begin with "minimum samples based on expected reasonable coverage . . . given the purpose of the study and stakeholder interests" (Patton 1990, p. 186). Once in the field, you will make a decision as to whether you need to expand your sample. Altering the subgroup composition in your design is justified in qualitative research if doing so will enrich your findings.

The qualitative researcher tries to collect information representative of the range of experiences, perspectives, and behaviors relevant to the research question. In contrast, quantitative approaches are more likely to result in samples that represent the distribution of these variables. The important thing to remember is that "the logic of purposeful sampling is different from the logic of probability sampling" (Patton 1990, p. 185). Small purposive samples are ideally suited to qualitative inquiry. A large random sample could not accomplish the objectives of an in-depth study, any more than a small nonrandom sample could accurately represent a large population. For the qualitative researcher, it is crucial to describe, justify, and explain small-sample selection so that others can judge its strengths and weaknesses. "Exercising care not to overgeneralize from purposeful samples, while maximizing to the full the advantages of in-depth, purposeful sampling, will do much to alleviate concerns about small sample size" (Patton 1990, p. 186).

RECRUITING PARTICIPANTS

Study participants are drawn from a community, any of its institutions (for example, clinics, schools, churches, workplaces, bars), or wherever people are willing to share knowledge and experience related to the research topics. In some studies researchers visit sites where potential participants gather; they chat informally with people and select an initial sample based on the apparent readiness of individuals to address the research issues. In other studies clinic records or membership lists serve as a sampling frame, particularly when individuals in the frame share a common characteristic of interest to the research. As in all sampling strategies, decisions must also be made regarding other selection criteria, such as age or marital status. In our study of new contraceptive users in Mali, researchers worked with clinic personnel to identify every married woman who had come to the clinic to begin family planning for the first time. But because this study used a longitudinal design, the invitation to participate was extended only to women who were geographically accessible for follow-up interviews.

In community-based studies, you may want to enlist the help of residents to identify and invite eligible individuals to participate. If so, select such recruiters carefully to avoid possible coercion or alienation of important subgroups. As we discuss in Chapter Five, incorporating local people into the field team at this point is especially useful in unfamiliar cultures or in communities with language barriers. It is important to orient helpers to the study's purpose, rehearsing with them how to introduce it, how to invite participation, and how to assure potential participants of confidentiality and freedom to decline.

SAMPLE SELECTION TECHNIQUES

Selecting a sample for a qualitative study is not haphazard, but neither is it bound by rigid rules of reproducibility. It should be systematic but flexible, guided by clear research questions as articulated in your theoretical framework. Because the purpose of qualitative design is to explore in depth, the investigator carefully selects cases that can typify or shed light on the object of study. Therefore, to identify and gain access to those who can teach you the most about your topic, it follows that sampling methods will generally be based on purpose rather than on statistical probability of selection. In qualitative sampling, purposiveness is a strategic approach, not a single technique. It means selecting participants for their ability to provide rich information. Purposive sampling should never be confused with sampling for convenience. The latter, motivated primarily by ease of access to respondents, may be economical but does not necessarily reflect the study's purpose; and it may weaken significantly the quality of the data.

There are many purposive strategies, each linked to the purpose of the study as expressed in the initial research question. Following one such typology (Patton 1990), we describe several strategies that in our experience have been useful tools for qualitative sampling decisions. Although we present these techniques separately, readers should be aware that many studies combine more than one.

Extreme Sampling Extreme, or deviant, sampling selects extreme cases in order to highlight and understand conditions or characteristics of more typical situations. For example, a study of reproductive health provider effectiveness selected two clinics known for high levels of client satisfaction and two with a poor reputation in the local community. By observing services and interviewing clients with experience in each setting, the investigators were able to identify and prioritize qualities that favored optimum use and those that discouraged it. In using extreme cases, the investigator must take care not to distort reality by making the unusual seem to be the norm. The purpose is not to generalize to all clinics but to magnify certain characteristics.

Intensity Sampling Intensity sampling focuses on excellent, but not necessarily extreme, examples of the phenomenon. Samples are small and rich in information but not unusual, such as in the case of people with particular experience in the topic or clinics that provide services relevant to the research problem. In a case study design, the sample may be a single case or multiple cases, or a unique or exemplary case for in-depth study (Yin 1994). In Bolivia (Paulson and others 1996) and Jamaica (Barnett and others 1996), researchers selected women-centered reproductive health services in order to demonstrate how health delivery can be sensitive to the particular needs of women. In any small exploratory sample, intensive exploration of selected issues with a few well-informed people or groups can add interesting, insightful, and reality-based perspectives and information.

Homogeneous Samples Whether to emphasize similarities or differences in selecting a sample again depends on the study's purpose. People in homogeneous samples have basically similar characteristics. This type of sample is appropriate if you are studying one or more groups in depth, for example, exploring the impact of an AIDS prevention program on male truckers at risk of HIV. A formative phase may be necessary to establish the criteria that determine risk. By limiting sample selection to individuals who meet these criteria, you are better able to focus on a central issue that is relevant to all of them. Focus groups typically use this approach, stimulating people with a common identity to discuss their shared experiences.

Heterogeneous Samples Heterogeneous samples, on the other hand, may be useful for studying issues that cut across individual or program variation. Qualitative investigators sampling from a diverse population may want to highlight variation in some complex phenomenon, for example, different perspectives on whether and how to intervene in the practice of female genital cutting. Or they may be looking for common themes that emerge even in the presence of other differences. A study of rural, urban, and suburban family planning clinics serving different socioeconomic groups revealed the common perception that providers were unwilling to discuss emergency contraception. The discovery of similar experiences, behaviors, or perceptions in an otherwise heterogeneous group may warrant further in-depth study in separate homogeneous samples.

Typical Cases Often in operations research or evaluation, it is useful to describe a typical case, program, or participant that serves as a profile for understanding the principal features of a group of programs or a class of individuals. The researcher may sample a typical case as illustrative or as a unit of analysis. Program planners and policymakers may be more interested in data on typical facilities, not services that are extremely good or extremely poor. What constitutes typical is a subjective judgment, but key informants who are especially familiar with the general category can likely identify examples that are average—not extreme in any sense related to the study.

Snowball Sampling Snowball sampling is a technique for locating informants by asking others to identify individuals or groups with special understanding of a phenomenon. The investigator asks each participant to suggest others with similar ability to address the issues, beginning with such questions as: Who knows a lot about . . . ? Where can I find good examples of what you're talking about? Thus, the "snowball" grows as it rolls, collecting an information-rich pool of resources for exploring the research question. Because informants with special expertise can likely identify other knowledgeable people, this technique can be a valuable one when the researcher does not know the field. It is also useful when individuals with the knowledge or experience to provide rich data are difficult to reach, such as secluded women, people whose behavior or lifestyle deviates from social norms, or anyone fearful of public exposure. When such individuals are willing to trust the researcher, it is especially critical to protect their privacy and confidentiality.

Opportunistic Sampling Because qualitative strategies can change in response to findings as they emerge in the field, you may need to select additional study participants—making an "on-the-spot decision to take advantage of unforeseen opportunities after fieldwork has begun" (Patton 1990, p. 179). In Mali we discovered that a small group of women had been using family planning for several years. We took advantage of this opportunity to look at contraceptive norms of experienced users, women who had successfully negotiated their way around cultural barriers in order to space or limit their pregnancies. This modification meant drawing a purposive sample of women who were coming to the clinic to renew their family planning methods.

Ethical Decisions for the Protection of Study Participants

Your ability to conduct a study while respecting research ethics will be linked closely to your research design. All human research should begin with the informed consent of participants, but how it is implemented depends on the nature of the research and the type and degree of risk that participation entails. At its most basic, informed consent means that study participants understand the following:

- Possible risks and benefits
- Voluntary participation
- Assurances of confidentiality
- The purpose of the research
- How they were chosen to participate
- Data collection procedures
- Whom to contact with questions and concerns

It is important to remember that potential harm to study participants is not just physical but can be psychological, social, economic, or professional. In fact, physical wounds may heal more quickly than wounds to a person's reputation or sense of security (Williamson 1995). In culturally sensitive studies, your ethical responsibility goes beyond the simple statement of informed consent. Moreover, many of the topics that commonly arise in public health research are likely to elicit delicate material—secret experiences, wishes, fears, even confessions—that the participant wants only the interviewer to hear. Avoiding deception, asking permission to record what they say, being willing to turn off the tape recorder, and being honest about the intended use of the research are all part of your responsibility to your participants, along with ensuring that they come to no emotional, physical, professional, or financial harm because they agreed to speak with you (Rubin and Rubin 1995). The common practice of coding participants to protect personal identity can be explained as further assurance of confidentiality. Researchers should also make sure they are not under any legal constraints, for example, requirements to report certain kinds of illegal behavior. If they are, they must inform participants of these legal obligations.

When you encourage people to talk to you openly, you incur serious ethical obligations to them.
(Rubin and Rubin 1995, p. 93)

RISK TO PARTICIPANTS

What kind of harm might come to a participant in a sensitive or controversial health study? In strongly patriarchal societies, subordinate women may be especially at risk in studies of contraception, abortion, female circumcision, domestic violence, or any reproductive decision that might conflict with norms of behavior. Clandestine contraceptive users in Mali feared rejection or divorce if their husbands discovered their pills. Women in Haiti feared physical abuse if they demanded that HIV-infected partners use condoms. Brazilian adolescents suffering the consequences of unsafe abortion might have been arrested if discovered. Providers who reveal actions by their superiors that compromise service quality may endanger their jobs. Injection drug users willing to participate in research on social networking and addiction bear a double burden of risk, not only for their own safety but also for that of any users and dealers they identify in confidential interviews.

Your first responsibility to your study participants is to assess the possibility that simply talking with you may pose a risk for some and to protect them from harm, even if it means changing the interview site or omitting material that might jeopardize the participant's safety. We discuss ethical considerations related to specific methods in Chapter Four.

THE SIGNED CONSENT FORM—DO YOU NEED IT?

How will participants indicate their consent? Most written study designs are expected to answer this question in detail. The signed consent form is a hallowed tradition of institutional review boards (IRBs) everywhere,[2] but in some cases oral informed consent may be a more appropriate format. Examples are studies in which a breach in confidentiality could have profound repercussions for the participant, such as clandestine users of contraception, men who have sex with men, women who have undergone unsafe abortion, or unmarried adolescent clients of a family planning clinic. For a study of adolescent women admitted to a hospital with complications of abortion, one

IRB ruled that the parental consent requirement for participation in the study was inappropriate, because it could put the participant at greater risk than the study itself.

U.S. federal regulations (45 CFR 46) include several different sets of potential waivers:

- Waiver of documentation of informed consent (that is, no signature needed)
- Waiver of particular items from the list of required elements for informed consent
- Waiver of informed consent (usually only used for things like chart review studies or lab studies using stored specimens)
- Waiver of parental consent for minors

U.S. IRBs are constrained in the extent to which they can grant each of these types of waivers.

Most IRBs can be expected to waive the signature requirement if all three of the following conditions apply:

1. The only record linking the subject and the research is the consent document.
2. The principal risk would be potential harm resulting from breach of confidentiality.
3. The research presents no more than minimal risk of harm to subjects and involves no procedures for which written consent is normally required (Williamson 1995).

As a substitute for signed consent, the interviewer may be asked to sign a statement for each participant confirming that the participant has read (or heard) and understood the statement and has given oral consent. However, regardless of the mechanism for obtaining consent, the study design should include a description of possible risk that could result from participation in the study, as well as the statement of informed consent exactly as it will be presented to the participant. Protecting human subjects should also include a referral plan or other response to possible harm should it actually occur in the course of the study. (See Appendix Two for examples of consent forms used in qualitative studies of reproductive health.)

Collecting Data

Designing the data collection process means making basic decisions about how you will build trust in the community, understand the cultural context, and create relationships with participants. Your design should include a plan for introducing the study to the community or site, enlisting local field assistance, creating a comfortable and secure environment for interviews or focus groups, and managing the data. How you will train and monitor field staff is also part of the design. We discuss these in Chapter Five.

Designing the study also raises critical decisions about what kinds of data you will collect and how to collect it in a way that best matches the purpose and flow of the research. Whether your data will come principally from observation or from interviewing or group discussion (see Chapter Four), plan the study in such a way that you will be able to alter or modify the process as new information and questions emerge.

An important decision at this point concerns the degree of structure in the questions you will ask participants. Although open-ended questioning is a basic tool in qualitative research, questions can be asked in many different ways. You will need to decide at the design stage how much structure is appropriate for your purpose (Patton 1990).

The first alternative, shown in Box 3.4 (see p. 43), is an informal conversation with little or no preparation and sequencing of questions. This option is appropriate if your purpose is to explore a topic on which you have very little information. You do not know exactly what questions you will ask until you are prompted by clues from the participants and the study environment. A less structured approach is well suited to some participant observation studies, because questions emerge naturally from what you are seeing and hearing (Patton 1990). Thus, one question or observation leads to another as you build your understanding of the situation. However, the flexibility of this kind of questioning also tends to make it time-consuming. Moreover, it assumes a great deal of experience on the part of the interviewer and may increase the difficulty of the analysis. For less-experienced observers and for most in-depth interviews and focus group discussions, we recommend the more structured, but still open-ended, alternatives that follow.

The second option, a topic guide or outline, helps you focus the interview or group discussion without prestructuring the questions. You decide in advance the areas you want to explore but not the questions' wording or sequence. The chief advantage of this technique is that data collection is systematic but gives you greater flexibility to adapt questions to participants and circumstances. It is a commonly used tool for gathering comprehensive information on specific research questions in a relaxed, conversational style. The resulting data are less comparable than in a standardized open-ended interview, but they may be more responsive to the way that participants naturally construct a situation. (We will discuss construction of topic guides in Chapter Four.)

A third strategy, asking a predetermined set of open-ended questions, is the most standardized approach to qualitative data collection. If you choose this type of questioning, you lose flexibility but gain comparability and more straightforward analysis. This approach is especially useful for comparative studies when it is important to maximize common features while remaining sensitive to cultural differences among the study groups (Knodel 1994). This format also lends itself to studies that are highly focused, for example, a program evaluation in which you want to interview several service providers with little time to spend on the interview (Patton 1990). Structured questions may be a good strategy if you have multiple interviewers or focus group moderators with varying experience and different interviewing styles.

Analyzing the Data

Chapter Six presents in detail the steps for analyzing qualitative data. However, certain aspects of data analysis will need careful consideration as you design your study. Specifically, you should determine the following in the design phase:

- Who will conduct the analysis?
- What level of detail will be needed to respond to your research questions?
- Will the analysis be computer-assisted or manual?

If a computer will be used, decide in advance on a qualitative software package for text analysis. If you are combining qualitative and quantitative methods, you will want to have a clear plan of analysis for each and a strategy for interpreting the results in an integrated discussion.

Qualitative analysis can be a deeply personal and subjective exercise. For this reason some qualitative researchers decide from a study's outset to use a team approach to analysis, involving data collectors as well as researchers more removed from daily field activities. The process of examining, negotiating, and incorporating multiple perspectives on data can strengthen their final interpretation. If using a team approach, anticipating the analysis process at the beginning is especially useful:

- Will all team members read and work on all the data, or will specific team members be responsible for different aspects of the investigation?
- Will team members work separately and then meet to share and reconcile their findings, or will the team conduct the analysis in group meetings?
- How will the team resolve differences of opinion?

For an expanded discussion of group analysis, see the field perspective by Woodsong titled Training Field Staff in Data Analysis in Chapter Five (p. 135).

If only one person will conduct analysis, it is important to review the data as they are collected. If not actually collecting data, the principal investigator or analyst must at least have access to interim data in order to identify areas for clarification or further probing.

Another decision to make at the design stage is the form your data will take. The purpose of your qualitative study will imply a certain level of detail. For example, you may be able to explore broadly the different personal, relational, and institutional barriers to use of dual protection from pregnancy and STIs by summarizing preliminary information from other observations or from interviews or group discussions. On the other hand, if you want to use qualitative data to design interventions that increase individuals' skills in negotiating dual protection, a formative problem, you will want to know exactly how people do and do not express themselves in such intimate circumstances. Fully transcribed tapes of interviews, in addition to notes about nonverbal or body language, would be more appropriate. If you are embarking on a mixed-method study, you will also need to decide in advance how you are going to handle the data from different methods and coordinate the findings in an integrated discussion.

Finally, the level of detail you anticipate and, to a lesser degree, the number of people involved in analysis will influence decisions about the use of computers. Manual analysis is sufficient when your goal is to map out broad categories of information or when the volume of data is small. As the analysis becomes more complex (that is, examining the nuances of language or comparing responses between a number of subgroups) and as the volume of data increases, a computer can greatly assist the analysis process. Again, if the analysts themselves will not be keying in data or operating analysis software programs, give some thought to how the data will be moved from field notes to data files to analysis procedures. Some software packages have special features to assist a team approach. (We will discuss specific advantages and disadvantages of different types of software packages in Chapter Six.)

Disseminating Results

In order for study results to be accessible to and used by others, you will need to build into your design a plan for dissemination, with a corresponding budget. Your study purpose has direct implications concerning how and for whom you will write your findings, as well as for your own role in their dissemination. (See Chapters Seven and Eight for a fuller discussion.) Likewise, as you focus your research questions, consider the eventual audiences for your findings and plan the length and detail of your report or presentation accordingly. When you sit down to write, "you begin a systematic inquiry of what you already know, what you need to know, and what you are looking for" (Wolcott 1990, p. 22). In short, outlining your study purpose and design can be done at the same time that you develop a tentative table of contents for your final report. This approach will sharpen your focus and help you sequence your material.

Conclusion

A well-organized research design is a strong argument for the relevance and integrity of the research. However, qualitative design is always a work in progress. Although a sound written design at your project's outset gives you and your reviewers a frame of reference, it is a plan, not a contract. It systematically details the problem driving the research and the strategy for solving it, but the design remains flexible to change, as repeated questioning and analysis in the field lead you to new questions and new ways to delve deeper. Such flexibility, ill advised in most quantitative research, is a necessary feature of qualitative methodology. The researcher's ability—indeed, obligation—to examine data as they arrive, throw out invalid assumptions, restate questions, and shape the design as the study progresses will ultimately contribute to the vitality and credibility of the results.

NOTES

1. For related formative work on nutrition and physical fitness among American Indian children, see Steckler and others (2003) and Gittelsohn and others (2000).
2. Institutional review boards (IRBs), or protection of human subjects committees, are mandated by governments and research institutions to protect participants in research by reviewing proposals for compliance with internationally recognized guidelines.

Field Perspective

Proposing Qualitative Research to the World Health Organization

Iqbal Shah, Ph.D.

World Health Organization

Since its inception in 1972, the Special Programme of Research, Development and Research Training in Human Reproduction (HRP) at the World Health Organization (WHO) has supported focused, in-depth social science research on issues related to family planning and, later, reproductive health. From 1985 to 2000 HRP launched major research initiatives on (1) contraceptive use dynamics; (2) the acceptability of condoms; (3) determinants and consequences of abortion; (4) sexual behavior and reproductive health; (5) the role of men in reproductive health; (6) adolescent sexual and reproductive health; and most recently, (7) quality of care in reproductive health. HRP has received and reviewed, cumulatively, over one thousand submissions and supported projects ranging from small qualitative studies to intervention projects with semi-experimental designs. A large number of these have included qualitative research methods, especially focus group discussions (FGDs).

Increasingly, HRP receives proposals for studies that intend to apply a battery of qualitative techniques, including body mapping, freelisting, in-depth interviews, case studies, and FGDs. Whereas these techniques can be enriching, little attention is being paid to the rationale and need for each one or to how the data arising from a mix of methods will be integrated, analyzed, or interpreted.

HRP's policy is to seek proposals of good scientific quality that incorporate a study design appropriate to the stated objectives. Many proposals describe use of a combination of cross-sectional surveys and FGDs. Although some qualitative research submissions have been of high caliber, many others have been weak, particularly when proposing FGDs. Based on many years of experience reviewing such proposals, I would like to offer some insights on avoiding common mistakes in such proposals.

Inappropriate Use

The single fatal flaw in any proposal is to set forth incorrect research methods to meet the stated objectives. We have received submissions proposing use of FGDs to measure the prevalence and incidence of contraceptive use or violence or to collect individuals' personal information and experience, for example, relating to sexual behavior. These proposals were not approved because FGDs are not suitable to measure prevalence or incidence. On the other hand, proposals that have suggested using FGDs to ascertain normative patterns, to develop a survey instrument, or to explain or expand on survey findings have frequently been approved. Also reviewed favorably are FGD proposals to understand community norms and attitudes toward specific reproductive health issues.

Design Concerns

Researchers frequently make mistakes related to the composition and number of FGDs, selection of participants, the focus group guide, and the conduct of FGDs. For example, one basic requirement of FGDs is that of homogeneity: you do not mix men and women in the same group nor adolescents and older women and so on. And it is inappropriate to extend the norms of quantitative research sampling to this technique. Nevertheless, we receive proposals that suggest holding enough FGDs to represent all age, socioeconomic, gender, religious, and ethnic groups.

Investigators may have a poor understanding of the appropriate number of groups to hold—we have seen proposals that ranged from one or two to over four hundred focus groups per study. Clearly, the rationale for an optimum number of FGDs was neither understood nor provided. Successful researchers suggest six to eight FGDs and understand that one must reduce or increase the number to avoid redundancy and to seek new information on substantive issues. Researchers often omit justification for the number of participants in each FGD. The majority of researchers suggest eight to ten members per group, which is normally appropriate, but we see proposals ranging from two to fifty.

Investigators frequently fail to provide enough information about other critical aspects of their studies. Sometimes they imply that reviewers should just trust them. Necessary information is often missing about how participants will be selected; where and how FGDs will be conducted; and how information will be recorded, compiled, and analyzed. In addition, concerns around confidentiality, informed consent, and storage and access to information are not always discussed. The FGD guide is rarely provided. This lack of information delays the proposal review as investigators are asked to provide supplemental information and assure reviewers that the structure of the questions is appropriate for an FGD.

A less common but equally serious pitfall is for investigators to propose using statistical techniques to analyze the results of FGDs, for example, chi-square or t-tests, with some going as far as to suggest multivariate analysis.

Other Precautions

Having now supported a number of scientifically sound qualitative research proposals, HRP has also accumulated experience on implementation and analysis. The implementation of FGDs does not usually present major difficulties, but some exceptions include holding mixed groups or allowing one or a few participants to dominate the group discussions. However, major challenges exist in the analysis and interpretation of focus group data. Most researchers find the amount of information they have collected overwhelming, and they often do not develop or follow a codebook or an analysis plan. The interpretation of FGD data is not always straightforward, and we receive reports from investigators who have reflected FGD findings with means, medians, and percentages. Finally, most researchers find it very difficult to summarize qualitative information in a succinct and meaningful manner.

Features for Success

- Articulate a clear and convincing rationale for the choice of the method of study, irrespective of the type of method (qualitative or quantitative or both).
- Provide complete details of the procedures to be used, including a draft questionnaire or guide, ethical considerations around informed consent and confidentiality, data management, and field procedures.
- Pay attention to the analysis and interpretation of data and to how information collected using more than one methodological approach, irrespective of the type, will be integrated.
- Include training of the staff and moderator for the conduct of the FGD, collection and coding of information, and analysis.

See World Health Organization 2000 in the references list. For further information about submitting research proposals to WHO, contact Dr. Iqbal Shah, Department of Reproductive Health and Research, World Health Organization, 1211 Geneva 27, Switzerland.

Field Perspective

Combining Methods to Understand Women's Positions in Their Households*

Sri Moertiningsih Adioetomo

Demographic Institute,
Faculty of Economics

University of Indonesia, Jakarta

The research literature indicates that lowering fertility increases women's participation in the labor force. Women who use contraception generally spend fewer years pregnant or rearing children and therefore have more time to work for income. Because the literature also suggests that working for income is associated with greater household autonomy, we decided to examine the assumption that working women actually have greater bargaining power in household decisions than women who are not formally employed.

To test this relationship, we conducted a secondary analysis of the 1993 Indonesia Family Life Survey (IFLS), a survey of seven thousand households in thirteen provinces of Indonesia.† Using logistic regressions, we found that family planning only partially explains women's work status. Completion of high school, a husband's low income, and urban residence were stronger predictors. And the link between work status and household autonomy was even less clear.

Although the IFLS is a rich data set for many purposes, it does not contain information about women's autonomy—that is, the extent to which a woman's daily household activities and economic decisions are free from her husband's control. Even if the survey questionnaire had included questions about household decision making, we could see that a structured questionnaire would not elicit the sensitive information we needed in order to understand women's domestic situations. To overcome this limitation, we decided to conduct in-depth interviews with women and separate interviews with their husbands, choosing a small sample of couples from the area where the IFLS was conducted. We selected eight couples from West Java and eight from North Sumatra for a total of thirty-two in-depth interviews. Purposive sampling took into account socioeconomic variations, culture and religion, and urban and rural residence. We were rewarded with a richer understanding of the relationship between family planning, labor force participation, and women's household autonomy in Indonesia.

As a quantitative methodologist, I found it unnatural at first to combine two such different methodologies in one study. Instead of specifying the variables and their relationships in advance of data collection, our understanding of key influences on autonomy emerged as we reviewed data from the interviews. However, our quantitative framework helped us to focus the problem for the interviews and to develop our semistructured interview guides. In the interviews we listened to women and men describing what family planning meant to them. Then we asked them to tell us in their own words how women and men make decisions in their households.

Women told us that family planning had indeed benefited their lives because with fewer children, they had more time to themselves. However, they did not make the connection between lower fertility and the opportunity to work for income; regardless of whether they used family planning, they felt free to work outside the home if they wished. Nor did they think that family planning determined their influence in household decisions and their use of family income for basic expenses. Couples felt that family planning had freed women's time for activities other than child care. Having smaller families also helped them stretch their limited resources to ensure that their children would have the food, health care, and education they needed. The qualitative research enabled us to conclude that family planning and women's employment are both elements of a common household survival strategy, which includes women's and men's joint participation in household decisions. Hearing couples talk about their lives enabled me to understand in a new way the association between family planning, working for pay, and household autonomy.

* *This study was carried out in collaboration with the Women's Studies Project of Family Health International, Research Triangle Park, North Carolina, from 1997 to 1998.*

† *Jointly conducted by the Demographic Institute at the Faculty of Economics, University of Indonesia, and the RAND Corporation, USA.*

Field Perspective

Integrating Qualitative and Quantitative Methods for Problem Solving in Research

Deborah E. Bender, Ph.D.

School of Public Health, University of North Carolina at Chapel Hill

In Bolivia, where breastfeeding initiation is almost universal and duration continues for as long as two years, we conducted a study to understand women's knowledge and preferences related to breastfeeding as a means of child-spacing. Our ultimate purpose was to garner information that could assist in developing guidelines for the promotion of the lactational amenorrhea method (LAM) of contraception at the community level (Bender and others 1990). In this study we wanted to examine the statistical interrelationships among infant feeding practices, contraceptive use, and lactational amenorrhea in a representative sample of childbearing women. But at the same time, we wanted to know more about how women understand the link between breastfeeding and LAM.

A total of 416 women having a child under eighteen months of age, living in a periurban community of Santa Cruz, responded to our survey. From survey data we learned that 60 percent had heard of LAM, although only 40 percent were aware that this protection lasts for only part of an extended breastfeeding period. Bivariate analysis also revealed that formal education was directly related to correct knowledge of the duration of LAM protection. Even among women who had completed primary education or more, only 45 percent correctly reported the duration of LAM's protection from pregnancy.

These findings raised questions concerning the rationale that led so many women to believe that breastfeeding could offer indefinite protection from pregnancy. Therefore, we invited sixty-three women who were outside the survey sample but lived in the same communities to participate in focus groups. The purpose of the focus group discussions was to explore in greater depth women's knowledge of breastfeeding as a method of contraception.

Although focus group participants were somewhat older than survey respondents, educational levels were similar, with approximately 60 percent of women finishing eighth grade or lower. On the question of LAM protection, we found even less consensus among focus group participants than in the survey. Women in six out of eight focus groups said they had heard that breastfeeding can prevent pregnancy and believed it to be true. However, most participants believed breastfeeding protected only some women and that lactational infertility was dependent on an individual's physical constitution. This belief, that a woman's fertility is related to her individual physiology, had not surfaced in the survey but is frequently reported anecdotally in Bolivia. According to traditional beliefs, a woman's constitution is an indicator of her health and marks her as either strong or weak. Many people believe that a strong woman has more blood than a weak woman and, therefore, can easily have many children without harming her own health.

Other focus group participants mentioned that they had heard breastfeeding could help prevent pregnancy but did not believe it. Note the lack of consensus in the women's responses:

> Well, if you are nursing and your period doesn't return and you nursed your child for a year or two, you are protected during that time.

> Yes, I have heard this, but I have also seen friends who are nursing become pregnant.

> It's a lie, because I became pregnant while nursing.

> Not all women have the same makeup or ovulation [sic]. Some people ovulate before menstruation, and there are others who ovulate after menstruation returns. In my case I ovulate before. The women who ovulate before and are breastfeeding become pregnant.

> I have heard that it protects you for only six months.

To elicit more detail on the meaning to participants of postpartum anovulation, we used a simple probe: "Why, what is happening?" Some women had no response, whereas others made various guesses.

As the focus group facilitator probed beyond the more superficial survey responses, it became apparent that women were making contraceptive decisions with little substantive knowledge of how breastfeeding relates to pregnancy.

Posing similar questions in two formats—the survey and the focus group discussions—allowed us to probe for depth of meaning in narrative responses as well as to understand the distribution of beliefs and practices by women's educational levels. It enabled us to hear some of the deeply held convictions that influence women's contraceptive decisions. Using both forced choice and open-ended methods for similar questions also gave us a set of checks on data reliability and validity.

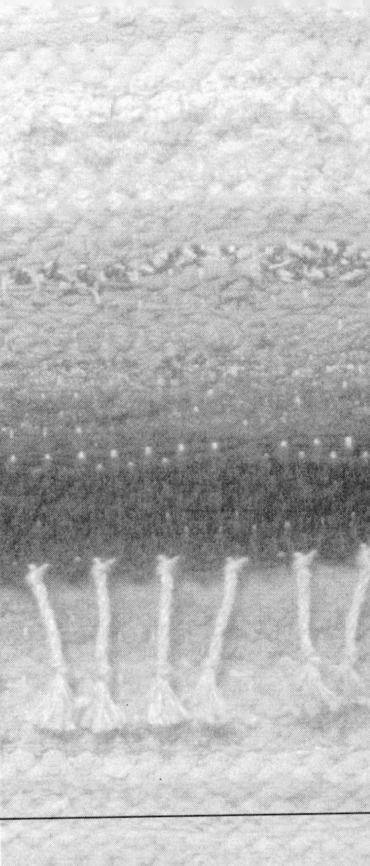

CHAPTER FOUR

Collecting Qualitative Data

The Science and the Art

Every interview is an interpersonal drama with a developing plot.

(Pool 1957, cited in Holstein and Gubrium 1999, p. 112)

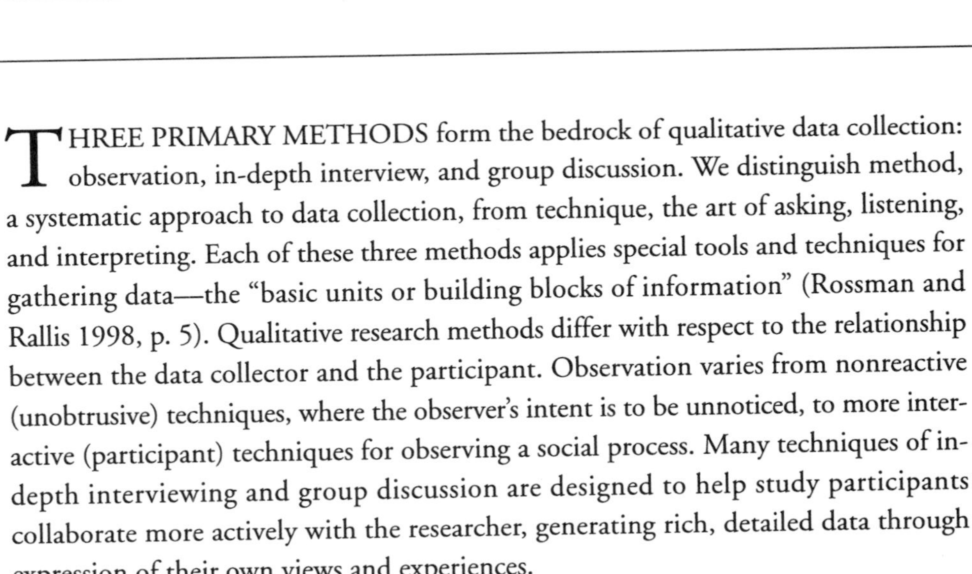

THREE PRIMARY METHODS form the bedrock of qualitative data collection: observation, in-depth interview, and group discussion. We distinguish method, a systematic approach to data collection, from technique, the art of asking, listening, and interpreting. Each of these three methods applies special tools and techniques for gathering data—the "basic units or building blocks of information" (Rossman and Rallis 1998, p. 5). Qualitative research methods differ with respect to the relationship between the data collector and the participant. Observation varies from nonreactive (unobtrusive) techniques, where the observer's intent is to be unnoticed, to more interactive (participant) techniques for observing a social process. Many techniques of in-depth interviewing and group discussion are designed to help study participants collaborate more actively with the researcher, generating rich, detailed data through expression of their own views and experiences.

This chapter describes the qualitative researcher as observer, interviewer, and group moderator. For each approach to research, we offer a variety of techniques; but our selection is not exhaustive. As you become more experienced in qualitative research, you will discover many more techniques of creative listening and learning. Working from an interpretivist or feminist perspective, you will focus on different issues, uncover new sources of data, and find more ways to enable people to tell their stories. But wherever you go, the basic principles of observing and interacting with individuals and groups will be the foundation on which you build your practice.

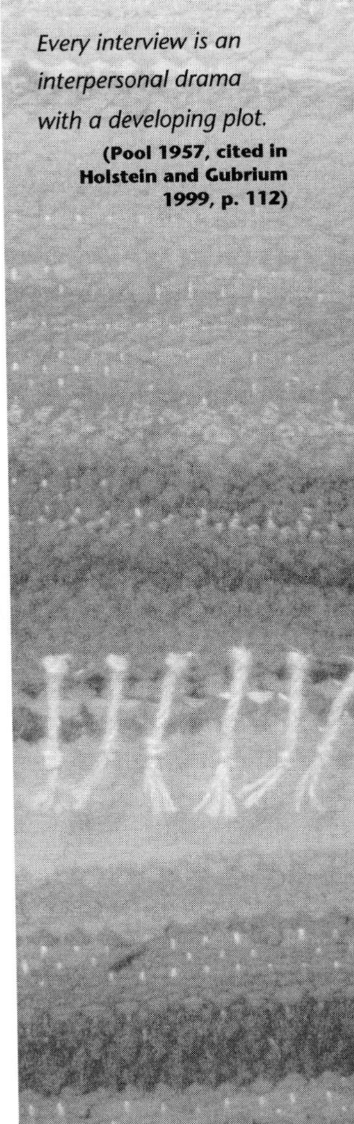

Observation

Observation is the oldest and most basic source of human knowledge, from casual understanding of the everyday world to its use as a systematic tool of social science. It is hard to imagine any field research, qualitative or quantitative, without an element of observation. Data collection does not begin and end with an interview. Interviewers and focus group moderators are also observers, noting body language, facial expression, and other nonverbal clues to subtle meanings. Qualitative researchers, particularly, must be acutely aware of context, observing the ebb and flow of activity around the study site. A chance conversation, an unexpected event, a spontaneous gathering—all may contain clues to understanding participants' expressions and meanings in the more formal interviews and discussions.

Depending on the purpose of your research, you will have to choose whether you are going to observe from an outsider's or an insider's perspective—or somewhere in between. Outside observers maintain distance in order to view events from their own perspectives. Inside observers reduce distance by joining activities and interacting with people in order to view events through participants' eyes and ears. Each approach has its place among the tools of scientific observation. As a researcher you are unlikely ever to be a true insider, but you can get insiders' perspectives from study participants. Your own perspective as an outsider enables you to listen, question, and interpret what they share with you. In this chapter we present these two ways to observe separately. But in practice most field observation involves skillful interplay of both. With experience you will learn to gauge the proper distance between yourself and your participants, knowing when to step back and when to join in.

Experienced observers use both qualitative and quantitative techniques, with qualitative observations differing from quantitative primarily in their focus on process rather than numbers. For example, counting the numbers of clients in different health center clinics could reveal variation in clinic use. However, it would not capture the qualitative interaction between clients and providers in the same clinics, a finding that might help explain different patterns of clinic attendance. Regardless of how and what you observe, observations become data only when they are guided by theory and conducted according to the rules and conventions of scientific inquiry.

NONREACTIVE TECHNIQUES

Observer as Outsider One strategy for observation is to remain on the fringe, watching people and events as unobtrusively as possible, observing without participating. Following the early work of Eugene Webb (Webb and others 1966), we have adopted the term *nonreactive* to describe techniques in which the researcher collects data without interacting or reacting visibly to participants' activity. Choose this technique if you want to see how something happens rather than how other people perceive it happening, gathering your own impressions by direct observation instead of through study participants' eyes and ears.

Program evaluation and operations research often combine nonreactive observation with other measures—for example, in quality of care studies—to observe firsthand the client experience, including the dynamics of interaction between client and provider. In such a setting, you might want to know how clients are received and how long they wait, who directs conversations, how information is offered, how questions are asked and answered, and whether providers initiate counseling on certain topics of interest to your research problem.

Nonreactive observation is sometimes used to validate interview data or other information that study participants report. For example, family planning counselors may have told interviewers that they always provide clients with information on a range of contraceptive choices—an insider perspective. Direct observation—the outsider perspective—could confirm their reports by the presence of a variety of contraceptives in half-empty boxes and colorful family planning posters on the walls, as well as actual counseling on the methods. However, several days of observation might reveal that in practice providers usually mention only one method to clients and have only that one in the supply closet. In the case of contrary evidence, the challenge to the qualitative researcher is to discover the reason for the apparent contradiction, for example, through in-depth interviews with clients and providers.

The quality of your data will depend on your ability to watch and listen without interrupting the natural flow of activity. An observer almost always has some effect on the study situation because unless he or she is hidden behind a one-way vision mirror, as in some laboratory-controlled studies, the observer's presence is noticeable. To minimize distortion of the observed behavior, an observer might be introduced simply as someone who is learning about health care in that area; the observer could then take a position behind the client-provider pair and observe silently from the sidelines. Longer periods of observation are usually more effective than shorter ones because they allow people to become accustomed to the observer's presence and return more easily to their natural interaction.

In most observation sites—a busy pharmacy, an active community center, a clinic full of people waiting for attention—the din of activity can be distracting. Beginning with a prepared list of things to watch for will help you focus your attention. The list may be as simple or as detailed as you wish, but it should be incorporated into your notes and revised at the end of each observation period. What you see and hear will almost always lead to new insights and new questions about relationships and events in the setting. Although taking notes on what you observe is essential, it is important to do so as unobtrusively as possible. Frantic scribbling of verbatim conversations and flipping notebook pages will only remind people that you are observing them and raise anxiety about your intentions. To minimize note taking, some observers use checklists with space for short, abbreviated comments. Others jot occasional notes on small cards, taking mental notes as much as possible. As soon as possible after each observation period, summarize your notes, incorporate mental notes and impressions, and reflect on what they have revealed about the research problem. Add interpretations, or tentative conclusions, to your notes and formulate new points to observe in the next session.

DOCUMENTARY RESEARCH

When observing human behavior, it is almost impossible not to intrude in some way. We include documentary research, also known as content analysis, under nonreactive methods because once the data have been collected and reported, the written record is the only totally unobtrusive way to observe a culture. It also offers other interpretations of the phenomena you are studying and in some cases a historical perspective that is available only through writings from the past.

In documentary research the material you are examining has been collected by others for other purposes; yet it can tell you a lot about how people think and behave in natural settings with no outsider influence. Large databases, such as epidemiological surveys, a country's Demographic and Health Survey, or the U.S. National Health Interview Survey, provide a wealth of information from which to learn about a study population. Documentary sources appropriate for research in public health also include hospital and clinic records, health education materials, newspaper stories, radio and television shows, magazine advertising, billboards, school materials (for example, health education curricula), religious writings, sermons, personal journals, diaries, and popular songs. Qualitative researchers also use this method for secondary analysis of transcriptions from interviews or focus group discussions conducted in the past.

Topics that might be addressed through documentary data collection include government policy on HIV/AIDS as presented in the press, violence in advertising, gender bias in radio and television drama, or differences in health information given to different social groups as documented in clinic records. For example, an AIDS activist in Kenya gathered information on adolescents' concerns about HIV/AIDS through their letters to an AIDS advice column for young people in a local newspaper (personal communication from L. Kimani to P. R. Ulin, Nov. 1990, unreferenced).

Documentary methods are similar to other qualitative data analysis. If you were studying gender bias in a series of radio comedies, you would start with an operational definition of gender bias and identify types of dialogue or situations that might contain bias toward men or women. Following the classic questions in communications research, you would focus on "Who says what, to whom, how, and with what effect" (Babbie 1998, p. 309). Creating a file of newspaper stories or taping and transcribing the radio series would enable you to code emerging themes and analyze the text, using rules of analysis like those for transcripts from interviews and focus group discussions, as we will discuss in Chapter Six.

As a secondary source of data, existing documents can add immeasurably to the researcher's understanding of the context of the research. Popular norms; cultural values and beliefs; and people's hopes, fears, and triumphs all can be found in materials they have created to express different aspects of their lives. However, like all research, documentary analysis has its limitations. Questions of credibility arise if one person interprets the data without benefit of multiple coders. Are the criteria that the original researcher selected valid representations of the key concepts in the present analysis? The same words or behaviors may have had different meanings at the time the document was created. Moreover, one can never be certain that the material reflects the views of a wider group, not just the voice of one author. The best strategies for ensuring rigor in documentary analysis are first, to keep a meticulous record of the analysis process, noting how you arrive at your interpretations and conclusions, and second, to work with multiple reviewers who conduct independent analyses and compare their results.

PARTICIPANT OBSERVATION

Participant observation brings the researcher into direct interaction with people and their activities. As defined by anthropologist H. Russell Bernard (1995, p. 136–137), participant observation "involves getting close to people and making them feel comfortable enough with your presence that you can observe and record information about their lives." As the foundation of cultural anthropology, this method has many uses in different domains of social science. "The thing to remember about participation," Bernard reminds us, "is that it belongs to everyone, positivists and interpretivists alike. . . . Whether your data consist of numbers or words, participant observation lets you in the door so you can do research."

Unlike nonreactive observation—in which you must be as unobtrusive as possible—in participant observation you will ask yourself: How can I get close to people? Will they share their lives, their thoughts, their activities with an outsider? In this more interactive approach, your responsibility is to stimulate conversation and behavior that will let you enter the culture as its members' guest. In initiating the observation, your challenge will be to adapt your interactive style to the participants' cultural style. For example, you would approach young schoolgirls differently from the way you might introduce yourself to commercial sex workers on the street. Experienced observers learn to present themselves in whatever way will put study participants at ease while simultaneously stimulating their interest in interacting with the observer. In some participant observation studies, the observer has adopted the lifestyle of the people observed, such as driving a taxi or working in a restaurant in order to study taxicab drivers or waitpeople. In some areas of research, including studies of sexual and reproductive health, the observer is more likely to remain an outsider on the inside, maintaining identity as a researcher but spending enough time in the cultural setting to know and understand people in the natural course of their lives.

The techniques for entering a culture are as many and varied as cultural variations themselves. The map-making exercise in Box 4.1 illustrates how, by starting with an activity that arouses curiosity, you can soon have a willing group of informants who want to participate because they find what you are doing interesting. The common goal is to enable people to accept you and interact naturally with you for sustained periods of time. As they get used to your presence, they will act almost as if you were not there (Bernard 1995, p. 136). Once accepted, you must continue to balance insider and outsider perspectives as you watch and listen to what unfolds. With practice you will respond naturally and flexibly to fluctuations in the research environment, always alert to unexpected events that could reveal important information on the cultural dynamics of the group.

BOX 4.1

Using Participant Observation to Introduce a Study

At the start of a multisite HIV behavior change project, a team of qualitative researchers set out to conduct some geographic-mapping exercises to learn about the social networks that would be targeted for an intervention. Researchers used this activity as an opportunity for community members to become familiar with the team, as well as for collecting the map data needed to begin the study.

After paying courtesy calls to community leaders, the researchers began to spend casual time in the communities, drawing their maps. Inevitably, they were approached by curious individuals. This enabled the researchers to start conversations and inquire informally about what they had observed in the course of their mapmaking.

As they became more interested in the maps, the community members began to offer advice and supply additional information. These interactions in turn led to informal invitations to share a drink or snack in a local eating place, which then offered more opportunities for observation.

Thus, as a component of a large research project, participant observation resulted in maps pertinent to social networks, which the research community then validated; introduction of the field staff to the community; identification of key informants, gatekeepers, and stakeholders; and the beginning of community trust and a foundation for community participation in the research project.

Source: Personal communication from C. Woodsong to E. T. Robinson, Aug. 2001, unreferenced.

To illustrate this process, imagine that you are going to study how women make health decisions for themselves and their families. Following preliminary introductions in the community, as described in Chapter Five, you obtain permission to join a local mothers' club. The group meets weekly to socialize and discuss their concerns as young mothers. At the first meeting you attend, you explain why you want to join them as an observer, sharing your own concern for issues the women believe are important. Until the women know and trust you, you probably do more listening than active participating. Remember that you are there as an observer, not masquerading as a mother in the group. As the women become comfortable with your presence, you might begin to ask a few questions or steer discussion toward topics related to their health decisions. Participating will give way to more listening, with occasional questions to explore interesting leads. Be open also to questions the women might have about you and be willing to reciprocate by sharing some of your own experience. However, avoid becoming an authority in their eyes. Emphasis on common experiences, values, questions, and concerns will help to minimize the effect of your presence on the views the group expresses.

Between the club's weekly meetings, you might arrange individual visits with some of the members at their homes or informal visits to other places the women gather, such as a church group or local health center waiting area. A process similar to snowball sampling (see Chapter Three) can enable you to reach out farther into women's networks. As you become known and accepted as a visiting member of the community, you will be an increasingly effective observer. As you piece together data from many conversations, you will notice how they converge around certain recognizable themes or perhaps reveal conflicting messages that suggest new directions to explore. In contrast to an interview, the participant observer's commitment to the study group is likely to be more intimate and sustained over a longer period. For understanding sequences and connections of events that contribute to health decisions, participant observation can be a powerful tool (Bogdewic 1992).

I want to understand the world from your point of view, I want to know what you know in the way you know it. I want to understand the meaning of your experience, to walk in your shoes, to feel things as you feel them, to explain things as you explain them. Will you become my teacher and help me understand?
(Spradley 1979, p. 34)

In this scenario the researcher is a woman, but there are equally rich opportunities for men to conduct participant observation. Examples might be studies of AIDS awareness among male assembly-line workers, HIV risk among truckers driving long-distance routes through countries with a high prevalence of infection, and knowledge and attitudes of health risk among men who are migrant farmworkers. Although on sensitive topics, participant observers of the same sex may be able to put participants more quickly at ease, same-sex research is not always a necessity. In numerous studies an observer has gained the confidence of both men and women in the study site, with skillful integration of different gender perspectives in the analysis.

Ability to communicate in the local idiom is a valuable asset but often not an option in cross-cultural observation. Although an experienced local assistant can help offset a language gap and offer cultural, as well as linguistic, interpretation, foreigners must realize that they are observing the scene through the eyes and ears of a person whose perspective may be quite different. (We discuss the use of field assistants in more detail in Chapter Five.)

MYSTERY CLIENT TECHNIQUE

In some situations the presence of an observer may cause participants to alter their usual behavior and consciously or unconsciously create what they believe to be a favorable impression. At such times researchers sometimes turn to a mystery client technique—a special form of participant observation that may combine qualitative and quantitative data collection. It has been used particularly in client-provider studies where the presence of an observer might significantly change the provider's customary behavior. Simulated clients or customers, trained to act out roles that reflect real-life experiences, present themselves to actual health providers in the natural setting. These actors may be professional data collectors or local people from the service area. After each encounter they typically record their experience on a structured form and report their observations to researchers in in-depth interviews. For this kind of research, an observation checklist is an important tool, because it enables the observer to assess the same factors in different settings.

A study in Nepal used the mystery client technique to examine interactions between clients and staff of family planning clinics (Schuler and others 1985). The simulated clients asked for guidance in choosing a method, including available alternatives and potential risks and side effects. The researchers found that providers' responses depended on their perceptions of clients' social and economic status, with lower-class participants receiving little information and brusque or rude treatment. Mystery client observation has also been used to compare information provided over the counter in different pharmacies, where the simulated customer asks for advice. Another application of this technique is in studies that explore health providers' attitudes toward adolescents, wherein the mystery clients are young people who present themselves to the clinic as sexually active adolescents seeking contraceptive information and service.

Note that in these examples, the provider is unaware of the visitor's real identity and purpose. We caution readers that the deceptive nature of this technique has raised serious ethical questions about its use. Some researchers have addressed this issue by obtaining informed consent from both staff and supervisors to use the technique at unannounced times over a period of several months. Nevertheless, a decision to use the mystery client technique should be made only after careful reflection on the purpose and ethical implications of doing so.

KEY INFORMANTS IN PARTICIPANT OBSERVATION

Ethnographers have always relied on key informants to help them make sense of their observations and interactions in unfamiliar cultures. Key informants are insiders with special knowledge, status, or communication skills, who are willing to share what they know with the researcher (Gilchrist 1992). They speak on behalf of others, expressing points of view that may be different from their own. They are not independent observers but rather "the voice of the people of concern" (Eng and Parker 1994, p. 207).

Although researchers ask all qualitative research participants to share their knowledge and perspectives, a key informant sometimes has a different relationship to the researcher, providing information, introductions, and interpretation, often on a day-to-day basis, as well as access to observations that an outsider would not normally have. In an ethnographic or longitudinal study, you are likely to have more personal involvement with a key informant who becomes your trusted adviser and guide to the culture. Although your relationship to interview and focus group participants is one of mutual trust and rapport, the key informant partnership often includes a degree of collegiality not typical of most data collection. Why should a qualitative researcher develop a special relationship with a few people instead of regarding all study participants as equal collaborators? Pragmatic limits constrain the researcher (Gilchrist 1992). One cannot be in all places at all times, observing everything and interviewing everyone. But more important, a researcher from the outside is unlikely to have the cultural perspective and community experience necessary to explore all aspects of the problem.

A personal relationship with a key informant, developed over time, helps to ensure more efficient access to rich information. For example, you might begin a study of gender influence on HIV risk with participant observation in a community known to have a high prevalence of sexually transmitted infection (STI). As you get to know people in the community, perhaps two or three stand out because they are particularly interested in the problem and are knowledgeable and articulate on topics concerning sexual risk. When you introduce yourself around the community, people often refer to such individuals as the ones who "know what's going on." You visit with each of them and find them willing to share what they know and take you to people and places that will help you understand gender relationships in relation to sexual risk in this community. These will be your key informants. They might explain cultural norms that govern partner relationships, including the meaning of sexual behavior that seems to deviate from the norm. They will comment on your interpretation of conversations with others in the community and help you synthesize pieces of information from different sources. They might introduce you to other potential key informants, such as a youth leader, a member of a women's advocacy organization, or a community health worker.

As in all qualitative data gathering, it is important to formulate a basic set of questions to start the process. Although these questions could be written, you should incorporate them casually into conversations with key informants. Accompanied by your key informant, you might start with a tour of the facility or workplace you plan to study or a community or neighborhood where potential participants gather. Initial questions might be as general as these: Who comes here? What do they do? To whom do they talk? As you begin to make connections, your questions will become more focused on specific issues related to the study's purpose and context: Why do certain things happen? How do people deal with a new event or a stressful situation? In this way a key informant can orient you to the study population in its natural environment.

Eng and Parker (1994) used key informants to evaluate a health promotion program serving a rural poor county of the Mississippi Delta. In order not to interfere with the community's broader goals for local empowerment, lay community health advisors were asked to select twenty-eight key informants for the study and conduct the interviews themselves. Speaking to familiar local people, key informants provided data on incidents associated with drug dealing. They also were able to identify related community-centered activity that demonstrated improvement in community competence to act on a public health problem.

Although we advocate use of key informants in most studies, quantitative as well as qualitative, we caution that there are limits to the information that informants usually can provide. Key informants are not infallible. A trusted informant may be reluctant to admit not knowing something or may try to please you by telling you what he or she thinks you want to hear. Key informants also may have their own biased interpretations, especially if they come from different ethnic, religious, or socioeconomic groups from the study population. Just as you look at a situation from different methodological perspectives, you would be wise to have more than one key informant so that you are not dependent on one person's interpretations. You can then raise and discuss contradictions or new ideas with other informants until you have consensus on an issue or perhaps decide to look elsewhere for different insight.

Be sensitive also to comments made by community members about your close interactions with key informants and take steps to correct misperceptions. Always ask yourself how any key informant will affect your acceptance in the wider group.

Although an informant may have much to offer, giving a single person extra attention could have negative consequences, engendering jealousy or suspicion in the group under study. Thus, it is always important to weigh the risks and benefits of developing a particularly close relationship with any individual in the setting.

MAKING THE MOST OF FIELD NOTES

The importance of good field notes—clear, detailed, and descriptive—cannot be overemphasized. New field observers often make the mistake of writing notes that are vague and imply judgment: "The unpleasant young man who came into the clinic was loud and impatient." Using descriptive terms can eliminate vagueness and reduce obvious bias: "The man who appeared to be in his early twenties approached the clinic supervisor and claimed in a loud voice that he had been waiting for three hours to see the doctor. The receptionist asked him to take a seat and told him the doctor would be with him shortly. The man shook his head forcefully and replied in a loud voice that he had been told the same thing twice already." The second note presents a more vivid picture of the scene without the overlay of observer judgment. In this case it would be equally important to include observation of objective facts such as the actual amount of time the man had been waiting, the number of staff on duty, and the number and behavior of others who were also waiting. Notes on comfort, noise level, lighting, decor, posters, health information, and other descriptions of the scene will help you analyze later the observed behavior in relation to the context. The extra effort to capture the moment in detail can provide you with rich observational data that will be meaningful when you review your large accumulation of field notes.

The journalist's query—who, what, when, where, why, and how—is also a useful guide to recording field observations. Make a practice of recording conversations and events as soon as possible after they happen, and set aside time every day to complete your notes. Start each note with the date, time, location, and a brief sentence about the purpose or circumstance of the observation. State clearly the ages, sex, and number of people you have observed or conversed with. Recall conversations, record thoughts and impressions, develop working hypotheses, plan next steps, and revisit and revise what you wrote on previous days. As you record observations, keep asking new questions, interpreting and reinterpreting what you have seen and heard. If you are also using audiotapes, enter summaries of the transcriptions into your notes. Gradually, interpretations take the shape of tentative conclusions that add structure to what you are observing. This running account will help you organize your search more efficiently, building from concrete instances to more general understanding—the process of inductive reasoning characteristic of qualitative research.

As we pointed out earlier, participant observation can begin from any theoretical perspective. It is important, therefore, to be keenly aware of your own orientation as an outsider and interpreter of the scene, documenting the distinction between what you see and what it means to you. Similarly, the observer's awareness of self in relation to the field of observation is critical to record. Qualitative researchers must frequently ask themselves two common reflexive questions, "What effect am I having on this scene?" and "How is what I observe affecting me, the observer?" Experienced participant observers learn to recognize the subtle interplay between the observer and the observed and to make it part of the record as they interpret what they see and hear.

As your field notes grow, keeping them organized may become increasingly difficult. In Chapter Six we will discuss techniques of coding text in large data sets, a process that can help the participant observer, as well as the interviewer, begin to analyze and interpret raw data while still in the field.

MANAGING BIAS AND MAXIMIZING RIGOR

Participant observation by definition entails subjective interpretation and therefore the potential for bias. However, there are a number of things you can do to keep subjectivity in control and maximize the rigor of observation data. Although it is important to become part of the group, be aware of the boundaries that distinguish your role as observer-researcher. For example, young staff conducting work in an HIV surveillance study were chosen in part because their youthfulness would help them blend in and build rapport with the young research participants. However, because their work would include observation of drinking and sexual behavior in bars, they benefited from careful guidance by supervisors on the limits of their participation (personal communication from C. Woodsong to E. T. Robinson, Feb. 2001).

Another strategy for enhancing the rigor of a participant observer study is the careful documentation we have discussed. At the end of a long day in the field, it is an easy pitfall not to document what you have observed. But by neglecting to take this important step, you risk losing what you may have learned or keeping valuable information only in your own mind, unavailable to the rest of the team. Lost data can have serious consequences in potential misinterpretation of other data and lead to erroneous or incomplete conclusions. It also leaves you vulnerable to claims that your research may not be reliable. By creating an audit trail (see Chapter Six), you will document your observations and conclusions in such a way that other researchers will be able to reconstruct the process that has led you to your results (Morse 1994). Participating in the creation of an audit trail can be a valuable learning experience for all members of the research team.

Other techniques to maximize the rigor of observation data include making comparisons among multiple observers or coders and verifying results with additional observations or semistructured interviews with other informants. However, as we emphasize throughout this text, discrepant findings do not necessarily mean methodological weakness; they may be a reflection of multiple realities, contradictory but valid perspectives and experiences in the study population.

IN-DEPTH INTERVIEWS

In-depth interviews are typically an exchange between one interviewer and one respondent. Although interviewing style is usually informal, guided by a few broad topics rather than a detailed questionnaire, there are many ways you can create structure without compromising the open exchange that is the hallmark of most qualitative techniques.

Scholars have called this kind of intensive, one-on-one interviewing a "conversational partnership" (Rubin and Rubin 1995, p. 10), "conversation with a purpose" (Burgess 1984, p. 102), and a "social encounter" (Holstein and Gubrium 1999, p. 106). These terms reflect the uniquely interactive nature of qualitative interviewing, differentiating it from the standardized survey interview. In most survey research, the interviewee is expected mainly to respond to structured questions. Qualitative researchers encourage study participants to take a more active role in determining the discussion's flow. Interviewer and participant are collaborators, "working together to achieve the shared goal of understanding" (Rubin and Rubin 1995, p. 11). In a relaxed and comfortable setting, the conversation generates empirical data by enabling participants to talk freely about their lives (Holstein and Gubrium 1999). A qualitative interview should not be a mechanical reading of standardized questions; collecting information-rich data requires mental agility, sensitivity, and practice.

FRAMING QUALITATIVE QUESTIONS

Whether in individual interviews or group discussions, qualitative questions are informal, nonjudgmental, and open. Speak clearly but casually, avoiding any suggestion that one answer might be more desirable than another. Inexperienced interviewers often use words that inadvertently suggest answers. The question "Do you believe all those things people are saying about immunization causing harm to young children?" suggests that they really are not true. Asking participants simply to comment on what they have heard about immunizing children is a more open invitation to express a candid opinion. Sometimes interviewers ask a yes-or-no question with an immediate follow-up question for more detail, but in general, it is advisable to avoid dichotomous wording and emphasize open-ended questions that encourage participants to interpret questions themselves.

Although we refer to qualitative interviews as conversations, most interviews and focus group discussions follow a pattern that comprises three kinds of questions: main questions, follow-up questions, and probes (Rubin and Rubin 1995; Patton 1990). The pattern is flexible but helps the interviewer or moderator cover the topics in sufficient depth to make the most of the rich information that participants can offer.

As Box 4.2 illustrates, the pattern begins with a clear idea of the topic or the direction you want the question to take. Because you will already have explained in a general way the purpose of the interview, you do not have to repeat the topic to the participant with each question. Main questions come from the themes and subthemes of the research problem. They introduce topics to be discussed in the form of questions. If one theme of a program evaluation is client perception of services, you might begin by asking, "What has been your experience with this health center?" Or for a study of women's vulnerability to HIV/AIDS, "How do you manage to protect yourself from infection?" Main questions are open enough to encourage spontaneous response but specific enough to keep the dialogue focused. If the discussion moves too far from the topic, you may want to repeat the main question, perhaps in a different way, to get back on track. On the other hand, be aware that getting off track may be

BOX 4.2

Levels of Interview Questions in a Qualitative Study of Emergency Contraception (EC)

Qualitative interviews typically begin with a few broad questions, then move to more specific questions, following participants' clues and encouraging depth and detail. The direction and pattern of movement can vary, depending on how the participant responds to the issues.

Topics	Main Questions	Follow-up Questions	Probes
Knowledge	Can you tell me what you know about EC?	What have you heard from others? In your opinion, are these things true?	Anything else about EC?
Source of information	Where did you hear about EC?	How did you happen to be discussing it? What did this person say about it? Who else is talking about EC these days?	Tell me more about that. Can you give me some examples?
Experience	Do you know anyone who has used EC? Have you used EC yourself?	Why did you decide to use it? What was using it like for you? Were you glad or sorry you had tried it? What made you glad or sorry?	Who influenced your decision? Why did you decide that way?
Opinion	What do you think are the advantages and disadvantages of EC?	How could EC help or harm someone like yourself? How do you think others would react to your use of EC? Do you think women you know would want EC to be available? Why or why not? Would you want EC to be available for yourself? Why or why not?	What are some ways EC could help or harm a person? What about your husband/partner/mother-in-law? What would women say if it were offered to them? What about men? What are some reasons that people you know might not want to use EC?

a clue to a different way of looking at the problem or an idea you might want to pursue or return to later in the interview.

Main Question Your main questions should reflect the logical flow you anticipate in the conversation, moving from easy and least threatening questions to more complex and interesting issues as you build rapport. However, as experienced interviewers know, this sequence may be logical only to the researcher. Participants often answer a main question before you have asked it. You must then decide quickly whether to continue with that topic or suggest coming back to it later. Or the participant may reconstruct the meaning of the question in a different way, requiring your flexibility to keep the discussion focused while encouraging participant perspectives and experiences. Interviewers and moderators often ask the most important—and perhaps more difficult—questions more than once, from different angles and at different points in the interview. Through experience you will learn how to move around among the main questions, pursuing each to its logical conclusion while not neglecting questions or new ideas.

Follow-Up Question A follow-up question moves the interview or discussion to a deeper level by asking for more detail. Follow-up questions are a natural part of any conversation. They suggest to the speaker that the listener is interested enough in what the speaker has just said to want more information. To some extent you can anticipate follow-up questions in advance, but even in a standardized open-ended format, you cannot know exactly what they will be until participants respond to the main questions. In the example in Box 4.2, a participant might have answered the first question by saying, "Well, I hear emergency contraception can prevent pregnancy." You would then ask for detail on what the person has heard and whether she or he knows it as fact (a knowledge question).

Probe A probe is a kind of follow-up question that takes the discussion into still deeper territory, with or without specific reference to the topic. For example, the interviewer might say, "Please tell me more about that" or "Then what happened?" or "I don't think I know what you mean—can you explain?" As you gain experience, you use these conversational devices naturally. They tell the participant that you are listening closely and that what she or he has said is important. They also indicate to the participant the level of detail you want and enable you to clarify points or pursue new ideas in a conversational manner. Note, however, the importance of maintaining a comfortable balance between too much detail and not enough. Insufficient probing could suggest boredom, but aggressive probing might be intrusive (Rubin and Rubin 1995). Through experience and careful listening, you will know how to probe sensitively and when to stop.

STAGES OF THE INTERVIEW

A particularly versatile format for in-depth interviews and focus groups in applied behavioral health research is the semistructured approach we introduced in Chapter Three. Interviewers typically use a written set of flexibly worded topics or questions that keep the conversation guided and on track but without imposing boundaries on the participant's style and expression.

Rubin and Rubin (1995) describe this type of in-depth interview in a series of stages:

- Creating natural involvement
- Encouraging conversational competence
- Showing understanding
- Getting facts and basic description
- Asking difficult questions
- Toning down the emotional level
- Closing while maintaining contact

Although these stages are presented here for in-depth interviews, they are easily adapted to focus group discussions as well.

Creating Natural Involvement Beginning with an informal chat is a good way to set the stage for the relaxed atmosphere you want to create for the interview. It helps to be able to comment on events or situations that are familiar and important to the respondent. If possible, link the purpose of the interview to some common experience, for example, "A young man in my office passed away from AIDS the other day. It has been hard for all of us who knew him." Or in a study of children's antisocial behavior and the mass media, the interviewer might begin, "I find it difficult to know how to respond to the violence my children see on television and on the streets." Sharing experience is a way of expressing the bond that you hope will develop into the conversational partnership that will generate the information you seek. Women interviewing women, or men interviewing men, may find common ground in gender, for example, in family relationships, childbearing, job seeking, or other experiences in the context of being a woman or a man. Expression of concern about the widespread prevalence of a common problem like adolescent pregnancy or a debilitating chronic disease may also be a springboard to the conversational partnership.

Early in the introduction, it is important to explain clearly what the study is about and why the respondent has been asked to participate. This is a good time to clarify the rights and responsibilities of participation and to obtain the individual's informed consent to continue. As you begin to develop rapport, you will move into a more formal introduction, explaining who you are and what you want to know. The respondent meanwhile will be assessing you, trying to decide what you really want and whether you can be trusted. It is important to show that you are genuinely interested, that you do not come with a judgmental attitude, and that you will honor his or her confidentiality and trust.

Encouraging Conversational Competence In the first few minutes of the interview encounter, you set the tone for the conversation that follows. People often agree to participate in an interview but are insecure or skeptical that they would have anything to offer. The interviewer's job is to give participants the sense that their opinions and experiences are important to the study. Starting with easy, nonthreatening questions allows them to feel sure about what they know and pleased to have an appreciative ear. Participants familiar with survey interviews may instantly adopt a compliant role, offering impersonal, monosyllabic answers to questions. It is therefore critical to dispel as quickly as possible the notion of passivity or subordination to the interviewer.

As you develop your own qualitative style, the language you use should help to establish you as a partner rather than an interrogator. "I'm hoping you will help me understand how women make choices about pregnancy." "I'd like to explore with you what it means to be the mother of a large family." "When it comes to housing and feeding the family, we men have a lot of responsibility. Let's talk a little about where the paycheck goes." "I know that as a grandmother you care very much about how the children are raised." And perhaps later: "I'm wondering how you feel about circumcising the girls." Whether or not you agree with the participant's views, your manner should reflect great interest and compassion. As they come to trust you and the confidentiality of the interview, participants will welcome a sympathetic listener; they will become more personally invested in the topic and will move with you to deeper levels of their experience. The interviewer-partner does not coax answers from the respondent but enters actively into the discussion in a way that explores incompletely articulated thoughts and encourages new directions (Holstein and Gubrium 1999).

The general way of approaching the reliability problem [in qualitative research] is to . . . conduct research as if someone were always looking over your shoulder.
(Yin 1994, p. 37)

Showing Understanding As the interview progresses, you can encourage openness and depth by showing that you understand and empathize with what the respondent is telling you. When a mother of six in a very poor village was telling the interviewer how hard it was to have so many children, the interviewer responded, "Yes, I can imagine life is very hard for you right now. How do you keep your children looking so healthy?" The question builds rapport by showing that the interviewer understands and by reinforcing the respondent's competence in her role as a mother. Emotional support comes through in a sympathetic tone of voice, responsive facial expression, murmurs, and gestures—all of which suggest acceptance of the person. It is not necessary to relate one's own personal experiences or to approve of everything the individual has done. Your role is to put the conversational partner at ease to share life experiences without fear.

Getting Facts and Basic Descriptions Once the partnership is established and conversation flows easily, you are getting into the heart of the interview. Now you can encourage longer answers by asking the partner to tell you about an incident or describe a typical encounter related to the topic of the research, following it up with simple, direct questions. At this stage of the interview, you focus on descriptive material, holding delicate or emotionally charged questions for later.

A topic to introduce at this stage might be how a young person gets answers to questions about sexual relationships. An adolescent will probably talk about conversations held with friends or questions asked of health providers, which will lead into details of the questions and perhaps reveal personal concerns about sexual matters. The exchange may prompt the interviewer to explore possible gaps in adolescents' understanding of health services or contradictions between the information young people want and the answers that providers are prepared to give. As a skilled listener, the interviewer will be alert to clues that the participant is ready to move to more sensitive levels of discussion.

Asking the Really Difficult Questions Save your most difficult questions until you sense that your conversational partnership is relaxed and trusting. Be aware not only of your partner's stage in the process but of your own comfort with the relationship and your readiness to raise issues that may take considerable skill to manage. Researchers in health behavior must frequently discuss topics that lie outside normal discourse with strangers. In varying degrees open discussion of sex is taboo in virtually all cultures; women, especially, may be socialized to strict norms of sexual privacy. As you enter this stage of the interview, it is important to respect the fact that you may be violating certain expectations of behavior and to be especially sensitive to the conversation's effect on your participant. Remember that you can ask and repeat important questions at different points in the interview. Repeating a difficult question later in a different way gives the participant a chance to think about it and offers you an opportunity to ask it from a different angle.

When the research problem requires you to ask difficult questions, there are ways to soften their impact. You may need to remind your respondent that the interview is confidential, that no names are recorded, and that identification will not be revealed. It also helps to acknowledge the sensitivity of the topic with a simple comment like "I know this is a hard thing to discuss—I really appreciate your sharing."

Another way to show responsiveness and empathy is to use familiar words and expressions in the conversation—an advantage of the informal style of qualitative interviewing. Telling a story or showing a picture that illustrates the topic is a way of depersonalizing a difficult area without sacrificing spontaneity. When you ask respondents to talk about an issue through fictitious characters, you are allowing them to control the extent to which they disclose information about themselves. If necessary for the research, the interviewer might ask if the picture or story is like anything in their own lives; but qualitative interviewers who have used this technique usually find that the respondent shifts spontaneously from the impersonal third-person to the first-person expression of self.

Hesitation may not mean embarrassment but may be simply a pause that reflects difficulty understanding the question. It can also mean that the respondent, especially if a woman, has never been asked her opinion on any topic. We have found that women in some societies are so unaccustomed to being consulted on matters of fertility that it may take several interviews before they are able to participate as partners in the interview conversation.

Toning Down the Emotional Level When participants have been open with you on sensitive or embarrassing topics, they may begin to feel uncomfortably exposed.

As the interviewer you may need to help restore the sense of privacy that enabled them to share their lives with you in the first place. Again you can simply remind them of the confidentiality of the information. When toning down the emotional level of the conversation, the researcher can turn the interview around and ask if the participant has questions to ask or has answers to other questions. By this time most participants will have identified themselves as partners and be able and eager to add clarifying information.

But sometimes it is difficult to move away from interview conversations that have stirred up strong emotions. If the conversation is upsetting to the participant, you can decide to change the topic or discontinue the interview. An alternative is to allow participants to ventilate their feelings until they become calmer or until you can shift naturally to a more neutral topic. A risk that qualitative interviewers often face is that they may learn more than participants want them to hear (Alty and Rodham 1998). The more comfortable the respondent is with you, the more easily she or he will disclose information not meant to be shared. You may hear such off-the-record comments after the interview or focus group has ended. The interviewer's ethical response to material that seems to go beyond the participant's original informed consent is either to interrupt the conversation at that point or to ask the participant whether those remarks can be included in the transcript. It might be important to have these comments in your personal notes to help you understand the meaning of broader issues. However, if the participant does not want them shared, your ethical obligation is to indicate clearly in your notes that they should never be quoted in full or described in publications.

To some extent we can predict topics that are potentially embarrassing or disturbing: drug or alcohol addiction, sexual preference if not in the open, deviant behavior, acts of violence, sexual intimacy, abortion, infidelity, and contraception that may be in conflict with religious beliefs or cultural norms. Other topics may evoke painful emotion, for example, loss of children or experience with rape or spousal abuse. Or a topic may have political sensitivity that you as an outsider have not guessed. In short, you need to be always on the alert for change in the tone of the interview conversation that could suggest that you are entering a vulnerable area. Rather than risk further discomfort for your respondent, avoid the question if it is not essential to the purpose of the research. If what you need to know is whether infidelity is a common experience for women in the community, it is not necessary to probe the marital relations of your conversational partner. If you ask her about women in general, she is free to illustrate her response with her own experience only if she wishes to do so.

On the other hand, qualitative researchers must be prepared to answer another important but often overlooked ethical question: What is the responsibility of the interviewer when a study participant asks for help? Even if violence is not the topic of the research, questioning women on gender decisions may suddenly evoke personal accounts of an abusive relationship. The interviewer must be prepared for such unanticipated disclosures, balancing the requirements of the interview with ethical responsibility for the participant's well-being. In one country where we experienced this scenario, we were able to refer vulnerable women to a local intervention program for abused or neglected women by handing all participants a card at the end of the interview with the name, address, and phone number of a women's counseling center. Other problems to note include a participant's fear of having an STI or disclosing recent untreated complications of an unsafe abortion. In such situations the interviewer's ethical responsibility is to refer the person to a sympathetic social service or health practitioner. Not all problems will have such convenient solutions, but interviewers must be prepared to identify distress and respond with empathy and appropriate referral.

Closing While Maintaining Contact Once the participant has accepted the role of conversational partner, it can be difficult to terminate the conversation. You will need to express thanks for the time taken to share valuable information, perhaps reiterating the confidentiality of the record. In case you need to return later to ask the participant to confirm or elaborate on a statement, it is wise to ask permission to call on the person again and verify contact information. Although the interview has ended, informal conversation usually continues. Be alert to casual banter, because it may contain unexpected clues or new leads to answering the research question. Unless participants indicate that parting comments are off the record, make notes on your observations at the moment or as soon as possible.

Focus Groups

"A focus group is the use of group interaction to produce data and insights that would be less accessible without the interaction found in a group" (Morgan 1988, p. 12). The key phrase here is *group interaction.* Unlike simple group interviews in which several people may be interviewed at once for convenience, focus groups depend as much on the exchange of ideas among participants as they do on answers to specific questions from the interviewer. The interviewer, in fact, is called a moderator, underscoring the role of guide and facilitator in the group process.

A focus group is the use of group interaction to produce data and insights that would be less accessible without the interaction found in a group.
(Morgan 1988, p. 12)

Moderating a focus group has much in common with in-depth interviewing. Introducing topics with main questions, asking more specific follow-up questions to elicit more detailed information, and probing the meaning of responses are as important in focus group discussions as they are in individual interviews. We will discuss this further in the in-depth interview section of this chapter.

The methodology of focused group interviews was first developed for social science during World War II by sociologists studying military morale and the impact of propaganda materials on public opinion (Merton and others 1956). Sociologist Harold Blumer (1969, p. 41) later used focus groups in a series of drug studies, remarking that "A small number of . . . individuals who are acute observers and who are well-informed . . . brought together as a discussion and resource group, is more valuable many times over than a representative sample." Focus group discussion has also proved a useful tool for marketers studying consumer opinion on commercial products.

WHEN TO USE FOCUS GROUPS

In recent years focus group methodology has been applied increasingly to research in population and health. Its use by researchers and consultants in these areas has shed new light on, for example, people's understanding of fertility and HIV risk, socioeconomic influences on health decision making, perspectives on health in the school curriculum, and attitudes toward community health intervention. Focus groups are equally useful for formative research and for evaluation of outcomes. On the other hand, indiscriminate use of focus groups by researchers with little experience in qualitative methods sometimes creates confusion about how and when to use them. In fact, in some circles their popularity has made focus groups seem synonymous with qualitative research. In practice, focus group discussions are only one of a growing number of qualitative methods, valuable in situations where the most rewarding data will come from interaction in a group (Morgan 1988).

As we discussed in Chapter Three, there are relatively clear indicators for choosing a focus group over an individual in-depth interview. Groups can be highly effective sources of data for studies that focus on social norms, expectations, values, and beliefs. Especially rich topics for focus groups are those that stimulate people to share their own ideas and debate others' views. Focus group discussions thrive on controversial topics. However, it is critical to the quality of the data that participants be well grounded in the topic, either through personal experience or a vested interest arising from a particular role or position. For example, a study of the acceptability of a new microbicide in a population at high risk of STI might suggest recruiting commercial sex workers who could speak from their experience of using the product with their clients. Or if the purpose of the research is to explore the feasibility of school-based health education for young people, it would be useful to hear not only from adolescents but from parents and teachers, as well as from religious, political, and other community leaders whose views on adolescent health and behavior could influence the program.

COMPOSITION AND SIZE OF FOCUS GROUPS

Most focus groups are relatively homogeneous, composed of people who are similar with respect to characteristics related to the topic. A family planning study might start with people of childbearing age. But it soon could become apparent that women feel uncomfortable speaking with men about reproductive issues. Or in some cultures, younger women are often reluctant to express their views in the presence of older women. Mothers may be unwilling to listen to women who have not borne children. Both sex and age often become defining variables when assigning people to discussion groups. Similar constraints may divide members of different ethnic groups, rural residents from urban, educated people from nonliterate, professional and technical workers from manual workers. Or it may be important to the research design to segment participants for the sake of stratification in analysis, the ability to compare and contrast the views of different subsets of the population (see Chapter Six). As the study progresses, you may find it advisable to expand the sample if emerging data suggest tapping new or different sources of information.

For most purposes groups of eight to ten participants are sufficient to stimulate good but manageable discussion for the moderator, who must keep the discussion focused while encouraging everyone to take part. The smaller the group, the less likely that discussion will express wider norms, values, or opinions. On the other hand, a large group is not only difficult to manage but may provide incomplete data if reticent members defer to their more voluble peers.

Although you hope that everyone in the group will contribute freely and openly, it is important to select individuals who will not dominate the discussion or inhibit others' participation. If the study design calls for the opinions of people in positions of authority—the company manager, a hospital director, or a community official—consider including them in individual interviews or as key informants rather than as focus group participants. Alternatively, you might decide to invite these authorities, or a subset of them, to take part in separate focus groups.

Should focus group participants be strangers or friends? Writers on focus group methodology often emphasize the importance of anonymity among participants, on the premise that one can speak more freely with strangers than with people one knows and will meet again. However, in many settings, especially in developing countries, it is neither feasible nor advisable to expect a group of strangers to participate in a discussion. It may be difficult to find participants who are not already acquainted. In some cultures women, and sometimes men, are uncomfortable sharing their perspectives with people they do not know. The investigator will base this decision on local norms of interaction. Under no circumstances should you ever allow observers or interested bystanders to listen to the discussion; doing so would violate confidentiality and possibly inhibit open discussion.

HOW MANY GROUPS?

The rule of thumb in deciding how many focus groups to form is to conduct at least two for each defining demographic variable. For instance, if the groups are divided only by sex, four groups may be sufficient. In practice, focus groups are seldom divided on only one variable, and the necessary number of groups quickly multiplies. If two age categories (younger and older) are added, the number of groups jumps to eight. Adding an education variable with three categories will bring you to twenty-four groups. And if you decide to conduct the study in three locales—rural, urban, and periurban—you will need seventy-two discussion groups, an unwieldy sample size for most field studies. The lesson many qualitative researchers have learned is that you have to balance the number of variable subsets (sex, age, residence) against the resources (time, money, personnel) available for transcribing, translating, coding, and analyzing the data. This equation takes you back to the study design. If you have more groups than you can handle, the chances are that your study design is too complex for the resources at your disposal. You may need to revisit the study objectives and focus them more tightly. Remember that establishing a comfortable balance between number of groups and available resources should take place at the design stage, not once you are in the field.

A normal rate for collecting data from focus groups is one group per day, including transcription. A two-hour discussion is likely to generate twenty-five to forty pages of transcript. A set of seventy-two discussions could yield as many as 2,880 pages to code and perhaps translate by the end of the study. Simple arithmetic demonstrates the importance of selecting criteria carefully to include variables essential to sound design while keeping the size of the data set within limits established by the research.

COLLECTING BACKGROUND INFORMATION

A brief profile on each participant can provide valuable information for later analysis and presentation of the findings. Knowing something about the individuals whose comments are recorded on the transcript will help you describe your sample, interpret what participants have said, and analyze emerging themes in the light of contextual differences and similarities. Background information can also enliven reports by highlighting the people behind the findings: "A thirty-year-old factory worker and mother of six commented that . . .". If included in a focus group study, this information should be brief and clearly related to the research problem, for example, sociodemographic characteristics such as age, education, occupation, marital status, or family size. In clinical research qualitative investigators sometimes use information from the sexual and reproductive history to help them understand their data: age at first pregnancy, use of contraception, number of pregnancies and live births, desired number of children, and so forth.

The rules in collecting background data for focus group analysis are simple:

- Keep it relevant.
- Keep it short.
- Keep it confidential.

If sociodemographic or other data will enhance your analysis, collect it with participants' informed consent before the discussion begins. Remember to keep the background form simple; one page or less of easy, short-answer questions is usually sufficient to record a few relevant facts. Participants may provide the data by completing the forms themselves or responding orally to a researcher. This is not a group exercise; it is done individually to preserve confidentiality and anonymity. The forms are identified only by codes that correspond to code numbers that the individual participants wear during the discussion. Store the completed forms securely, accessible only to the researchers and their assistants. Of course, the researchers will respect the preference of any participant who wishes not to be so identified. However, in our experience, most participants like their coded tags. They are a reminder that a system is in place to protect the anonymity of anything they say. Sometimes participants refer to each other by the numbers they are wearing, even when they know each other by name: "I agree with eight that . . .". In the following pages, we will describe how note takers can use participant code numbers and enter them into the transcript for analysis.

CONDUCTING THE DISCUSSION

As we have seen earlier in this chapter, qualitative interviewing requires a high level of interpersonal skill to develop a conversational partnership. Similarly, the focus group moderator's special task is to create a group of conversational partners, listening with nonjudgmental interest while keeping the discussion focused and moving. Whether in the individual interview or group discussion, the responsive interviewer or moderator shows interest, curiosity, empathy, and encouragement but also must be flexible, creative, and able to tailor questions and comments to each person's unique responses. A topic guide, introduced later in this chapter, is an important tool for keeping the discussion centered while encouraging participants to speak naturally and spontaneously.

As in the in-depth interview, a sensitive topic like reproductive health is likely to be more acceptable to members of a focus group if the moderator is the same sex as the participants. If women are not accustomed to expressing their views to men, even the most skilled male moderator may inhibit discussion. Other characteristics will depend on the topic of discussion and cultural norms that prescribe who can discuss what with whom. Similarly, respondents in developing countries who have had little opportunity to know Westerners may be uncomfortable with a U.S. or European interviewer. An effective partnership may therefore depend on cultural similarity and the ability of researchers and participants to understand each other's language and perspectives.

THE MODERATOR AND NOTE-TAKER TEAM

To ensure accurate data and to facilitate analysis, qualitative researchers usually tape their focus group discussions. Although videotaping would capture more nonverbal expression, participants may find the camera more intrusive than a simple tape recorder. For most data collection, we therefore recommend audiocassettes. Even so, overreliance on the tape recorder is a common pitfall with negative consequences when technology fails. The most efficient organization is a team of two trained moderators, one to guide the discussion and the other to monitor the tape recorder while recording on paper as much of the discussion as possible (Hogle and others 1994). Although verbatim text from transcripts will be of great value in the analysis, notes on the discussion are also important. The skilled field researcher learns to take good notes unobtrusively and to quickly expand them after the interview, regardless of whether the discussion has been taped. In case of an inaudible recording, a power failure, or lost tapes, the researcher will have recorded on paper enough of the discussion to preserve the raw data. In addition to copious notes on the verbal process, the note taker also enters observations that will enrich the transcript with nonverbal messages that have a bearing on the discussion. For example, notes might state that "Participant A appeared angry and left the group" or that "The group seemed much amused by this remark."

If the researcher has collected background information, it is usually the note taker's responsibility to assure that identification codes on information sheets correspond to codes that participants wear. The note taker follows the discussion carefully, indicating the code number or letter assigned to each speaker. The code and the first few words of each comment are usually enough to identify the speaker when the note taker's observations are transferred later to the transcript. It is not essential to identify every comment; and in fast-paced discussions, such precision is often impossible. However, to the extent you are able to identify who said what, you will have a richer analysis and a livelier presentation, because you can amplify comments from the transcript with information about the speaker. (We discuss integrating participants' comments and characteristics into the report in Chapter Seven.)

With the note taker in the role of recorder-observer, the moderator is responsible for creating a comfortable climate for open exchange, encouraging participation, and guiding the discussion. As participants enter, the moderator seats them in an informal circle with the note taker just outside the circle to avoid distracting the group. The tape recorder is placed where it can easily record the discussion but with as little distraction to participants as possible. We generally do not recommend passing a microphone around to each speaker, although this approach has been used when the meeting place has a lot of background noise or the centrally located recording device is weak.

The moderator welcomes the group and introduces herself or himself and the note taker, explaining the role of each. The moderator also explains the purpose of the tape recorder: to enable the researchers to capture ideas that emerge from the discussion without identifying the speakers by name. Participants are assured that written reports will not include names and that tapes will not be shared outside the research team. In the process of administering informed consent, remind participants of the group's responsibility to guard the confidentiality of the discussion. Participants should also understand that there are no right and wrong answers and that all opinions are welcome.

It is important for participants to understand the general goals of the discussion, but "clarifying goals does not necessarily mean revealing . . . the questions under study. Clarifying goals does mean communicating to participants what you want to know from them" (Basch 1987, p. 416). Indeed, in an overly informed group, members may obligingly supply the answers they think you want to hear, regardless of their truth. Once the participants generally understand the topic and procedure, the moderator may then ask them to introduce themselves, although if anonymity in the group is important, introductions can be replaced with informal conversation and nonthreatening questions to put the group members at ease and encourage them to talk among themselves.

The moderator then asks participants to accept ground rules, such as speaking one at a time, not interrupting each other, and speaking clearly and slowly so that the tape can pick up the words. Participants should be asked to suggest additional ground rules, which will reinforce the idea that their contributions are a valuable part of the research process. The moderator encourages participants to speak freely, addressing questions any way they want, while at the same time reminding them that discussions sometimes wander off track and may need to be refocused. This can be a difficult course to steer but may be greatly facilitated by a well-designed yet flexible topic guide, as we will discuss later in this chapter.

Following this warm-up period, introduce the first topic. The moderator should observe the group closely, watching for signs that some participants might merely be agreeing with others rather than voicing opinions of their own. Other signs of potential problems in the group process are participants who are unenthusiastic, aloof, confused, overly positive or excessively negative; are highly critical of others; or attempt to control the discussion with their own points of view. Early identification makes it easier to respond effectively to these problems. For example, a domineering participant might be seated next to the moderator to discourage eye contact, or the moderator might remind the group that ground rules include respectful listening.

ENDING THE DISCUSSION

At the end of the discussion, the moderator may ask the participants to summarize what they have said, adding any comments they want to include. Or the moderator might supply the summary, beginning with "Since we are almost out of time, I will try to summarize what you have told me." The summary is a chance to clarify issues and give the group a sense of work accomplished. Participants are able to restate points and correct any misunderstanding the moderator may have. The note taker then turns off the tape recorder. Most groups conclude with light refreshments, which local assistants can organize.

Some researchers include a debriefing with participants at the close of the discussion, inviting feedback on the discussion experience. Did they feel included? Were they comfortable with the topics? Do they think the group fully explored the topics? Were there topics or questions that the group should have discussed but did not? Can they think of how the discussion should have been conducted differently? Debriefings can be useful not only for evaluating and revising the discussion protocol but also for providing additional context in data analysis. They also are an important learning resource for the field team.

The question of reimbursement to participants frequently arises in focus group research. Should participants be reimbursed for the time they contribute to discussing the research questions? Projects that pay focus group participants sometimes come under criticism for raising expectations that future researchers may not be able to meet. A compromise is to offer each participant a modest gift that expresses the researchers' appreciation without setting an unrealistic precedent. A rule of thumb on this issue is to take local customs and expectations into consideration. If people have come to expect payment, then it is appropriate to pay them according to the local scale.

Appendix Four elaborates on the steps in managing a focus group discussion. These steps can also help guide your preparation of a budget. Appendix Five gives an example of costs to consider when proposing a focus group study, from the planning stage to interpretation of the data and final presentations.

Structured Data Collection Techniques

It is often the case that individuals or groups will be able to organize and articulate their thoughts more easily if they have a concrete reference point. There are a number of ways to add this kind of structure to interviews and focus groups without compromising flexibility and spontaneity. Centering a question on an image or task adds a tangible dimension to an otherwise abstract issue. Framing potentially uncomfortable issues in a less personal context also is helpful. The interview or focus group guide might start a topic with a statement of presumed fact: "We have heard that women are not going to the clinic for prenatal care. Can you comment on that?" or "A woman in another village told us that she had been beaten several times by her husband. Are you familiar with such a problem in your own community?" This indirect structure is likely to elicit a more open response than "Why did you not attend the antenatal clinic?" or "Have you ever experienced domestic abuse?"

The following techniques for adding structure to data collection can be used with almost any qualitative method, particularly when you are interested in helping a group to center on specific research issues, as in focus group discussions and participatory action research.

FREELISTING AND PILE SORTS

An old technique with application to qualitative research in public health is freelisting, combined with pilesorting, in which the researcher asks participants to make a list of all instances of some phenomenon. Items on the categories list are then transferred to cards that participants sort into piles according to their own criteria and labels. This approach is based on the principle that people make sense of their worlds by grouping their observations and experiences in classes known as domains. A *cultural domain* is "a set of items or things that are all of the same type or category" (Schensul and others 1999, p. 115). How people assign items to domains indicates to the researcher how they interpret the meanings of these items in their own lives. For example, if you are interested in popular perceptions of STI, you might ask participants in a study to list all the diseases and symptoms they can think of and organize them in groups according to common characteristics. The common denominators they use can tell you a great deal about the meanings people attach to STI symptoms. You may discover that people classify symptoms according to traditional notions of cause and effect, attributing some to supernatural causes, whereas others sort the cards into piles that represent biomedical, environmental, or political explanations.

To take this example a step further, you might want to explore possible links between cultural definitions and choice of provider. You could ask participants to group the items in help-seeking categories, including different types of healers as well as peer consultation, self-help, or no action at all. Whether you are collecting data from individuals or groups, this technique lends itself well to qualitative exploration, because in probing the logic behind participants' assignment of items to categories, the researcher may uncover reasons for popular perceptions and behaviors that might not otherwise be apparent.

The lists that participants create are themselves an important linguistic tool if they provide insight into cultural expression on topics related to the research problem. For example, public health researchers conducting a formative study of neonatal mortality in Guatemala wanted to understand how local people expressed the topics and feelings surrounding the loss of a child in their idiom. Inviting women to tell their stories, the researchers identified a list of words. They asked women then to sort the words into like piles, explaining similarities and differences among them. The result was a taxonomy of indigenous expressions that the researchers could use to develop culturally sensitive tools for collecting data. Through a better understanding of linguistic expression, they learned, for example, that many of their participants associated neonatal deaths with the lunar eclipse, referring to the lost child as *"el nino eclipsado"* (Patricia Bailey 2004, personal communication with P. R. Ulin, unreferenced). Most participants enjoy sorting items into categories and then talking about their decisions. The process itself can be interesting and the outcome motivating, as people begin to reinterpret familiar experiences in new ways.

PHOTO NARRATIVE

The interviewer may present a visual aid such as a poster or photograph and ask participants to talk about what it means to them. In a study of Latina women's perceptions of the quality of prenatal care, participants were shown photographic prompts—pictures taken in a clinic setting with staff and client actors (Bender and Harbour 2001). An interviewer asked participants to describe each photograph, including how the woman in the photo was feeling. She then asked the participant if the photograph reminded her of any experience she had had and, if so, to tell the story of that experience. As these researchers point out, photographic prompts allow the participant to talk about herself in the third person, projecting experiences and opinions that may not be socially desirable onto the subject in the photograph.

Also known as photo voice (Bender and Castro 2000; Wang 1999; Wang and Burris 1997), the photo narrative technique is well suited to feminist inquiry because as documentary evidence, it has the potential to give "voice" to people on society's margins. Researchers have put cameras into women's hands, enabling them to capture scenes that reflect their own lives and to communicate their perceptions and experiences more effectively than by words alone. The photographic record empowered the women to enter into critical dialogue on issues that affected their everyday lives and to present their concerns directly to policymakers.

STORYTELLING

Another way to introduce structure is by telling a story, one that is fictitious but designed to include issues at the heart of the research problem. A focus group study of sexual decision making and HIV/AIDS risk in Haiti presented the topic through the story of an imaginary young woman, Joujou, who believed she was at great risk of acquiring HIV from her partner, René (Ulin and others 1995). Issues to be explored were embedded in a culturally familiar context of women's economic dependence and sexual subordination. When she discovers that René has other sexual partners, Joujou must decide how to protect herself. The interviewer then opens the discussion to the group, inviting their ideas and suggestions, while prompting them to think beyond their initial reactions with such questions as "How do you think René would react to that?" or "How can Joujou support herself and her children if she leaves him?" Participants in both men's and women's groups quickly recognized Joujou's dilemma and entered into vigorous discussion of alternatives and their consequences for women's lives. As in Bender and Harbour's photo narrative study (2001), storytelling relieved the pressure of self-disclosure by asking people to comment on the problems and decisions of another person, albeit like themselves.

Note that, used in focus groups, these techniques elicit participants' perceptions of cultural norms, views, and behaviors of people like themselves and are not a dependable record of case-based behavior. As discussion builds, speakers frequently identify with the photo or story actors, switching easily from third-person to first-person narrative. Nevertheless, in most instances only the individual interview and similar techniques, with or without additional structure, can fully capture individual perceptions and behavior.

BODY MAPPING

Body mapping is a projective technique in which participants draw maps of the human body. It is particularly useful in studies of people's perceptions of reproductive anatomy and physiology, fertility awareness, and other reproductive health issues. It may also be a more comfortable means of expression for participants who are reticent to speak openly about sexual matters. As a visual representation of the participant's understanding of reproductive function, the participant's drawing, or body map, can then become the focus for in-depth conversation with the interviewer.

A participatory action project in Zambia used body mapping to understand how Zambian youth conceptualize the reproductive system (Shah 1999). The researcher asked small groups of adolescents divided by age and sex to make simple sketches of the human body to show how the reproductive organs function. The researcher then asked each group to label the body parts and explain their functions, prompting them with questions such as "How does a woman get pregnant?" or "How can pregnancy be prevented?" Researchers were able to identify gaps and distortions that could be addressed through intervention. As the author of this report points out, body mapping can be combined with other qualitative methods or expanded into picture stories, or cartoons, as the basis for discussing sexual relationships. Although semi- and nonliterate people will not be able to write labels on their maps, research has shown that they can participate in a body-mapping project, interpreting their drawings orally to the researcher (Shah 1999).

In similar uses of body mapping, researchers sometimes chose this technique to study women's perceptions of maternal morbidity. Women will express themselves more easily about reproductive risk if they can talk as they draw in organs on a female figure. As the women describe each organ, how it works and how it can fail, researchers are able to identify, for example, cultural perceptions of cause and effect, as well as local patterns of help seeking for symptoms that participants identify.

SOCIAL NETWORK ANALYSIS

Social network analysis is based on the premise that individuals seldom make decisions in isolation. Through network research we are able to explore attitudes, beliefs, and actions of individuals in the context of group affiliations. Tracing a person's social network helps the researcher understand what people do and think in relation to group norms and expectations. It also reveals how people, as well as ideas and information, circulate in and among different groups. Discovering the social network can be a first step in developing effective interventions to reduce behavior that puts people's health at risk.

Social network research has been used extensively to study risk behavior associated with sharing drug injection equipment and engaging in unprotected sex with HIV-infected partners. For example, a network study of heroin injectors found that many were introduced to hard drugs by, or regularly shared drugs and drug-using equipment with, relatives (Pino and others 1999). Moreover, cousins and other close relatives were heavily represented in the drug-using networks of people who had started injecting heroin as adolescents. Such findings suggest that to be successful, interventions designed to prevent hard drug use among adolescents must address issues in family addiction as well.

Network analysis begins by identifying not only the network itself but also its members:

- What sets these people apart from nonmembers?
- What qualities do they share?
- What brings them together, and how strong is the bond?

The task is to determine the criteria for inclusion or exclusion and establish network boundaries. This process may be as easy as obtaining a class roster or list of employees; it may be as difficult as patiently tracking down individuals through participant observation and key informant interviews. Researchers can discover clues to network boundaries by asking people what makes a member. Having defined the network and identified its members, the investigator proceeds by in-depth interviews and participant observation to explore the meaning of the relationships among network members.

In northern Thailand, where unwanted pregnancy and STI rates among young people are high, researchers turned to social network analysis to help develop new programs to reduce sexual risk (Bond and others 1999). The research team used snowball sampling to identify networks. The team randomly selected two young women at each of three locales—public dormitories, workplaces, and entertainment venues—and asked each to name five friends they frequently went out with at night. These friends were contacted and asked to name five more friends. When no new names were mentioned, the process stopped, yielding three networks of affiliated youth at each site. In-depth interviews with individual network members explored cultural norms and behavior related to friends and romantic partners. Discovering sexual linkages led to identification of youth subcultures, communication channels, and patterns of risk behavior that varied among the networks. With this information as a base, program planners could then work with natural peer leaders to establish an outreach program that focused on healthier sexual decisions among different categories of youth at risk. Although the number of members in any one network may be small, the Thai example illustrates that knowing the network's characteristics can help researchers and program planners understand the health risks of its members.

Social network studies often combine qualitative and quantitative techniques in the same research design. From a quantitative perspective, investigators use surveys and statistical analyses to measure relationships within, and linkages between, networks. Computer software for quantitative network analysis enables the researcher to characterize, quantify, and create visual images of these relationships (Borgatti and others 2001). Qualitative analysis takes a more holistic approach in order to explore the meaning and context of the network relationships in their natural setting. Combining quantitative and qualitative methods is a powerful strategy, not only for studying network characteristics but also for understanding the diffusion of ideas and behaviors within and among networks.

Participatory Methods

Participatory research (PR) is not a specific method but rather the use of multiple methods to solve a problem through group action. There are several ways to incorporate participatory action in a study, but all have in common the objective to help work groups or communities analyze their own situations and develop strategic interventions. Methodology depends on the research problem and the group's or community's skills and resources, but the important factor is *local* participation in decision making and in implementing the study process (Díaz and Simmons 1999). Participatory approaches to problem solving appear in many contexts, including education, agriculture, and community development, under terms such as participatory action research, rural rapid appraisal, participatory rapid appraisal, and participatory learning and action.

The concept of subject as participant in the research process is basic to qualitative design. However, PR takes the concept a step further to cast participants as problem solvers in their communities. The choice of topic therefore depends as much or more on a problem the participant group wants to solve as it does on the researcher's interests. Participants typically are community groups that collaborate with the researcher to define a problem; identify information needed; collect, process, and interpret the information; and take action consistent with the results. Roles tend to blur as researchers and participants pool their knowledge to arrive at concrete solutions to problems.

A PR project can use any qualitative method, usually multiple techniques and sometimes combined with quantitative methods. A common PR tool is geographic

BOX 4.3

A Participatory Action Model: The PALS Program in Zambia

In 1996 CARE International in Zambia was planning to start a new project (Shah 1999) in adolescent sexual and reproductive health. Its goal was to reduce sexual and reproductive health morbidity and mortality by promoting behavior change and encouraging more adolescent-friendly health services.

Having had little experience with adolescents, the planners began by asking adolescents themselves to share their perspectives on reproductive health needs and concerns. Before making any programmatic decisions, all CARE staff took part in a training workshop on the methodology of participatory learning and action. A participatory appraisal with adolescents in one Lusaka community followed formal training. The results led to establishment of the Partnership for Adolescent Sexual and Reproductive Health (PALS) Project and twelve more appraisals in Lusaka, Livingston, and Ndola, where the PALS Project was subsequently implemented.

Using results from the participatory appraisals, CARE submitted a proposal to donors and received funding for the PALS Project. The field methodology developed for PALS included an appraisal tool kit that adolescent participants could use in their own communities. The tool kit consisted of seventeen participatory activities, including interviews, group discussions, pictures and storytelling, role-playing, mapping, and other techniques. With the support of clinicians and CARE staff, the teens used these techniques to identify problems and motivate peers to evaluate their own sexual decisions. Sharing and disseminating results from their appraisals also created an effective climate for helping young people work with health providers, teachers, and other community members on a peer education program that ultimately led to increased condom use and more effective use of family planning and pre- and postnatal services.

mapping. For example, a PR study to strengthen the link between an underused rural health center and the community might begin by mapping the community to identify geographic constraints such as the distances people have to walk to get to the center. Participants might then use their map to sample local residents for informal interviews, gathering information on experiences people had when they attended the health center and reasons they did or did not return. Their study would be likely to include direct observation of the health center itself aided by a semistructured guide. Based on their interpretation of these data, participants would arrive by consensus at a plan of action directed to specific policymakers or providers willing to discuss and help implement the proposed intervention strategy.

PR clearly has both rewards and challenges. On the one hand, PR builds knowledge from the ground up, involves stakeholders in defining problems and identifying solutions, links research directly to action, and increases local self-reliance through experience in systematic problem solving. However, to make PR work, you must adopt attitudes and expectations that may be significantly different from standard professional norms of scientific research. You will have to make the transition from researcher to facilitator and trainer, stepping back from the dominant position, sharing ownership of the project, and encouraging participants to take an active role in project decisions. In fact, "the key difference between participatory and conventional methodologies lies in the location of power in the research process" (Cornwall and Jewkes 1995, p. 1667). Your skill as facilitator-trainer may be more important for the project's success than your credentials as a research scientist. You may have to make compromises on the choice of methods, arbitrate differences among participants on interpretation of the data, or find alternative solutions to a problem when the group's recommendations are inconsistent with available resources. Finally, because any participatory study by definition has a specific activist agenda, it is important to understand that resulting grassroots social action may be as important as—or even more important than—publishing the findings in professional journals.

Topic Guides

Experienced qualitative data collectors often gather meaningful data with little more than a set of topics as a guide; the research questions are clear in their minds, and the techniques of qualitative data collection are their normal ways of working. In the course of designing the study, researchers may also have spent time getting to know the people and the setting through preliminary participant observation or other formative research. By the time they are ready to conduct interviews or focus groups, topics flow easily from the research questions, aided by familiarity with the study population's language. Interviewers may also have memorized the list of topics to cover and can direct conversation spontaneously from one to another, stopping to clarify points or probe comments or perhaps return to earlier questions as needed to ensure that participants have gone as far as they can with each topic.

However, many who collect qualitative data are new to these techniques and will benefit from a more structured set of guidelines. Many researchers prefer a semistructured topic guide with questions that reflect the initial themes and subthemes contained in the basic research problem. This kind of tool may be a set of standardized open-ended questions, but more often it shows examples of how questions can be worded, as well as being a reminder of the material to cover (see Box 4.4). The topic guide can also suggest follow-up questions for various possible responses and examples of probes to elicit information at greater depth. If you will be presenting stories or other scenarios to stimulate ideas, you should include them in the guide.

Interviewers are encouraged to use their own words in the interview but to keep firmly in mind the purpose of each question and its relation to the research problem, referring to the guide as needed. Interviews and group discussions can take many paths, moving toward and sometimes away from the key problem. Organizing the topic guide around a few central questions can help keep you oriented in the right direction, following possible new leads but always returning to the study's purpose.

Although we urge all interviewers and focus group moderators to state questions in a natural way and not to read semistructured guides as they would the questions on

BOX 4.4

Constructing a Topic Guide

Compose search questions. Reread the research protocol at least once, concentrating especially on the research objectives and associated problem statements. Turn the statements into a short list of broad questions that reflect what you want to learn in the study. Interviewers should commit this list to memory. For example: "I want to know how people in this community would react to a campaign to promote dual method use (DMU). Do they see themselves as needing protection from both pregnancy and STI? What factors would encourage or discourage DMU?"

Identify topic and subtopics. Subtopics are variations on the more general topics. There may be more than one topic in a single research objective, and each topic may have several subtopics. Topic: Acceptability of DMU. Subtopics: Understanding of DMU, experience with DMU, perception of partner's opinion.

Decide on a sequence. Arrange topic and subtopics in a logical sequence that suggests a natural flow for discussion. The pattern and sequence of themes do not have to follow the proposal's order of research objectives.

Develop sample questions. Each topic or subtopic may have three kinds of questions: a main question, follow-up questions, and probe questions. The main question introduces the topic. Follow-up questions get more specific and take the discussion to a deeper level. Probe questions go even deeper, seeking clarification, asking for more detail.

Select projective techniques. Decide whether the addition of projective techniques will help participants identify with the issues. Examples are stories, photos, posters, and role-playing. Projective techniques are especially useful for encouraging expression on sensitive topics, such as sexual norms or illegal abortion, or on abstract issues, such as quality of life, self-esteem, or empowerment.

Prepare opening and closing statements. Compose sample statements that let participants know that the interview or discussion group is beginning or has ended. The opening statement includes an explanation of the project and information for informed consent. The closing statement thanks participants for sharing their insights and experiences and reminds them again of the confidentiality of the data.

For examples of detailed topic guides on sexual risk, men's health, and other issues, see Appendix Six.

a structured survey instrument, many will feel more confident with some specific questions to help them manage the interview or discussion. Several examples of topic guides are shown in Appendix Six.

Conclusion

Collecting qualitative data is a process of bringing what you want to learn together with what you observe and what participants know and have experienced (Rubin and Rubin 1995). This chapter has emphasized the concept of partnership in participant observation, qualitative interviewing, and focus group discussion. Although we advocate a semistructured topic guide to help the interviewer or moderator keep the research problem in focus, flexibility is critical. Successful data collectors are prepared to adapt the tool and their personal styles to the discussion's natural flow, wherever it takes them, as long as they are learning. Qualitative interviewing therefore demands versatility and sometimes quick change when the mood of the interview shifts or unexpected but important content interrupts the planned sequence. Similarly, participant observers return to the field each day open to new and possibly surprising discoveries.

Whether in observation, interview, or group discussion, researchers often feel bombarded with stimuli. Participants eager to share their experiences and ideas can quickly overwhelm an inexperienced data collector with valuable information. Careful planning and meticulous record keeping can help the investigator manage information overload. The conceptual framework, imprinted in the mind of the interviewer or observer, is a valuable compass, helping to keep a firm grasp on the research's purpose and main questions and to locate what participants say or do in the emerging picture. And even the most experienced qualitative researcher does not expect to remember all the details of what happens in the field. Clear transcriptions and detailed field notes are key to skillful management of large amounts of information that otherwise will be lost to science.

Each interview, each focus group discussion, each trip to the field can be an adventure. You will not know in advance exactly what will emerge; but with a clear sense of direction, flexibility, and enthusiasm for the unknown, your discoveries can become valuable contributions to qualitative understanding of many public health issues.

Field Perspective

Ethical Dilemmas in Development Research: An Anthropologist's Perspective

Nancy Stark, R.N., Ph.D.

Bowman Gray School of Medicine, Wake Forest University

Anthropologists disagree about the extent to which social scientists should become involved in the decisions and choices of the people they study. The notion of cultural relativity is central to anthropological research. Embracing local viewpoints is considered essential if one is to accurately understand and represent a society. Yet anthropologists have always had to contend with ethical dilemmas in the field, at times witnessing what they might consider discrimination, cruelty, unfair practices, and even crime. In each situation they must decide how to respond. In general, the anthropologist in the role of participant observer attempts to be transparent, participates in the culture, and observes but does not attempt to lead or initiate change.

More recently, some applied anthropologists have challenged the notion of cultural relativity. The contradiction between the principle of cultural relativity and the researcher's role as a change agent has been especially apparent in international development, where applied research often accompanies interventions to improve health care and reduce mortality.

When the researcher is also a nurse or a physician, there is the added complexity that the study community may expect the medically trained researcher to respond with medicine, technical advice, information, and care. The researcher is therefore caught between the standards of her academic discipline for rigorous research and the ethical responsibility of her caring profession to help people in need.

As a registered nurse with a background in obstetric nursing, I had the opportunity to conduct fieldwork for my Ph.D. in cultural anthropology through the International Centre for Diarrhoeal Disease Research (ICDDR) in Bangladesh from 1989 to 1990. In an effort to reduce maternal and neonatal mortality, the center had recently implemented a program in which nurse midwives were trained to respond to obstetrical emergencies. Because my research addressed decision making among families who would have access to these nurse midwives, my fieldwork included observation of deliveries. The question of how I might respond in an obstetrical emergency became a key issue that affected both my research practice and the expectations of the international staff at the ICDDR.

In order to understand how families make decisions about obstetrical complications (when to call for assistance, whom to call first, who makes the decision that care is needed), the anthropologist does not intervene in the decision-making process. However, as a health professional my own ethical code and the views of my colleagues at the ICDDR compelled me to decide that I would intervene if necessary. At the very least, I planned to notify the nurse midwife in emergencies should the family resist seeking care in a timely manner or fail to call for help. I also decided that I would take action only in the most dire circumstances. When the first delivery I observed presented a complication, I was surprised, in retrospect, at how I reacted.

A lay midwife had invited me to be present at a birth. Childbirth in the village is a very private matter: to protect the mother and child from spirits that come through the wind to cause birthing complications, the windows and doors of the house are kept shut during childbirth, and the laboring woman is expected not to cry out, so that others will not know that a child is being born. Thus, the family did not invite me; in fact, the mother of the woman who was having her first child was not pleased that I had come with my research assistant.

As the woman's labor progressed, I observed without comment the midwife's technique. Even lay midwives in the ICDDR communities have received training in safe delivery techniques,* but I saw little sign of any such instruction and worried that a complication could result from unsafe practice. Labor seemed to be progressing normally until prior to the birth, I noticed meconium staining in the amniotic fluid. Without hesitation I put down my notebook and pen and attempted to clear the baby's mouth as he was delivered. My action brought a cry from the lay midwife: "Stop! You could kill the baby!" I did stop, still concerned that the infant might aspirate meconium. But the baby cried spontaneously, and all was well.

I, in contrast, was exhausted from the ordeal. Now that the infant was breathing normally and crying, my concerns turned to how I might have damaged a fledgling relationship with the lay midwife, an individual central to the success of my research. I was concerned about the mother's reaction and how her experience might affect community attitudes toward me, possibly undermining my ability to conduct the research. Finally, I worried about my relationship with the ICDDR, the institution that had made my research possible. It occurred to me that if something were to go wrong during a delivery, I risked being held responsible by everyone.

I overcame those worries and attended other deliveries. As time passed, I became more familiar with delivery customs in the village and with the lay midwife, and I no longer felt the need to intervene. As I became more comfortable with the village culture, my attitude about the need to act softened, and my stress subsided.

These are a few of the lessons and insights that I gained from this experience:

- The researcher must (or perhaps will, in spite of herself) be true to a personal ethical standard.
- Belief systems can change. What the researcher considers an ethical dilemma at the beginning of research, she may not consider a problem later.
- Multiple cultures frequently converge in applied social science research, and all must be respected—the researcher's culture, the culture of the supporting institution, and the culture under study.
- Prior to initiating a research project, it is important to anticipate, as much as possible, the ethical challenges that may arise and to discuss them with others who have conducted similar research. What worked for them? What failed? And why?
- And finally, be ready for surprises.

**The instruction included techniques such as wearing gloves when performing vaginal exams, avoiding cervical massage or pulling the umbilical cord, and cutting the cord with the sterile razor provided in a safe birth kit that is routinely supplied to the pregnant woman by a community health worker.*

Field Perspective

Using Qualitative Research to Understand How Providers Spend Their Time

Barbara Janowitz, Ph.D.

Family Health International

Qualitative research offers important methods for use in cost analysis that go far beyond poring over figures provided by the finance division of a reproductive health program. To analyze reproductive health program costs, we concentrate on how resources are used to provide services. One of the most important resources is labor. If programs are to understand whether their workers are being used efficiently and whether there is a way to reduce costs, then programs need to find out what workers are doing.

To study how workers use their time, Family Health International has used participant observation, or activity sampling (also known as time and motion studies). We started using this methodology in 1993 during a cost study in Bangladesh (Janowitz and others 1997). In one component of that study, we accompanied workers to the field and noted how they spent their time, including traveling to the field, traveling between households, and talking with clients. In addition, we used a checklist to note the activities that providers carried out with clients. Our results showed that the costs of expanding family planning services to households could be greatly reduced if fieldworkers increased their level of effort. In addition, our findings indicated that interactions with clients often involved no more than the dispensing of pills or condoms when these were needed. But when they were not, little effort was being made to counsel women about the potential benefits to them of using family planning.

In similar studies we have observed staff members at clinics that provided reproductive health services. Instead of measuring the duration of each activity, we used a technique called activity sampling. This involves obtaining information about exactly what a staff person is doing during a defined sample of time. Using a beeper that went off every three or five minutes, we noted on a checklist what activity the person was engaged in at that moment. Activities were grouped into categories that included client contact time; client-related activities; general administration; tea, coffee, and lunch breaks; and unproductive time. The latter included such things as coming to the clinic late or leaving early, talking with friends in person or on the phone, or simply waiting for clients to arrive at the clinic.

We used this information to determine whether providers might in fact have time to expand their interactions with clients in order to increase the quality of their services. If they could do this without reducing the number of clients that they saw, then there would be no cost to the clinic in terms of a reduced number of women obtaining services. We found that on an average day, providers had a considerable amount of time that they could be using to expand their contact time with clients. This time was mainly clustered very early in the morning or in the late afternoon, in large part because providers arrived late and left early. We concluded that it could be difficult to get providers to be at the clinic for a full day and for them to be busy during late afternoon hours.

Our findings generate a number of other questions about how services are organized. More qualitative research would help us in the following ways:

- To better understand what providers actually want from their jobs
- To learn why they arrange their schedules as they do
- To determine what interventions would work to change time allocation
- To find out how clients feel about waiting times in the current model of service provision
- To ascertain whether clients might prefer to get services at some other time than midmorning if it meant they would not have to wait

Field Perspective

Clandestine Contraceptive Use: A Prospective Study

Sarah Castle, Ph.D.

London School of Hygiene and Tropical Medicine

Although family planning has been available in Africa since the 1960s, many couples today are becoming acquainted with it for the first time. In Bamako, Mali, only about 16 percent of married women use a modern contraceptive method, and the discontinuation rate is high. In order to understand the experiences of new contraceptive users, the Centre d'Etudes et de Recherche sur la Population pour le Développement, in collaboration with the Women's Studies Project of Family Health International, conducted a prospective study of fifty-five first-time contraceptive users in Bamako (Castle and others 1999). Three in-depth interviews were conducted over a period of eighteen months with each participant who remained in the study.

When the study was designed, the theme of clandestine use was not high on the research agenda. However, it became clear in the first round of interviews that a high proportion of women, seventeen out of fifty-five, were using contraception without their husbands' knowledge. All but seven of these women had attempted unsuccessfully to discuss family planning with their husbands before resorting to secret use. A feature of qualitative research is that it allows a certain degree of flexibility in the research content and methodology. Therefore, once we discovered this phenomenon, we were able to modify the interview guide to explore it in greater depth in the second and third interviews.

The use of repeated in-depth interviews, conducted at a location of the participant's choice, enabled interviewers and participants to develop relationships of rapport and trust. It also enabled the research team to follow the family planning process over time, to build on information as it emerged, and to test our interpretation of what contraceptive use meant for these women. The topic guide for each subsequent interview with each woman thus reflected the discussion of the previous interview.

In the second round, three of the seventeen original clandestine users' husbands had found out about their use. Two had directly told their husbands. One husband had spotted his wife's appointment card but had not commented on it. Thus, although spousal communication has now become a key theme in family planning research, this study indicates that there may sometimes be nonverbal communication about family planning use. These two women, who guessed that their husbands were likely eventually to accept their action, left clues that would present their decisions as a fait accompli.

However, most of the women feared dire consequences of divorce or physical violence if they were discovered. We asked why they thought their husbands and others in the family were opposed to family planning. The most common response was that the husband simply wanted many children. Three believed their husbands' objections were related to their understanding that the Islamic religion opposed the practice of family planning. Two women said their husbands were afraid family planning would make them unfaithful. Several clandestine users related their secrecy to their perception that their husbands had neglected or treated them unfairly, and they did not want to risk obligations in an unstable union.

All the women had confided in someone, most often a sister-in-law. Informal support groups for family planning seemed to exist among younger members of the family, illustrating how within households typified by the dynamics of cooperative conflict, those with vested interests form allegiances. Because many of the clandestine users interviewed lived in extended families in which older female marital relatives monitored and controlled young women's time and movements, they had to employ cunning strategies to deceive not only their spouses but also their older marital kin.

As the study progressed and the women's experiences unfolded, their strategies to obtain contraception and to maintain secrecy became central themes. The transcribed texts were coded and analyzed using the computer software Ethnograph. Clandestine use became a main (parent) code during the overall analysis, whereas aspects of clandestine use, such as type of method, techniques to ensure secrecy, social consequences of discovery, and so on, became subcategories (child) codes.

A major methodological problem in this study was the number of study participants who could not be found for the second and third interviews—seven of the original seventeen clandestine users. Given the secret nature of their behavior, this was perhaps to be expected. In most cases they had given fictitious addresses at the time of the first interview, which was conducted at the clinic. Fear of discovery may have made them unwilling to participate in the research, although some clandestine users remarked that the discretion and sensitivity that the interviewers showed encouraged them to continue. Nevertheless, we cannot say whether there are fundamental differences between the clandestine users who dropped out and the women who were using contraception openly. The study did indicate that among those who remained in the study, a higher proportion of clandestine users had stopped using contraception by the end of the study period compared with overt users. Methodologically, the high dropout rates did present some problems that could only be resolved by not generalizing the results to all women in the study. The study methodology points to the importance of flexible research methods, careful interviewer training, and recognition of the limitations of results from small samples.

Field Perspective

Research Versus Support: Focus Group Participants Living with HIV/AIDS

Michele G. Shedlin, Ph.D.

National Development and Research Institutes

Focus group discussions offer an opportunity for individuals to exchange ideas and validate personal experiences. This interaction is one of the methodological goals of such discussions, but it can also benefit the participants, who enjoy the opportunity to be heard and valued. However, two things are crucial: first, that facilitators anticipate potential problems that could arise from discussion of sensitive topics; and second, that they have the skills to prevent, control, or process such problems effectively.

Whether participants are discussing their own experiences or their perceptions of others, raising stressful topics such as risk behaviors, illness, dying, and loss can trigger powerful emotional reactions. Facilitators need guidelines to help them respond sensitively and appropriately to these situations. They also need to know when it is appropriate to continue the discussion or terminate it. At issue is the dilemma that can arise when the need for scientific rigor and systematic data collection are not possible without compromising the well-being of the group or an individual.

Because focus group participants must be willing to share their experiences and perspectives openly with the researcher and the group, an experienced facilitator will be aware of the following possibilities:

- Emotional distress can emerge from the discussion at any point.
- Some or all participants may have prior experience with group sessions for support or education; and these—rather than research—may be their only points of reference for group discussions.
- When people are experiencing the stress of chronic illness, mutual empathy and support are a natural aspect of any group process.
- When a group responds spontaneously to the emotional needs of any member, the facilitator's first priority is to the well-being of all of the participants; the second priority is to the research objectives.

Twenty years of work with marginalized people have brought me in close touch with the urban poor, the incarcerated, people living with HIV/AIDS, and affected individuals. To help focus group facilitators understand and resolve potential contradictions between the emotional needs of the group and the objectives of the research, I have developed the following guidelines:

1. Establish ground rules for discussion, especially that people respect and listen to one another.
2. When introducing the session, stress the purpose of the discussion, which is to teach the researchers. Remind participants that they are the experts and the reason for their recruitment is to share their knowledge and experience. Explain clearly that it may be tempting to become a support group, but that if possible, they should maintain their roles as teachers and advisers. This acknowledgment of the possibility clarifies the participant role and encourages both focus and thoughtfulness. Reinforcement of their role as teachers is always empowering, a role that many participants have not previously experienced.
3. Be aware of body language as well as what people are saying. Participants give nonverbal signals of distress, which the facilitator can often handle in a supportive way before the group intervenes. This may save a participant from experiencing (unwanted) temporary loss of control and the embarrassment of tears or outbursts, and it may help them to continue to participate.

4. If an individual is not able to continue, acknowledge their distress and give them a quiet moment to regain composure; ask them what they need and what they would like to do. Most often the individual wants to continue, and the group supports this verbally and nonverbally.
5. If the person is not able to continue, either (a) allow group members to provide support and encouragement and continue; or (b) allow the group to provide support; the facilitator then acknowledges the member's need and group's response and ends the session.
6. You should have three major concerns:

   That the person in distress has appropriate support and a referral if necessary

   That the experience is processed with the group so that the participants are not discouraged or frustrated and so that their supportive reaction is validated as the most important issue

   That if the individual and group want to continue, the research focus has not been lost and the collection of valid data is still possible
7. If you decide that the research focus has been lost, thank the group members for what they have accomplished and minimize the early termination. The session should not end abruptly but be allowed to have appropriate closure with discussion that may or may not be relevant to the research but is necessary for the participants.
8. To respond appropriately to emotional distress, you must be thoroughly informed on HIV/AIDS issues and should have access to a list of the local referral services available. Ideally, you should have familiarity and access to a local HIV/AIDS service agency or point person wherever the research is being implemented.
9. Unless you have appropriate professional training and credentials, as well as prior permission from the facility or program within which the discussion is taking place, the support group mode should never become the session's objective.

Responsible focus group research with persons living with or affected by HIV/AIDS adds an important way to gather the qualitative data that inform our response to the epidemic. The focus group method also can be an interesting and positive experience for participants. I believe the researcher's highest priority when conducting focus groups should be to see that all participants have a positive experience and do not leave the session in distress or frustration. Our research objectives should always be secondary to participants' well-being. With good planning it is possible to ensure that both participants and researchers are satisfied with their collaboration.

Field Perspective

Exploring the Birth-Weight Paradox with a Photo Narrative Technique

Deborah E. Bender, Ph.D., and Dina Castro, M.P.H., Ph.D.

School of Public Health, University of North Carolina at Chapel Hill

In the United States, prenatal care is positively associated with improved birth outcomes, particularly the reduction of low birth weight. However, birth weights of Mexican-born Latinos tend to be higher than those of Latinos born in the United States. This relationship is surprising, because recently arrived Latino immigrants are less likely to have received timely or adequate prenatal care (Scribner and Dwyer 1989). The birth-weight paradox has remained constant regardless of the mother's age, marital status, or educational attainment (Cobas and others 1996).

The idea of resilience offers a conceptual framework for studying the birth-weight paradox. *Resilience* has been defined as a universal capacity that allows a person, group, or community to prevent, minimize, or overcome the damaging effects of adversity (Rutter 1993). Gaining understanding of what generates resilience offers an opportunity to develop initiatives that will help people to be less vulnerable in the face of adversity (Werner 1993).

We wanted to know why birth outcomes to newly arrived Latinas were better than those of their U.S.-born counterparts. Through focus groups and photo narratives, we explored topics related to pregnancy, prenatal care, and social support with Latina women, using their pregnancy experiences to probe for their perceptions of which factors are protective—give them resilience—and which pose a risk to their health status.

After the focus group discussion, women were invited to assist in the collection of data by serving as community photographers. Their two-week assignment was to take pictures of people, places, and things they considered important to their health and well-being (Williams 1984). Each woman selected six to eight photographs to illustrate her personal story, which she elaborated in an individual, in-depth interview. For each photograph the woman described who was in the picture, what was happening, and why the picture was important to her.

The following themes of resilience and risk were identified through analysis of the focus groups and photo narratives transcripts:

- Access to health care services and self-care during pregnancy
- Strong family relationships, especially with one's mother
- Aspirations for a better life in the United States
- Education for one's children
- Dreams of eventual return to Mexico
- Unanticipated hardships of life in the United States, particularly related to language barriers

Examples of the concerns the women expressed follow.

Catalina delayed initiation of prenatal care due to the pressure of work. She felt that the quality of care was compromised by language differences. She explained: "Well, when I arrived [at the hospital] here, they began to treat me a little badly. I don't speak English, but I speak a little. Then, when they saw that I could speak some English, they began to treat me better because I was trying to communicate with them."

Maintaining strong family relationships was a theme that the women expressed repeatedly. Angélica was pregnant with her first child in this country. Her sister was nearby, but she still found it necessary to call her mother in Mexico to discuss her fears. Her mother reassured her that her pregnancy was normal. Angélica explained: "A mother always listens; a mother always helps; a father protects you. Here, no. Here, nobody protects you; nobody listens; nobody pampers you."

One woman's photograph of a telephone hanging on an otherwise blank wall spoke to the importance of regular phone contact with absent family members. The photographer, Carmen, explained her selection: "The telephone is very important for communication. You can communicate with your family [in Mexico]. It is not considered a luxury in this country but a necessity. It is not like in my country; here the lines go to everywhere."

Carmen also described a photograph of herself with her language teacher and talked of the importance of learning English to be able to manage one's own daily life: "Knowing English, you can solve problems that happen to you better. Before, my husband had to go with me to the doctor, the dentist, the bank, and the post office. He was losing time from work. Now, I do not have to depend so much on him."

When the women spoke of returning to Mexico, some of their words hinted that their dreams might not be realized. Opportunities for work and economic gain in the United States seem to take priority. Luisa already knew that her husband had little intention of returning: "When I ask my husband, 'When are we going back to Mexico?' he answers, 'I am not going to put myself in the position of working in Mexico, having to resign myself to earn two hundred pesos per week while here I earn that money in a day.'"

Although economic opportunity in the United States has enabled the families of the women who participated in the focus groups to create a better life, each woman spoke of unanticipated difficulties. Elena took a photograph showing the wrought iron staircase in an otherwise dark apartment entrance. Three women are ascending the stairs; the viewer sees only their backs. She explained that although living conditions are better in the United States than in Mexico, there are risks here too. In Mexico everyone knew everyone else; it was safe. In the United States, women were afraid to go out. She summarized: "Here, we live in a cage of gold, but it never stops being a prison." Elena's eloquent but simple words describe the paradox of life in the United States for Latino immigrants.

These photographs represented everyday situations. Their importance lies in what they meant to the women who took them. When we asked the women to photograph people, places, and things that were important to them, we hoped they would select themes that could be classified as related to resilience or risk. In fact, the photographic choices of the women were exquisite, their stories poignant. The women were able to articulate clearly how the people or objects they had photographed were important in their lives. It was apparent that the factors they identified had contributed, negatively or positively, to how they evaluated their health in pregnancy. Spontaneously, they selected themes related to demographic characteristics and medical and behavioral risks that are recognized to have an impact on health status during pregnancy.

CHAPTER FIVE

Logistics in the Field

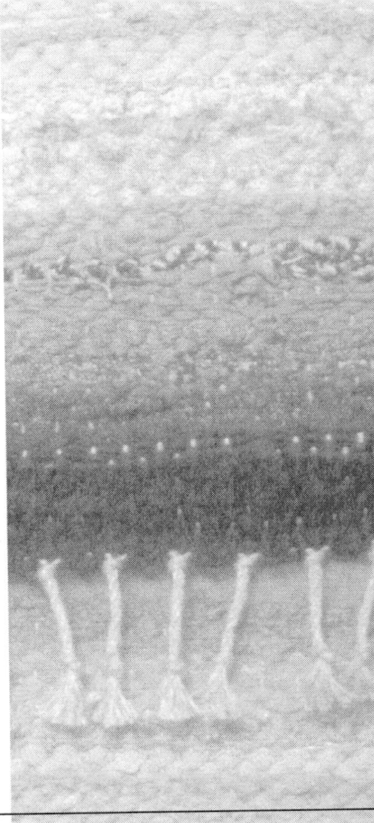

Reason and logic are needed to chart your way through the woods . . . painstaking planning, analysis, and execution, testing the ground every step of the way. [But] human compassion and understanding are also necessary throughout the journey.
(Fetterman 1992, p. 87)

DRAWING ON THE EXPERIENCES of many qualitative researchers, this chapter bridges the transition from study design to implementation in the field. In the following pages, we help you create a research-friendly environment by anticipating some of the pivotal decisions and tasks that will launch your study: establishing contacts and involving key stakeholders to assembling a field team; training and monitoring interviewers; protecting confidentiality; developing and testing materials; organizing equipment and supplies; and recording, transcribing, translating, and storing data.

Most qualitative research is interactive—composed of many face-to-face, often intimate, conversations with study participants. Ideally, we would spend long periods of time in the community or other setting, getting to know the people informally in their everyday lives. Researchers who are able to live in the research site during the study have found that participating in local events, observing both the routine and the exceptional, adds a great deal to their understanding of the social context. Yet practical limits on time and resources may be constraints. In large studies you may also be supervising the work of trained assistants who collect the data. In such circumstances it is crucial to find ways to stay as close as possible to the field by, for example, paying frequent visits to the site, talking with local people, reviewing transcripts, and questioning data collectors about their observations and progress. If you are working across national, cultural, or language barriers, you may have a counterpart who will be your interpreter and guide. In any case, you or that colleague has to be there—listening, questioning, hearing, observing.

Although in this chapter we cover day-to-day issues in implementation, every field experience has its unique challenges, some predictable and some not. With careful planning, however, you will be able to identify and manage many of the risks and resources that will influence your study's outcomes. And once you have become familiar with people at your study site and they with you, you will have no end of on-site expert advice to help you negotiate a successful field experience.

Contacts: Introductions and Approvals

Research textbooks that go from study design to data collection often fail to provide directions through the maze of introductions and permissions that stand between the researcher and the study participants. Yet how you approach these challenges may be key to the success of your whole project. In most situations the researcher needs to be highly visible: an active participant, known and trusted in the community. In addition, a critical facet of interpretive understanding is knowing the study participants' world or the social context in which they live. You are more likely to be welcomed into that world if you have presented yourself and your study in a culturally appropriate manner. Pay attention to district medical officers, community officials, heads of organizations, and other local leaders, because they may have their own vested interests in your presence as well as your findings. Some may be protective of their constituents; others may fear possible negative consequences from your research. Still others may expect unrealistic support from you on some local issue. Take the time to explain the purpose and implementation of the study, turning potential adversaries into partners. Keep in mind that community leaders not only control access to the study site but can also help you understand local culture, customs, and personalities.

INTRODUCTIONS TO STAKEHOLDERS

Most investigators start with introductions to district administrators, medical and nursing directors, women's advocates, religious leaders, teachers, or others invested in the program or community. Is the political climate in this community or agency authoritarian, or do individuals generally make their own decisions on matters that would affect their participation in the study? Try to identify influential leaders whose views could potentially affect others' decisions on whether or not to participate. Do not overlook informal leaders, including influential women in the community and people who may not occupy positions of formal authority but tend to be consulted by others who know and respect them.

Visit these individuals, making appointments if possible, to introduce yourself and your study. In some communities you may be expected to present yourself to a governing council who, along with the mayor or administrative head, will decide whether to approve the activity you propose. Similarly, a clinic director might ask you to explain your ideas to a board or to the clinic staff. Community leaders and local officials frequently take their cues from their constituents in deciding what stance to take on a proposal coming to them from the outside.

Remember that getting appointments and permissions can be time-consuming. The data collection schedule you developed for your study probably has little relevance in the time frames of most community leaders and administrators. Take possible delays into account when you plan the study, and regard this introductory phase as a vital part of the research process. Approached this way, an otherwise frustrating delay can become an opportunity to become better acquainted with the research site.

FAMILY INFLUENCES

Individuals' decisions to participate in your study may also depend on family members' influence. Many research problems in sexual and reproductive health contain culturally sensitive material; women whose independence is limited by their subordination to more powerful family members may be fearful of consenting to participate in such a study. If they do consent, they may feel limited in how much of their lives they dare reveal without danger of recrimination. The same caveat applies to women in casual unions with sexual partners. In authoritarian relationships like these, the researcher may have to present the purpose of the study to a head of household, whether husband, father, mother-in-law, or unmarried partner. If so, the presentation should be honest but relatively general, with firm insistence on the privacy of the interview. Another approach to winning cooperation of powerful family leaders is to invite them to share their own views on the topic in separate, and equally confidential, interviews—whether or not such an exchange is part of your study design. Showing respect for the opinion of an otherwise resistant person not only involves him or her in a positive way but may offer interesting insights that you might have missed.

On the other hand, in studies of particularly sensitive issues, full disclosure on the topic of the research may put the participant at risk in her family or community. In such a circumstance, your ethical priority is to protect the participant. In our study of clandestine users of contraception in Mali, researchers and providers alike were careful to help participants maintain secrecy from husbands who, the women felt, might punish them for attending a family planning clinic or even participating in the study (Castle and others 1999).

Involving Policymakers and Change Agents

Research can often influence policy or the way services are delivered. If your intent is to link your study results to local policies and programs, it is important to include policymakers, service providers, and nongovernmental organizations (NGOs) early in the design and implementation. For example, ask staff of the ministry of health to orient you to particular resources and needs of the study population; meet with a member of parliament who has a special interest in the problem you plan to study; introduce the study to the district commissioner or other local authority; or discuss the study with medical and nursing officers in charge of health services in the area. Invite suggestions for implementation, and be open to possible new ways of articulating the research question for a better fit between the purpose of your study and policymakers' goals for improving the population's well-being.

Establishing reciprocity by including stakeholder questions not only facilitates access to the study population but also may result in a stronger research design with findings more relevant to the problems and the institution's policy needs. As cited earlier, when one of the authors introduced a proposed study of contraceptive decision making among women to the administrators of a family planning clinic in Bamako, Mali, they said they would like to know more about how women involve their husbands in the decision. The research team therefore introduced partner negotiation as a major topic in the interviews and later shared the results with the entire staff. Similarly, NGOs often can use research findings to develop advocacy messages. Invite leaders of local women's or youth advocacy organizations to contribute to the research design by suggesting questions that would help them serve their constituents' needs. You are not obligated to use stakeholders' questions, but if they are relevant to the basic research problem, you will win cooperation and respect by finding ways to obtain the information they need.

PROJECT ADVISORY COMMITTEES

An effective vehicle for mobilizing the interest of policymakers and community leaders is the project advisory committee. Depending on the nature of your study, you may want to establish an advisory group of influential people who will meet periodically to review progress on the study and advise on implementation issues. Such a group might include representatives from local and central government, schools, churches, women's advocacy organizations, youth groups, and other organizations. Because advisory committee membership may imply special privilege, it is best to include as broad a representation as possible so that selection of members does not seem to favor only one segment of the community.

Advisory committee members customarily do not participate directly in the design and conduct of the research. Their role is to advise. It should be clear from the outset that their purpose is to provide valuable consultation and review, not to make research decisions. Different members of the committee may take on different roles related to their interests and expertise; but typical activities might include reviewing protocols, suggesting culturally appropriate ways to ask questions, identifying key messages in the findings, linking results to recommendations, and participating in dissemination plans. You can help to ensure that these influential people will promote and use study findings if you begin by formulating clear research questions that address policy or programmatic issues, explaining or demystifying the research methods, and providing a role for stakeholders in the process.

Developing the Field Team

Never underestimate the value of local assistance. Including people from the study site in your field strategy not only helps in day-to-day management but also enhances community rapport and increases the professional team's understanding of the site. Professional data collectors and local assistants will work well together if they appreciate the complementary roles that each can play.

FIELD ASSISTANTS

The Local Team When introducing the study to the community, identify a few local people who are especially interested in the project, who know the community, and who are willing to work with you. They will be your local field team. In Chapter Four we discussed the role of key informants, people with special knowledge and insight into the phenomenon you are studying. The local assistants who help you implement the study should also be honest informants on the local scene and channels of information to their peers. But whereas a key informant is primarily a confidante and guide to the culture, local assistants are there mainly to help you with practical arrangements. They might be lay church leaders, community workers, or simply individuals who are well known and respected by their peers. As a general rule, it is advisable not to seek assistance from people who are controversial or in positions of authority in the group. Examples of people not to include on the field team might be the mayor or a member of his family, a prominent traditional healer or shaman, or the medical officer in charge of the health center. These individuals might provide valuable information, but other participants may perceive them as intimidating or coercive. Confidentiality issues may also arise.

The role of the local field team might include interpreting the study to people in the community, helping identify respondents who meet the sample selection criteria, welcoming participants (focus group members or interviewees), organizing refreshments, distracting curious visitors during interviews or focus group discussions, providing child care, or reminding individuals in the sample to come on time to the interview site. Local team members must not be present during interviews or focus group discussions and must not have access to data in any form. They should be strongly encouraged to respect the privacy of people in the study sample who have agreed to participate.

BOX 5.1

Characteristics of a Good Interviewer or Moderator

- Ability to feel at ease and to put others at ease
- Ability to project unconditional respect and acceptance of others
- Ability to convey warmth and empathy
- Good verbal and interpersonal skills
- Good listening skills
- Ability to project enthusiasm and genuine interest in others
- Awareness of own nonverbal reactions, using body language to project positive response
- Ability to interpret and explore what people say in light of the research problem, versus rote response

Source: Adapted from Debus 1986.

Local team members will know they play a vital role, especially if they are welcome to attend meetings of the whole team and if they receive a stipend consistent with the local pay scale. They may also appreciate a simple certificate or letter that documents their experience on your project. The certificate might be used to secure similar positions in the future.

THE PROFESSIONAL FIELD TEAM

Field Supervisor As researchers we usually are outsiders, educated in research methodology but naive to the sociocultural matrix in which we conduct our studies. The gap may exist not only across countries but even within a country, where socioeconomic, professional, or other differences can create communication barriers. When this situation occurs, a field supervisor can be an invaluable counterpart, a skilled assistant who understands the cultural context, is fluent in the local language, and has experience in qualitative techniques. Working closely with the researcher, this individual can help coordinate and supervise much of the data collection. Needless to say, the field supervisor must be a person whom interviewers and other members of the team, as well as participants and community leaders, like and respect. A field supervisor who helps you gain access to information and serves as a cultural interpreter can also be a valuable key informant.

Interviewers In the best of all worlds, interviewers are trained in a social science and experienced in qualitative data collection. Unfortunately, such individuals often are in short supply, because few universities around the world provide training in qualitative research. However, we have found that less-experienced people with strong interpersonal skills and readiness to apply new interactive techniques can learn to collect excellent qualitative data. Because the task of a qualitative interviewer is to become a conversational partner with the participant (Rubin and Rubin 1995), personal attributes are important. A warm, empathic manner; sensitivity to different perspectives; and an ability to listen carefully and ask insightful questions are characteristics of a good interviewer, whether educated in the social sciences or not.

It is also important to know where potential interviewers would fit in the community structure. If interviewers or supervisors differ significantly from study participants with respect to distinctive characteristics such as education, economic status, or religious affiliation, they must be able to minimize the difference in status through an interpersonal style that is friendly and nonjudgmental. Would-be interviewers who, for whatever reason, are unable to put participants at ease, accept individual differences, or respond appropriately to the changing dynamics of the interview or group discussion will not be effective.

Training

Unless you are collecting all the data yourself, you will need to conduct a training workshop for your interviewers, focus group moderators, observers, or other field staff. Most teams will benefit from at least one week of comprehensive training before they enter the field, but training and monitoring are a continuous process, even as data collection proceeds.

You may find that your study is the first time that otherwise experienced field staff have been exposed to qualitative principles and techniques. Survey interviewers are available in most countries, but we have often noticed that those with more experience with structured protocols have the most difficulty being effective as in-depth interviewers and focus group moderators. When interviewers have been trained to phrase questions exactly as written and assign answers to preconceived response categories, as in a multiple-choice format, they do not easily adapt and modify questions, probe answers with new questions, and control—but not dominate—a guided conversation or focused discussion. A tendency of experienced survey interviewers is to use a topic guide as if it were a questionnaire, asking questions verbatim, shifting topics too quickly, and forgetting to follow leads to deeper and richer sources of information. Similarly, field staff who have been reared and educated in relatively authoritarian families and societies may need considerable guidance in nondirective, nonjudgmental interviewing styles. This task is made all the more difficult by the same cultural constraints on participants who may have trouble being conversational in an interview. The interview may seem like a formal interaction or even a duty. (See the field perspective by Woodsong at the end of this chapter titled Anticipating Strengths and Weaknesses When Training Data Collectors.)

In addition to orientation to the research objectives and materials, training must therefore include instruction in the elements of conversational style and nondirective interviewing, with ample demonstration and practice. A goal for successful data collection will be sufficient familiarity with the research questions that the interviewer can engage a participant in creative dialogue without having to read aloud from the guide but without losing sight of the central research problem. Experienced qualitative data collectors can also benefit from a refresher course on the use of qualitative techniques, including formulating questions, following leads, noting silences, and identifying field problems. Trainees will catch on to the conversational style more quickly if they can keep the main research topics in their heads.

We have found that the best training approach is practical and experiential, with liberal use of role-playing and simulated data collection. A typical training program might take a week or longer if the field schedule allows, depending on the complexity of the research problem and the trainees' skill level (see Appendix Seven). It usually begins with a thorough orientation to the research problem and purpose and careful review of the interview guide or other protocol. Topics are likely to include the roles of the interviewer or moderator and note taker, adapting what trainees have learned from survey research to qualitative data collection; different moderator or interviewer styles; the art of probing data; ways to encourage participation; instruction in observing nonverbal cues; training in managing problems that arise in the interview or group; and methods for closing the interview or discussion. Interviewers should also receive training in the mechanics of taping and transcribing the sessions, including a backup plan for the occasional malfunctioning tape recorder or other mishap. Important elements of training are sensitivity to issues surrounding vulnerability and confidentiality and the protocol for obtaining informed consent.

Devote several days in the training program to practice of interviewing and observation skills, beginning with role-playing and group feedback. As trainees become more proficient, consider bringing in outsiders to play participant roles in mock interviews or discussions. Actor-participants could be prompted ahead of time to simulate problems that commonly arise in interviews or groups, such as the argumentative participant, the silent participant, or the focus group member who dominates the discussion. Feedback from the group will help trainees gain confidence in handling these and other, often unanticipated, situations. If the team includes interviewers with qualitative experience, these individuals can assist with training, helping the less experienced at the same time they are reviewing qualitative techniques themselves. You might pair new interviewers with more experienced partners in role-playing, switching roles as the less-experienced person becomes more comfortable with interview skills.

As you observe these practice sessions, take notes on the process to share with trainees. For example, note when an interviewer misses a cue to another question or fails to probe a provocative comment. Trainees can also listen for gaps in the interview and prompt each other. If possible, tape and transcribe the practice interviews and distribute copies to the trainees to illustrate the interviews' strengths and weaknesses. Group critique of both novice and experienced interviewers' practice sessions is also helpful. Exercises like these can build confidence, at the same time underscoring the importance of attentive listening and flexibility in adapting the guide to the interview's conversational flow.

Also include in the training sessions a brief overview of data analysis and in some settings special training for staff who will help with the analysis. Understanding how the data will be analyzed reinforces for interviewers the importance of rapport in the interview partnership, as well as careful probing and flexible use of the interview or focus group guide. A simple explanation of coding and searching (see Chapter Six) will help interviewers understand that information will not be lost if it emerges out of the expected sequence of the interview.

A critical component of interviewer training in sexual and reproductive health is recognizing and responding to clues that a participant may be at significant risk. Survey interviewers typically are trained to be relatively passive on matters not related to the actual conduct of the interview, but in qualitative research the interviewer as conversational partner cannot be impersonal and uninvolved. Confronted with disclosure of domestic violence, child abuse, or any threat to participants' well-being, interviewers who collect sensitive data must learn how to give a caring and helpful response without jeopardizing the quality of the interview. They can also be prepared to offer referral for participants in need of counseling or other assistance. (See Chapter Four for the interviewer's responsibility when a participant asks for help.)

Field Materials

Provide members of your field teams, both professional and local, with written instructions and summaries of the steps in the data collection phase. Such written communication might include the following:

- An overview of the project
- A summary of ethical standards for the study
- Detailed task descriptions for the local field team and for each professional role (for example, focus group moderator, note taker, in-depth interviewer, field supervisor, or translator)
- A calendar with daily activities such as team meetings, training, pretests, and scheduled interviews or focus group discussions
- An activities schedule, including a time frame for collecting data and completing transcriptions or translations if done in the field
- A sample introduction to the project
- Names and phone numbers of researchers who can answer questions and provide additional information about the project

You might also give copies of some of these materials to interested local leaders, especially if they are supervisors of individuals on your field team and have granted them time off for participation in the study.

Pilot Testing

The pilot test is a dress rehearsal for all members of the field team in a mock venue with characteristics of the actual research setting. As in all social research, it is important to ensure that a research team has tested interview and focus group guides or topic lists, observation guides, photographs and stories, or other tools of data collection in a group of trial participants similar to the participants in the actual study. If the study design includes subsamples of the population, each should be represented in the pilot test. Held at the end of interviewer training, a comprehensive pilot test gives data collectors additional hands-on experience and even more familiarity with the project. Interviewers who participate in this phase often add valuable suggestions for strengthening data collection materials and processes.

Pilot testing informed consent materials is as important as finding out whether participants will understand the interview questions. The pilot should therefore include an introduction to the project and explanation of informed consent, worded as data collectors will present it to study participants. Is the language clear? Do participants understand the purpose of the research and the part they are expected to play? Are both women and men sufficiently assured of confidentiality to participate without reservation? If not, revise the statement until the researcher is confident that no one is taking part in the study without adequate knowledge of its purpose, expectations, and possible risk.

Ideally, pilot interviews or focus group discussions should be recorded and transcribed exactly as they will be in the study. If possible, allow time to analyze the data using whatever computer software or other approach you have chosen. Analysis of test data will point to any need for further revisions of the topic guides, instruments, or data collection process. It also enables the researchers to assess interviewing skills and retrain interviewers.

As part of the pilot test, researchers should also conduct a trial run of administrative procedures for managing data and protecting the confidentiality of interview or focus group discussion tapes or other raw data in the field.

On the basis of these trial results, rethink your data collection techniques. Are you tapping the issues most relevant to the research problem? Are trial participants understanding and responding openly to these issues? Are interviewers tactfully probing responses, giving participants opportunities to think creatively about the questions? Review of pilot data can be an excellent team-building exercise, involving all members of the professional team in reviewing and revising the data collection process.

Supervision and Monitoring

Have a plan for monitoring data collection and providing continued support to the field team. The researcher or a field supervisor should review all taped records or transcripts as soon after the interview as possible to pick up potential weaknesses that could jeopardize the quality of the data. If the researcher's or field supervisor's presence is not distracting to the participants, he or she should also sit in on some of the interviews, perhaps in the role of note taker, in order to provide consultation later to the interviewer or moderator.

Even the most experienced qualitative data collectors will benefit from field supervision. Because the qualitative interview is not bound by a structured questionnaire, the interviewer is responsible for guiding the conversation, responding creatively to clues to new information and helping each respondent to express him- or herself openly. Unless you are doing your own interviewing, you will need to review tapes and, if feasible, observe interviews from time to time. If you are not fluent in the language of the interview, your field supervisor can be an invaluable aid in the monitoring process.

To ensure protection of study participants, review with the entire team, including local field assistants, the importance of respecting privacy and confidentiality. Pilot testing and discussion of the informed consent process is a natural way to remind data collectors of possible risks of participation. Moreover, interviewers and moderators who come from the same culture as participants may be able to heighten the researcher's awareness of sensitive areas in which participants might be especially vulnerable. Discuss with data collectors how they will resolve situations that arise in the field, for example, family members who insist on being present in the interview or individuals who seem not to respect the confidentiality of other participants in a focus discussion group. Although you cannot control what focus group participants tell others after they leave the site, most will welcome a basic rule for trusting and respecting each other's confidence, especially if they have helped to formulate the statement. Asking participants as well as staff to sign a confidentiality pledge will reinforce the message.

Researchers in the field must be always on the alert for ways to help data collectors improve or alter the process for more relevant information. Reviewing fieldwork as it happens helps you ensure quality and enables you to modify the process or address possible new questions or interesting ideas as they emerge. For most interviewers and moderators, probing beneath the surface is an especially difficult aspect of data collection. Valuable information can be lost if data collectors miss opportunities to probe significant comments. Appendix Eight summarizes some of the common errors that occur in moderating focus groups and how the moderator might have avoided them.

Generating Data Files

Take seriously the adage "Your research is only as good as your data." Because how you document your data will be a clue to their trustworthiness, we advise great care in creating and managing data files. You can record an interaction with handwritten notes while or soon after it happens, but audio recordings may provide a more complete account. Others will be able to review the tapes and decide whether they would draw the same conclusions from them. Using a computer to store and manage text facilitates the process of revising and updating your coding system as you review the data. You should also consider mechanisms for protecting the integrity of electronic data once it is cleaned and finalized for analysis.

Yet despite the value of recorded data, you must also collect it in as unobtrusive a way as possible. We try to use a small table microphone that we place slightly out of the line of vision between interviewer and respondent. As soon as you introduce yourself and the study, explain the purpose of the microphone and ask permission to use it. We have found that participants usually forget the microphone quickly and may even be pleased that the researchers value what they have to say enough to record it. However, if at any point during the session a participant requests not to be recorded, you should turn off the tape recorder and resume taping only when the participant agrees. Good note taking would obviously be an important alternative at this point.

Although tape recorders are very useful, they should not be the only data record. The field notes that you generate from your observations or spontaneous conversations are also valuable data, complementing the records of interviews or focus group discussions that you transcribe from audiotapes. Notes entered in brackets in the transcript are a good way to flag interesting observations or draw attention to contradictory responses. Analogous to the numbers generated in quantitative research, data from all these sources may be handwritten, typed, or entered in a computer file. But be cautious: observations that remain in the researcher's mind will not be part of the research.

Transcription and Translation

Transcribe audiotapes as soon as possible after the interview or discussion. When tapes accumulate on the shelf, to be reviewed only after fieldwork is over, you surely will miss subtle, nonverbal points as well as the opportunity to clarify ambiguities, investigate new leads, and follow up emerging hypotheses. Transcription services are available to take the drudgery out of this often lengthy and tedious process, but only the researcher can add nonverbal data, like a tone of voice or facial expression that could affect how you interpret the text.

Interviewer input is especially important in transcribing group discussions. In our experience it works best for the moderator and the note taker to transcribe each tape together, putting the spoken messages together with coded speaker identifications and nonverbal clues that the note taker has recorded as the discussion develops. The note taker's skill as observer and recorder of group process is obviously critical to the transcription's quality.

When scheduling your fieldwork, allow two to three hours of transcription for each hour of focus group discussion; or plan to conduct your interviews or discussions in the mornings and work on transcription in the afternoons. Immediate recall is essential for capturing subtle nuances, verbal and nonverbal, in qualitative responses.

Good transcription is time-consuming, and inexperienced researchers are sometimes tempted to cut corners by summarizing, rather than transcribing, the data. But language gives us important clues to meaning. How people say things is often as important as what they say. For insightful and powerful analysis, we advise taking the time to create verbatim transcriptions. A question often arises whether the transcription should faithfully replicate slang, jargon, obscenity, or incomplete or ungrammatical sentences exactly as spoken on the tape. For the purposes of most qualitative research, the transcript should be a faithful reproduction of the popular idiom, because that is how people express themselves. Even a pause in the conversation may be worth noting, because it may mean that the participant is tentative or unsure about what he is saying. And what about those grunts, sighs, and barely audible murmurs that punctuate most conversations? Researchers vary on this issue and must decide whether such utterances are extraneous or might be further clues to the meaning of the data.

Notes and bracketed comments on the data collection process can be very useful. For example, the researcher might note in brackets that a particular question was loaded—phrased in such a way as to elicit a specific response. Methodological notes are red flags that alert the researcher later to points at which bias may be influencing the data and questions might have to be modified.

Translation of vernacular expression is always challenging. Ideally, transcription and translation will be done at the same time, with input from the interviewer who collected the data for the transcript. Even if this degree of coordination is not feasible, the translator should work closely with the transcriber, trying to stay as close as possible to the original meaning. However, some words simply have no translation. Many idioms and metaphors are culturally specific, and concepts that fit one culture's conceptual framework may have no parallel in another. Describing symptoms and diseases is a case in point, because even when similar terms are used for an illness, they may have different meanings in different cultures. The best solution is to use the word or phrase that comes closest and include the original word in parentheses. If you have more than one translator, it helps to develop a vocabulary list so that there is agreement on terms to be left in the local idiom and to ensure that all staff fully understand the meaning of each term. Inclusion of particularly expressive terms from the original language enriches the transcript and may lead to discovery of new themes or ways of constructing familiar concepts. If meaning is not easy to understand in a long, discursive response, the translator might then paraphrase it and enter it in the transcript in brackets with a note. Chapter Seven provides more detail on transcribing and translating data.

Data Management and Storage

The researcher or field supervisor's job will be facilitated by a well-articulated plan for handling data as it is collected. Someone must be in charge of assigning identification codes to all individual records, including audiotapes, transcripts, demographic information sheets, and quantitative data if collected as part of the study. Store the documents in a secure location with access only by the researcher or field supervisor.

Preparation for efficient data management includes setting up a filing system with a place for each component of the study, for example:

- The original proposal
- Protocols developed for data collection
- Field notes
- Maps of the study community
- Topic guides
- Informed consent forms
- Sociodemographic data sheets
- Codebooks
- Instructions for data collectors and local field assistants
- Interview or focus group transcripts
- Other study materials

A good filing system will help ensure that important documents are not lost and that all materials will be at hand when you need them for analysis and writing results.

Timelines

Achieving an accurate estimation of time needed for data collection is never easy, but in qualitative research it is especially challenging. First, a qualitative interview or discussion is by definition flexible and open-ended. A session of one to one and one-half hours is a comfortable time frame for most participants; but as experienced interviewers know, much depends on how the guided conversation develops. On the one hand, even with skillful encouragement, participants occasionally have little to contribute. More often, however, as trust builds, so will the momentum and intensity of the interview or discussion. Participants will become more animated, and you will begin to hear the experience you are seeking and possibly the emergence of new themes in your inquiry. The interviewer must also be alert to participant fatigue, including distractions or loss of interest, and conclude the interview while it is still a positive experience. A thorough pilot test will help you gauge how long to stay on any one topic and how to move ahead without rushing participants. But however carefully you plan, expect to find many variations in the ways that different individuals and groups will respond to the study.

Other issues to consider when estimating your time in the field are the supervisory needs of data collectors, the time required to transcribe data tapes, and the importance of preliminary data analysis. The less experienced the interviewer is in qualitative techniques, the more time that person will need with a supervisor. Additional assistance may be needed to ensure accurate and ethically derived information.

Inexperienced qualitative researchers sometimes pack each day in the field with more interviews or focus groups than they or their interviewers can comfortably manage. If the team will be doing transcription or translation in the field, you may need to allow several hours for this task on the same day as the interview, depending on the interviews' length and the team's experience. A common time frame for a focus group study calls for one group discussion each morning: approximately one and one-half hours of discussion with time left for gathering and concluding activities. The afternoon is then devoted to transcription and translation, a process that typically takes three to four hours for each recorded session. On the other hand, if participants are employed outside the home or otherwise occupied during the day, it may be more convenient for them to meet in the late afternoon or evening. In that case, use the daytime hours for transcription, translation, and review of data. Be flexible to adapt the schedule to the needs of the men and women in the study. Remember also to include in your estimate an interviewer fatigue factor. Qualitative interviewing is intense and tiring; too tight a schedule may exhaust interviewers or moderators, with a negative impact on team morale and the quality of the data.

Finally, as we will emphasize in Chapter Six, the researcher should try to plan time in the schedule to listen to tapes or read transcripts while still in the field. Preliminary review and analysis are important elements that distinguish qualitative research from other, more structured, investigations.

Conclusion

Many texts about research methods offer their readers copious instructions on what to do and relatively little advice on how to do it. Their argument might be that because no two field experiences are the same, each investigator must negotiate the terrain individually, tailoring implementation to available resources. This caveat is important. However, the prudent investigator anticipates and detours as many potential roadblocks as possible. Knowing how to introduce oneself, use local resources, and build an effective team are fundamental to successful implementation. Success in the field demands diplomacy, respect for cultural differences, and an uncompromising code of ethics for the protection of participants and their families. A strength of qualitative research is that the researcher is continuously reviewing and evaluating the work in progress, clarifying questions, sharpening tools, and adapting techniques to new discoveries. We therefore urge researchers to keep ahead of the data collection, listening and observing, reviewing notes and transcripts as they are generated, being constantly on the alert to correct possible weaknesses, ask new questions, and strengthen the research process as it unfolds.

Field Perspective

Working with Drug Abusers: Lessons from the Street

Lorie Broomhall, Ph.D.

Family Health International

Since the 1980s the epidemiology of AIDS has shifted; the majority of new infections in the United States now occur among poor, inner-city minority populations. To develop effective interventions to reduce infection rates, health professionals need accurate, descriptive, and contextual information about the people at highest risk: injectors who use contaminated "works" and their sex partners, commercial sex workers, and others whose risk behaviors span more than one category. For the most part, these groups tend to live in run-down, dangerous neighborhoods in inner cities.

As an anthropologist, I started studying HIV risk behavior in a northeastern U.S. city in the late 1990s. Working as an ethnographer for a small community-based research organization, I intended to use participant observation to learn as much as I could about HIV risk among Puerto Rican injection drug users and pathways to hard drug use among inner city youth. Three years on the street turned out to be valuable training for the science and the craft of ethnography. The following lessons have served me well as I continue my career as a qualitative researcher, now directing and collaborating on studies on reproductive health and HIV/AIDS in developing countries.

Lesson One: Be Yourself

This lesson seems so obvious; yet when I first started to interview addicts and sex workers, I wondered how I could ever develop strong enough rapport to put them (and me!) at ease. I was a middle-class, middle-aged white woman who looked more like a social worker than a neighbor. What could I possibly have in common with my informants? As it turned out, plenty. Instead of focusing on differences—ethnicity, drug use, income, education, and work—I learned to find common ground with the people I interviewed. For example, I am a woman, a single parent, and a sibling. Most of my informants shared these characteristics or relationships. As a researcher, I could draw on common experiences to connect with people on the street. I did not have to attempt to be someone I am not. If I had tried to adopt "street" language, clothing, and attitudes, to be "down with the people," I would quickly have become an object of ridicule, not a trusted observer. The masquerade would have made the participant uncomfortable and eroded the trust I needed to build.

Lesson Two: Be Nonjudgmental

When signing their consent to be interviewed, participants did not agree to be judged, criticized, or looked down upon. Addicts well understand, and are frequently reminded, that no one is lower in the social hierarchy than a street junkie. I did not need to reinforce that perception. My purpose was to listen to them tell their stories without appearing to cast judgment or blame. Sometimes collecting data among these participants was not an easy task, listening with respect to their tales of past—and sometimes present—criminal activities or particularly graphic descriptions of violent behavior. There were times, however, when lesson one (be yourself) and lesson two (be nonjudgmental) clashed. During my fourth interview with an addict who had sold heroin at a local high school, he revealed how he had befriended lonely, disaffected teenagers and convinced them to shoot up with him as a way to get them "hooked on dope." Inwardly disgusted, I continued to maintain my neutral expression as the story unfolded. When he finished, he stopped and watched me closely and then asked what I thought of his actions. Deciding to be honest, I told him that, as a mother of a teenage son, I was horrified. He nodded with what appeared to be relief, telling me how ashamed he was of the things he had done to feed his habit and revealing his intimate feelings about addiction and its consequences. In this case, my honest response was the right one, but I'd like to think my nonjudgmental approach during the previous three interviews established the rapport this participant needed before he could trust me completely.

Lesson Three: Be Respectful

The few dollars study participants receive for interviews can never adequately compensate them for the wealth of critical information—often very private, sensitive, and sometimes painful—that they generously provide. It was easy to forget, especially when rushed for time and distracted by my own problems, that the disheveled, street-hardened addict sitting across from me was doing me a favor. Nevertheless, I made a habit of offering participants a cup of coffee or a soda, and sometimes a light snack, before starting the interview. That small sign of respect is especially meaningful to those used to getting no respect at all. I also tried to show my respect by being attentive and asking appropriate questions instead of rushing them through their answers to get to the next topic on the interview guide. Sometimes that practice yielded great rewards, as when a participant would bring up unexpected information critical to the investigation.

Lesson Four: Have Realistic Expectations

This last lesson was in some ways the hardest yet most important one to learn. It would have been easy to idealize study participants as innocent victims of an unfair world. A "savior complex," however, can do more harm than good when researchers compromise their objectivity by involving themselves too deeply in participants' personal lives or by putting themselves in dangerous and sometimes compromising positions. Besides, that perspective is inherently condescending. Drug injectors and sex workers are like the rest of us, except that circumstances of addiction and years of hard living on the street too often compel them to engage in criminal activity, deception, and manipulation. One young addict I interviewed seemed to revel in increasingly colorful stories of drug and street life, and it was only after several such interviews when I realized he was lying. Initially outraged and a little hurt, I came to understand that his deception was not personal; rather, storytelling was a clever and easy way for him to get cash to buy more heroin.

Being realistic also means recognizing that you will always be an outsider on the street. Though my street smarts vastly improved over time, they were not always adequate to alert me to potential danger. For that reason I always worked with an outreach worker, a local resident and former drug user who was a constant barometer of impending danger. In any situation, when Cal said, "Time to get out of here," we left.

Street ethnography can be exciting at times, and I felt some pride in my ability to work in a setting others would find difficult. In the end, however, I learned far more from my participants than they ever learned from me. They taught me about the values of compassion, generosity, honor, and loyalty—and that these qualities are found among people who can least afford to express them. For that I am grateful.

Field Perspective

Using Qualitative Research Methods to Empower NGOs

Suzanne Smith Saulniers, Ph.D.

Academy for Educational Development

In Pakistan, nongovernmental organizations (NGOs) working in public health service delivery have played a passive role as providers of information to donors. Donors, on the other hand, typically request, analyze, and use the information they get from NGOs but generally do not reciprocate by communicating back new information. For the past ten years, middle-sized family planning community service NGOs have received no written feedback from external monitoring teams or from the government agency that acts as the grant manager.

The role of local NGOs is confined mainly to collecting monthly and quarterly data on door-to-door family planning service delivery. They seldom analyze their own program evaluation results and are not taught how to use data they collect for program planning and assessment. Donor and government fund managers neither expect NGOs to assess service delivery problems nor encourage them to develop their own solutions to such problems. The result is that NGOs have become powerless to make fundamental changes and are discouraged from initiating improvements in reproductive health programs.

In 1998 the Asia Foundation, concerned about increasing decentralization of leadership and management capacity building of NGOs, decided to adopt an innovative approach. The resulting research and intervention project, initially funded by the William and Flora Hewlett Foundation in 1996, aimed to promote the well-being of families and to advocate for smaller families by strengthening men's role in family planning and women's reproductive health care. The project included a two-part formative research phase and a phase in which we tested an intervention model that used qualitative tools.

The remarkable empowerment of NGOs that took place during the research phase of this project convinced me that introducing qualitative techniques is an important capacity-building process in its own right. I believe this had as much to do with learning how to use the qualitative techniques—semistructured interviewing, focus group discussions, and direct observation—as it did with the social responsibility that the program promoted.

Our research used the trials of improved practices (TIPs) methodology, a social marketing approach in which members of the affected groups implement the trials. TIPS can be used to evaluate behaviors, motivations, instructional information, and approaches to overcoming barriers to a proposed change (Dickin and others 1997). Five middle-sized NGOs were selected as participants, along with a four-member core research team of Pakistani health specialists.

Empowerment started from the beginning of the research. The key elements of empowerment were the following: a rigorous and closely supervised participatory training process, peer exchanges and collaborative support, and promotion of the message that the research teams were learning skills new to NGOs in Pakistan.
I learned that when NGOs are directly involved in implementing research, they assume ownership and responsibility for the results of the data.

Three of the five NGO providers had been trained in TIPs research methods as part of a previous qualitative study. This project gave them an opportunity to reinforce their skills in focus group discussions, in-depth interviews, direct observation, and NGO research management. The team worked collegially, benefiting from a nonhierarchical structure and mutual exchange during training sessions. When focus group discussions needed stronger researchers, not only would a core research team member step in, but also an experienced interviewer from another NGO might be invited to assist with discussions or refresher training of the interview team.

We found that peer learning and reinforcement secured team members' skills in asking questions or knowing when to seek solutions to irregular use or nonuse of modern family planning methods. They also learned how to engage in gender-appropriate needs assessments of female and male clients. This interactive peer approach and the qualitative results that emerged encouraged all the NGO participants to look critically at their current programs and to review their relationships with government.

Questioning the effectiveness of their current service delivery approach, the NGOs noted the absence of male involvement in their delivery design. They were surprised at how far removed they had been from their clients—delivering health messages without really understanding how people made reproductive decisions. They wondered why they had meticulously collected quantitative data without understanding their clients' attitudes, problems, and criteria for personal health care decisions. In fact, NGOs were so optimistic about what they were learning that several approached the government minister to discuss service delivery policy.

They asked if they could receive funds to engage in self-monitoring, continue qualitative data collection, and collect quantitative data less frequently. They requested that greater attention be given to the role of men in decision making about family planning. And they asked that the government and donors also send them regular government monitoring reports on their activities and performance. Until this qualitative research experience, they had never considered raising questions to government or donors, nor had they considered themselves qualified to undertake program monitoring. Since then this group has started a reproductive health network among middle-sized NGOs. Today they are continuing their qualitative research training, applying for grants through the network and seeking funds to train others in qualitative methods.

Field Perspective

Anticipating Strengths and Weaknesses When Training Data Collectors

Cynthia Woodsong, Ph.D.

Family Health International

Previous experience of field staff charged with data collection can vary widely within and between projects, with implications for training, monitoring, and supervision.

In providing training to field staff in international multisite ethnographic studies focused on HIV/AIDS behavior change, I have found it helpful to take into account the trainees' professional backgrounds and the way these might bias data collection. Field staff often come from the following backgrounds: health care workers, survey researchers, or data collectors.

Health Care Workers (for Example, Nurses, Health Educators, or Social Services Providers)

Strengths: (1) Health care workers may be more comfortable talking about reproductive health issues, sexual behaviors, and the body than most people; (2) participants may be more willing to discuss these things with someone they know is a health worker, a person whom they see as legitimately privy to such talk; and (3) health care workers know how to engage people, build trust, and offer reliable confidentiality.

Weaknesses: (1) Health care workers may find it difficult to elicit data that are at odds with medical knowledge, feeling instead a need to correct misinformation; (2) they may be considered authoritarian, thus blocking free discussion of behaviors that the respondent knows the health profession does not consider correct; and (3) participants may only endure the interview in order to receive treatment. Their expertise may inadvertently bias responses as well as make participation potentially coercive.

Health care professionals enter the qualitative interview from the perspective of someone trained to provide for people, not to learn from them. In training and supervising health care workers, I have found it helpful to remind the trainees that the respondent (patient) is the expert on the issue being discussed. Such trainees often need practice letting the respondent do most of the talking and remaining neutral to the content of what the respondent is saying. Although it is common practice to correct misinformation at the end of an interview, I learned that if a health worker interviewer says, "I can tell you more after we finish the interview," she may find it difficult to convince respondents that their opinions and beliefs are important. Additional skills training is often necessary to avoid a situation in which the respondent views the interviewer as the expert.

Survey Researchers (Usually Trained or Experienced in Quantitative Pencil-and-Paper Surveys)

Strengths: Survey researchers demonstrate (1) an appreciation for adherence to protocol and conscientiousness in covering all topics included, (2) an awareness of the potential for biasing responses through additional explanations, and (3) efficiency and careful documentation.

Weaknesses: (1) Survey researchers can be rigid and have a tendency to follow protocol in an almost robotic style, and (2) they may have difficulty in grasping the concept of appropriate probing.

Survey researchers who have internalized the importance of staying closely within a structured protocol with strict question-by-question specifications are probably excellent interviewers and rightly proud of their expertise. However, they often find it challenging (if not unscientific) to switch to a conversational style of interviewing, with the extensive probing and disruption of question-flow order so common in qualitative research. When training survey interviewers, I rely heavily on role-playing as a training tool, with trainees interviewing me as well as each other. Reviewing verbatim transcripts of practice and initial interviews is an essential training tool. Such review allows the trainer to point out more clearly missed opportunities to probe and to provide guidance on leading probes and questions, while also reassuring trainees of things they have done well.

University-Trained Social Scientists (in Anthropology, Sociology, or Psychology)

Strengths: Social scientists have (1) a strong theoretical background; (2) appreciation for and training in qualitative, in-depth interviewing; (3) an awareness of cultural assumptions and worldviews of both respondent and interviewer; and (4) skills in careful (sometimes excessive) documentation of the research process and data.

Weaknesses: Social scientists may (1) spend too much time per data collection task, (2) lack awareness of the nuances of applied research, and (3) be devoted to favorite theories that may not be essential to the project.

Data collectors with university training in the underlying theoretical perspectives of social sciences and public health can be wonderful to work with. However, their solid training can be a hindrance if they are so vested in a particular theoretical perspective that they cannot adjust to the fast pace and practical requirements of applied research. In these situations firm time limits, deadlines, and deliverable schedules help to keep the data collection on track.

With appropriate training and supervision, data collectors' different skill sets can be productively harnessed as an asset to qualitative data collection. Even novice field staff completely new to social science research may provide surprising abilities to connect their life experiences with data collection. If the research team leader and those involved in training field staff are aware of the trainees' potential strengths and weaknesses, they can move more quickly to spot and solve problems and to organize data collection efforts to make best use of appropriate skills.

Field Perspective

Training Field Staff in Data Analysis

Cynthia Woodsong, Ph.D.

Family Health International

Analysis of qualitative data usually requires a minimum of three steps: coding the data, running the coded data, and analyzing the data runs. In a truly iterative process, the final step usually leads to further coding, running, and analysis. The most common models for division of labor for data analysis are the following:

- Staff who collect the data send it to other staff for analysis (most often based in the United States) and are not involved in the analytic process.
- Junior staff code the data (which they may or may not have collected) using a qualitative software package, and more senior staff (again, often in the United States) then run and analyze these data.
- The same staff who collect data are involved in coding and analyzing data.
- The same staff who code the data are responsible for analysis.

The realities of conducting applied reproductive health research often preclude field staff's participation in data analysis. Still, it is advisable to look for ways to involve those responsible for data collection in at least some aspects of the analysis.

Previous experience is probably the most important issue to take into account when making decisions about who should do which analysis task. Other factors include language and translation issues, the analysis approach, budgets, and timeliness. Whichever model you choose, your decision will have important implications for field staff training.

If staff are responsible for their own transcription and translation of data, it is reasonable to train them to do at least some basic high-level coding—that is, organizing data into broad topic domains. Take care to provide training and supervision for this high-level coding; when in doubt, have data double-coded. I have had good results training junior staff to use basic analysis software; their ability to quickly code pages and pages of transcripts is a real time-saver. When using junior staff, however, periodic inter- and intracoder reliability checks after initial training are necessary. It is becoming standard practice to perform routine checks for agreement between different coders to ensure that they are coding similarly, as well as to check decisions made by the same coder to ensure the coding designations do not drift over time. These intra- and interreliability checks may need to be carried out more frequently with junior staff until their skills have been validated. Such quality control checks provide not only quality assurance for the research project but also opportunities for further iteration and modification of the coding scheme.

Timeliness is, unfortunately, often the biggest driver in making decisions about whom to involve in analysis. Because fuller participation and inclusion in analysis takes more time and more extensive training of field staff, inclusion usually falls by the wayside. For example, staff responsible for data collection in a Uganda HIV study recently told me that they would welcome the chance to be involved in computer analysis of the data. I was pleased to hear this until I learned that they did not have basic word processing or typing skills. Due to time and budgetary constraints, as well as quality control issues, teaching them the analysis software to be used in the study would have been impractical.

At a minimum field-based researchers should be asked to review summaries of data once they are run. When those who have been involved in data collection are members of the culture from which the data were derived, they are in a unique position to make meaning of the data and advise on its application. Furthermore, by strengthening field staff capacity to serve more fully as partners in research, these staff members can be better involved in seeing that the results are put to good use. An inclusive, learning approach is not only the correct thing to do, it also potentially increases research quality, especially for qualitative research.

Example: Two Coders, Two Coding Decisions

Software can facilitate intercoder reliability checks in different ways. The following text section was coded by two staff members with visible differences in coding decisions.

Coder 1

Well, I used to think that once I was married that I could be safe and not have to worry about catching anything. I mean, you trust your husband, but I caught him with a condom and I know he's having sex with someone else. He even admitted it, but he says it's natural for a man to have a little on the side. He says I should be grateful that he does the right thing and uses a condom with her. That way he won't give me anything. I know he hates to strap up, so I had to believe him about that, but still . . .

married

men, extramarital

beliefs

Coder 2

Well, I used to think that once I was married that I could be safe and not have to worry about catching anything. I mean, you trust your husband, but I caught him with a condom and I know he's having sex with someone else. He even admitted it, but he says it's natural for a man to have a little on the side. He says I should be grateful that he does the right thing and uses a condom with her. That way he won't give me anything. I know he hates to strap up, so I had to believe him about that, but still . . .

married

men, extramarital

gratitude

terms

Field Perspective

Learning to Listen: How Qualitative Research Affected Novice Interviewers

Naveeda Khawaja, M.Sc., M.P.H.

United Nations Fund for Population and Development, Nepal

A seldom-acknowledged benefit of qualitative research is its impact on the people who collect the data. When interviewers are also health practitioners—for example, clinic staff or community-based family planning motivators—learning to listen and ask sensitive questions can open their eyes to the worlds of their clients and thus help them provide understanding and more sensitive care.

This is something we experienced when studying male involvement in reproductive health care in Pakistan.* The study's purpose was to learn more about the roles of men and women in family planning and reproductive health and ways to help men understand women's reproductive health needs. Data collection was carried out in all four provinces by five nongovernmental organizations (NGOs).† A four-member core research team trained the interviewers in the field for in-depth interviewing and focus group discussion. Male interviewers collected data from male participants and female interviewers from female participants. At the conclusion of the study's first phase, interviewers provided oral feedback to all the researchers, the NGO managers, and the donor. Interviewers also completed an evaluation questionnaire to assess what they had learned from taking part in a qualitative research project.

Our careful examination of the questionnaire responses revealed that the interviewers had benefited professionally and personally from participating in what was for them a novel form of research. Their participation in qualitative research training and data collection had built self-confidence. The research process had enhanced their ability to think reflectively, which in turn had led them to question many of their own firmly held assumptions about how people live and manage their lives. Learning the skills of interviewing also made them better listeners, able to maintain greater objectivity in interpersonal interactions, build rapport, and know when and how to probe. Some who had come recently to their respective agencies with little technical background gained specific knowledge about family planning and reproductive health.

Without exception the interviewers reported that working together as a research team was satisfying and enjoyable. They described their participation in the project as a metamorphosis in their understanding of the relationships in marriage, between parents and their children, and between mothers-in-law and daughters-in-law. Field experience had caused them to dismantle many of their own assumptions about sexual, reproductive, and family life and to give up stereotypes. One interviewer noted, "I liked doing focus group discussion with mothers-in-law. My assumption regarding them, that is, mothers-in-law not cooperating and fighting with us, proved wrong. They talked so sweetly that I enjoyed talking to them."

Commenting on how field experience had increased their ability to listen reflectively to others' views, an interviewer said, "It was my opinion that I am correct in whatever I say or think. Now I give importance to conversation and thoughts of people and try to learn from them."

Another interviewer remarked, "Because of this research, I feel a change in myself. My skills of listening, understanding, and making others understand through the process of a two-way communication have improved." And another described the research process as "similar to peeling an onion. We peeled each layer till nothing was left inside."

Speaking about the training itself, researchers agreed that the experience of learning together had increased their motivation and their commitment to the whole research process. "The work and enjoyment went together," said one, "the newness and novelty of the experience."

What they found novel seemed to be the access that qualitative interviewing gave them to people's private thoughts and personal lives. Within the comfortable exchanges of the interviews, they heard sensitive details that most people do not share even with their closest confidantes. The interviewers realized, too, that this information was available to them because they had indeed been successful in creating the trust and rapport that enabled the study participants to share their lives.

Another unanticipated benefit for some was the way that the research seemed to be working toward positive social change, especially around issues of gender. One interviewer said, "In this male-dominated society, this research was needed."

As rewarding as the interviewers found the research, there were also challenges to overcome. They had difficulty finding volunteers, and men in particular were often reluctant to be interviewed. Each team evolved a strategy to overcome this problem. In one case, women who agreed to participate were asked if they could persuade their husbands to be interviewed as well. Another team enlisted the help of a male colleague to recruit husbands of female participants.

Over the course of the research, the interviewers developed skills in crisis management, learning to be patient and persuasive, and to reduce heightened emotions. For example, as one interviewer reported, "In one or two focus group discussions, participants exchanged heated words and at times came close to a fistfight. We just changed the topic to cool the matter." Another interviewer found that "during the research we had difficulty asking questions because some women would hardly [ever] agree to give answers to questions. After a long wait, they would give an answer, but we would be patient and give them time to relax and answer."

Teamwork was one of the most valued aspects of the research design. Interviewers commented that working in teams prevented mistakes and contributed to completeness, reduced tension and anxieties, provided the opportunity for constructive feedback, and generally made the work better and easier. Because men and women worked together, they had the opportunity to question their own gender stereotypes.

As a result of their experience on our research team, clinic staff gained technical skill and personal confidence as interviewers in the field. But perhaps even more important, they acquired new interpersonal skills and understanding of common reproductive health and family problems in their communities. Their discovery of their own abilities as listeners and new respect for the people they serve in their health centers will add immeasurably to the quality of care they can provide.

**The formative and qualitative study of men's role in family planning and reproductive health formed part of a larger program funded by the Hewlett Foundation and executed by the Asia Foundation Pakistan.*

† The five NGOs' names are followed by the province name in parentheses: Mother-Child Welfare Association of Pakistan (Lahore, Punjab Province), Lyari Community Development (Karachi, Sindh Province), MEHAC Trust for Community Development and Welfare (Quetta, Balochistan), Anjumune Taraqiya Tanzeem Khawateen (Quetta, Balochistan), and Community Council Mardan (North West Frontier Province).

CHAPTER SIX

Qualitative Data Analysis

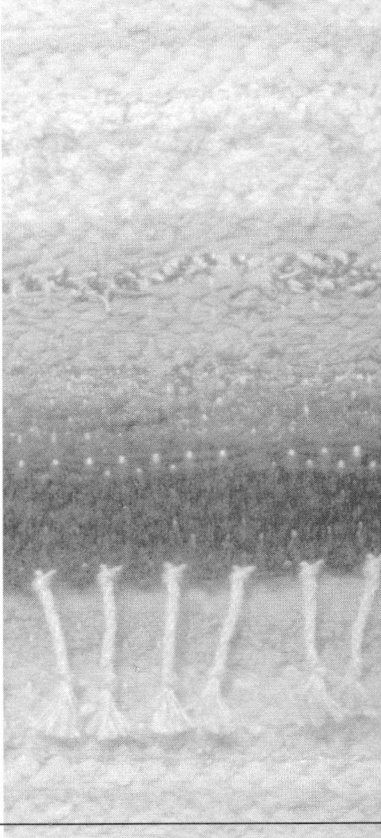

IN ALL SOCIAL RESEARCH, whether qualitative or quantitative, the investigator systematically examines data to discover patterns and in some cases, to identify cause-and-effect relationships. The process must be well documented so that others can follow it, understand the decisions that have been made along the way, and independently verify the results.

In other ways qualitative and quantitative data analyses diverge. In quantitative studies researchers carefully focus their questions, identifying key explanatory variables and expected outcomes in advance. They either identify and control for contextual variables or consider them outside the study's scope. Data collection and analysis remain distinctly separate phases of research. Analysis emphasizes prediction and testing of relationships between variables using statistical processes.

In contrast, qualitative studies are designed to explore the broader psychological, social, political, or economic contexts in which research questions are situated. As earlier chapters have emphasized, qualitative researchers typically begin with more general, open-ended questions, moving toward greater precision as detailed information emerges. Though previous research and theory may suggest that certain constructs will be important to include in a conceptual framework, their definitions may still be only tentative at first. As data are collected, the meanings of these ideas or concepts begin to take shape, making preliminary analysis a necessary part of data collection. Qualitative analysis begins with the first field activities and may lead to revisions or refinements in research questions as the study proceeds.

This chapter shows the reader how to process and interpret raw data—perhaps several hundred pages of transcripts, field notes, or other written materials—to

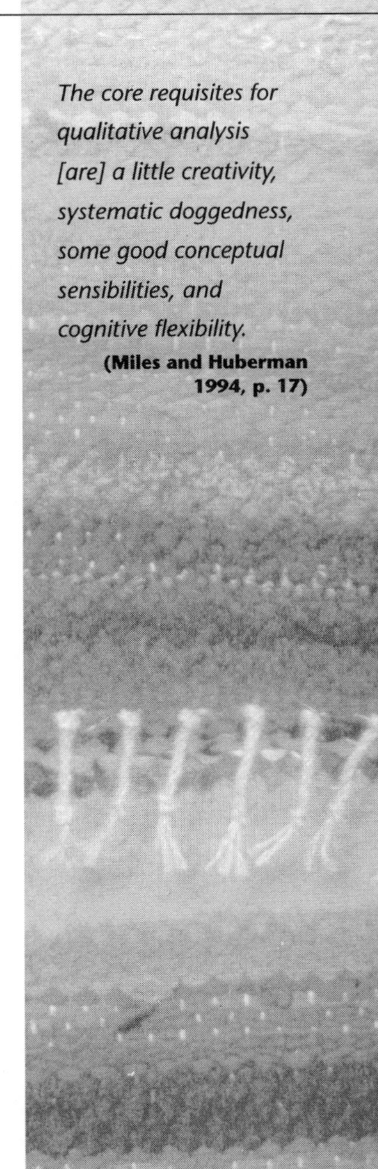

The core requisites for qualitative analysis [are] a little creativity, systematic doggedness, some good conceptual sensibilities, and cognitive flexibility.

(Miles and Huberman 1994, p. 17)

answer important research questions and address theoretical issues. It covers the following topics:

- Principles of qualitative analysis
- Terms used in describing the analysis process
- Processes used to analyze qualitative data, including reading, coding, data display, and data reduction
- Choice and use of software for qualitative analysis, as well as data management and logistical issues, more generally
- Interpretation of data—moving from the minutiae of study results to the main ideas
- Integration of qualitative findings in mixed-method designs

Principles of Qualitative Analysis

Following are five principles that guide qualitative analysis.

- People differ in their experiences and understandings of reality; how participants define a situation may not reflect the researcher's assumptions. This principle is as central to qualitative analysis as it is to designing the study and collecting the data. Other chapters have highlighted the premises that social reality is complex, that participants often have different understandings of reality, and that their perspectives may differ substantially from the researchers' assumptions. In analysis, too, it is important for us as researchers to recognize and account for the cultural lens through which we inevitably view our research populations (Kelle 1997).

  Learn to recognize and become aware of your own perspectives during the data collection and analysis process. Account for them in field notes and bracket them in transcripts. Note what you think might be emerging explanations and check them against raw data. Be open to surprising findings but not too quick to explain them. Always be ready to return to your study participants to understand better what you have learned. Actively seek out alternative explanations and see which ones stand over time. Understanding the world that your study participants have presented to you takes patience and perseverance.

  It is important to pay attention to the language we use in our dialogues with study participants. Even when speaking the same dialect, we may in fact be speaking from different vantage points—attaching different meanings to the common words we are using.

  As we noted in Chapter Five, language can pose a serious challenge. If the researcher does not speak the study participants' language, he or she will rely on others' translations of what they said. It is important to work closely during the analysis with key informants who are familiar with the languages and underlying perspectives of both researchers and participants.

- A social phenomenon cannot be understood outside its own context. By *context* we mean not only the physical setting in which a behavior, attitude, disease, or process takes place but also the historical, social, and political climates and the organizational or individual characteristics that influence the phenomenon. Qualitative researchers do not assume that they can examine such aspects of the context independently from one another. Rather, dependence and interdependence of phenomena are the working assumptions. We bring context into analysis by considering how informants' stories are shaped by their social position, economic opportunities, or religious convictions and how narratives are embedded in the broader physical, social, economic, and political environments in which informants live. For example, when investigating clandestine abortion practices, we might analyze context by seeking explanations in what we can learn about individuals, families, institutions, communities, or policies and events at regional and national levels. Documentation of past and present abortion legislation would provide insight into historical trends affecting access to abortion and ways in which the government might seek to influence popular opinion. Stories covered in the local media could provide important information about the key institutions involved in supporting or opposing abortion practices. Separate focus group discussions with clinicians, policymakers, and religious leaders, as well as groups of men or women can provide a community perspective on abortion practice. Confidential interviews with abortion practitioners and recipients focus at the individual level on the economic, relational, and personal circumstances that influence how abortion is provided. Through analysis of information from many sources, you will identify the ways in which different groups' views converge or diverge and seek to explain what contextual factors lead them to do so.

- Theory both guides qualitative research and results from it. As we introduced in Chapter Two, substantive theory offers a systematic explanation for some aspect of life, an explanation that has been tested and stands in multiple research settings. It does so by specifying a set of general or abstract concepts and their relationships to one another—the whole of which can be used to explain or predict the behavior, attitude, disease, or process under study (Glanz and others 2002).

  Qualitative analysis can be informed by theory, or it can generate theory. If the study is grounded in a theoretical framework, your plan for analysis should begin with the concepts and categories that have guided the research design. In other study designs, researchers avoid imposing a theoretical framework, letting theory emerge from the data analysis. (See the example of grounded theory in Box 2.3, p. 20.) In either case, qualitative data lead to a rich, textured analysis and always the possibility of new theoretical understanding.

- Exceptional cases may yield insight into a problem or new leads for further inquiry. Although analysis may seek common ground or consensus across different individuals or groups, it is equally important to understand how and why individuals or groups differ with respect to issues under study. Identifying and tracking exceptions may yield important insights and lead to a better understanding of the research problem.

  In research involving sensitive topics, the individual who appears to be atypical or unique may in fact represent a much larger group of study participants who were unwilling to express themselves fully. Such might be the case if a physician were willing to relate circumstances and outcomes of clandestine abortions that are commonly conducted but rarely discussed. For some qualitative researchers, an important goal of such research is to make visible those whom society has overlooked. Recording the voices of minorities and others whose voices are seldom heard in the scientific arena is an important contribution of qualitative research.

- Understanding of human behavior emerges slowly and nonlinearly. As in design and implementation, qualitative analysis typically follows an iterative path. A flexible and integrated approach is therefore essential if the researcher is to understand complex issues from the participants' perspectives. It may, in fact, take numerous rounds of questioning, reflecting, rephrasing, analyzing, theorizing, and verifying. We emphasize again that qualitative analysis should begin in the field, continuing through (and beyond) the data collection period.

Sometimes analysis in the field can lead to unanticipated but consistent findings that the investigator will explore with related questions. In a study of new contraceptive users in Mali, participants often mentioned conversations they had with sisters-in-law about family planning. This clue led the investigators to introduce questions about the influence of different family members in the decision-making process (Castle and others 1999). Field analysis can also lead to inclusion of new participants. Looking at the data after every observation, interview, or focus group session keeps you alert to new discoveries and the potential for modifying the research process to strengthen the data.

BOX 6.1

Terms Used in Data Analysis

characteristic A single item or event in a text, similar to an individual response to a variable or indicator in quantitative research. It is the smallest unit of analysis.

coding The process of attaching labels to lines of text so that the researcher can group and compare similar or related pieces of information.

coding sorts Compilation of similarly coded blocks of text from different sources into a single file or report.

concepts or themes Idea categories that emerge from groupings of lower-level data points.

indexing Process that generates a word list comprising all the substantive words and their locations within the texts entered into the program.

theory A set of interrelated concepts, definitions, and propositions that presents a systematic view of events or situations by specifying relations among variables.

What Are Qualitative Data?

Qualitative data may come from direct interactions with participants; observation or secondary sources, including numeric or textual data from clinic records; or summaries or full texts from newspapers, popular literature, academic reviews, and other sources. In this chapter we use the term to refer primarily to textual data in the form of expanded field notes or transcripts of recorded interviews. We do so with the understanding that even images or sounds must eventually be interpreted and their meanings noted on paper, to be systematically incorporated into analysis.

Text can be read at many different levels. As you become more experienced, you will begin to recognize and incorporate these different levels in your analysis. Among the characteristics to note when analyzing a segment of text are the following:

- The primary message content
- The evaluative attitudes of the speaker toward the message
- The content of the message and whether it is meant to represent individual or group-shared ideas
- The degree to which the speaker is representing actual versus hypothetical experience

Consider, for example, a text excerpt from a thirty-four-year-old woman in Mali who works as a telephone operator and uses an injectable contraceptive: "I don't have a child on my back; I leave him playing with the other children. I leave him at home, and I work until my lunch hour. Then I come back and work until the late afternoon and then go home. If I had a child on my back or if I were pregnant, do you think I would be able to do this job? Rather, I would always be worrying about the state of the children, and I'd be the laughingstock of everybody" (Castle and others 1999, p. 243).

From the text we can assume that this woman has at least one child but a child who is old enough to be left at home. Her main message is that contraceptive use has enabled her to work—something she feels would be difficult if she were pregnant or caring for an infant. We see the emotion in her words with her use of rhetorical questioning: "do you think I would be able to do this job?" The phrase, to "have a child on my back" (referring to the West African tradition of carrying young children piggyback, supported by a large piece of cloth), evokes the constant attention, the burdensome quality of early child care. We sense a kind of relief from the speaker that she is not experiencing it now. The speaker also alludes to both psychological constraints and social expectations that could prevent her from working outside the home. Though she is expressing her opinion in this paragraph (rather than speaking for a larger group of working mothers), it is not clear whether she speaks from personal experience, from observations of others who have tried to work with young children on their backs, or from a more hypothetical stance. The most we can say is that she believes she would have a hard time concentrating on her job if she were caring for a young child and would be ridiculed for trying to do both.

Basic Steps in Qualitative Data Analysis

Qualitative analysis emphasizes how data fit together as a whole, bringing together context and meaning. There are many approaches, but one way is simply to use the research questions to group your data and then look for similarities and differences. This approach may be particularly appropriate when you have limited time or resources for a more in-depth analysis or when your qualitative research is a smaller component of a larger quantitative study, conducted to provide further depth in predefined areas of interest.

A more in-depth and inductive approach to analysis is also appropriate. Box 6.2, which outlines a qualitative data analysis process, identifies a sequence of interrelated steps in data analysis: reading, coding, displaying, reducing, and interpreting. The process begins with immersion—reading and rereading texts and reviewing notes. As you read, you listen for emerging themes and begin to attach labels or codes to the chunks of text that represent those themes. Once your texts have been coded, you explore each thematic area, first displaying in detail the information relevant to each category and then reducing this information to its essential points. At each step you search for the core meaning of the thoughts, feelings, and behaviors described in your texts—that is, you interpret the data. Finally, you provide an overall interpretation of the study findings, showing how thematic areas relate to one another, explaining how the network of concepts responds to your original study questions, and suggesting what these findings mean beyond the specific context of your study.

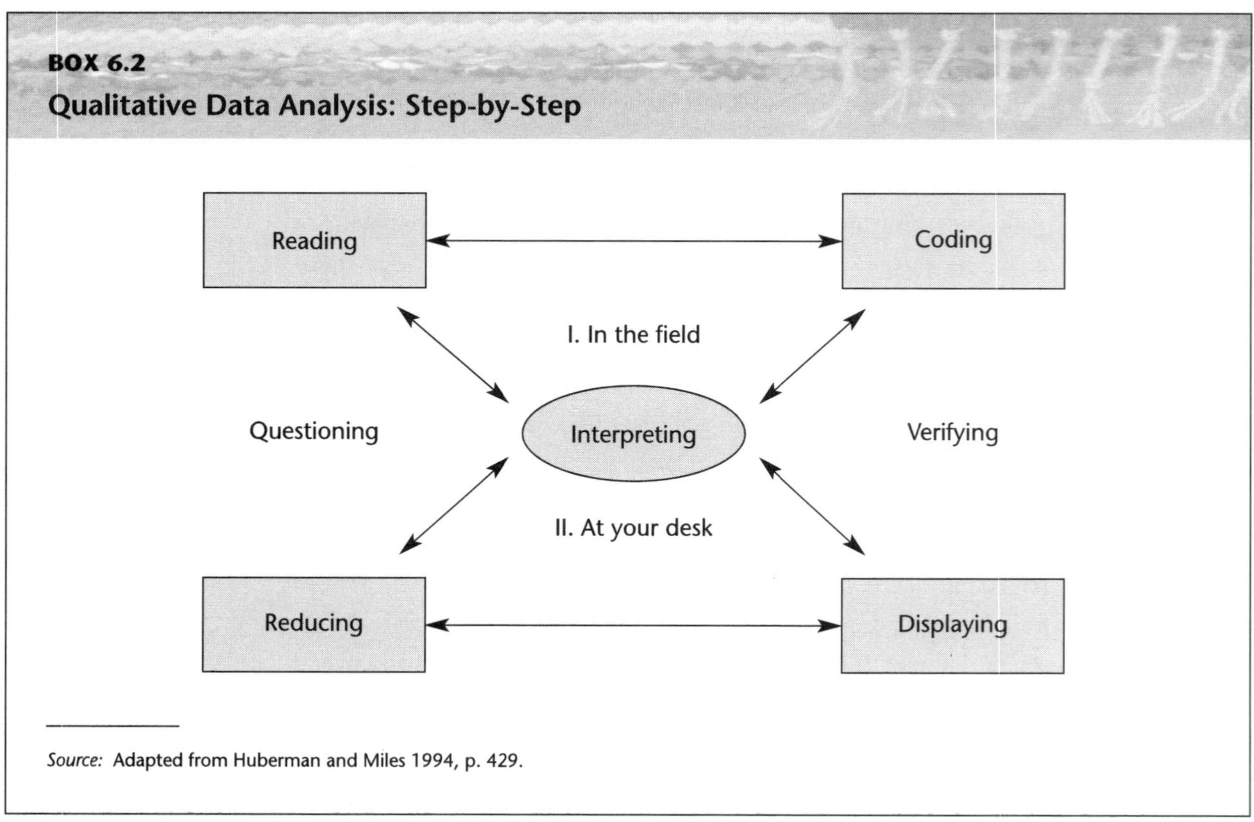

Source: Adapted from Huberman and Miles 1994, p. 429.

The five steps relate to one another in a way that is both structured and flexible. It is structured in the sense that each of these five steps builds upon previous ones. In general, you first carefully read your field notes and transcripts and then begin to code the data. You should initiate reading and coding while the data are still being collected in the field. The data display and reduction processes are often conducted at your desk once all the data have been collected, but they may be initiated earlier. However, even during these later steps in the qualitative analysis process, researchers may loop back through earlier steps to refine codes, reread texts, and revise certain aspects of the analysis.

We now discuss the five steps in data analysis, illustrating these steps with examples from the qualitative component of one multisite clinical trial of a vaginal microbicide product in development to prevent HIV transmission. The goal of the trial, designed and conducted by Family Health International, was to determine the microbicide's safety and acceptability among women in four countries. The qualitative component explored the experience of using this microbicide from the perspectives of women in the trial and their male partners (Bentley and others 2004). Because many women at high risk of HIV may be unable or unwilling to obtain the approval of male partners to use risk-reduction products (like condoms or microbicides), a key question in the qualitative investigation was whether the woman could insert this product, a vaginal gel, without her sexual partner's knowledge. We take the reader step-by-step through this qualitative analysis, using it to help the reader visualize and apply a technique for turning raw data into credible, publishable results. Although presented in the context of a clinical trial, the analytical framework developed for this study by one of the authors (Tolley) is applicable to almost any social and behavioral health research.

Reading: Developing an Intimate Relationship with the Data

Most qualitative researchers would agree that qualitative analysis begins with data immersion. This means reading and rereading each set of notes or transcripts until you are intimately familiar with the content. As we have emphasized, the researcher does not wait for all the data to return but starts gradually immersing him- or herself with progressive review as data are being collected. The process is analogous to wading into a lake instead of diving headfirst.

READING FOR CONTENT

What do you look for as you read? First, you should read for content. Are you obtaining the kinds of information that you intended to collect? Are the responses full and detailed, or are they superficial? These first data may not be as rich or as topical as you would like. Perhaps the questions are not adequately framed or sequenced. Maybe the interviewers are not following up important leads with appropriate probes (see Appendix Eight). Other aspects of the interview process may be inhibiting data collection—the venue, composition of groups, or the interviewer's style or characteristics. It is important to discuss these issues with data collectors or make note of them if you are the one gathering the data.

As you review the data, begin to identify emergent themes and develop tentative explanations. Make a note of any topics that the research has not adequately addressed up to the present and ones that have emerged unexpectedly in the transcripts. You may find undeveloped or surprising new topics to explore in continued fieldwork. As recommended in Chapter Five, you might type these ideas directly into your transcripts, taking care to put them in brackets or italics so that you can distinguish them from original text. Or record your ideas in a field journal or type them in separate memos. Some qualitative software programs, such as QSR N6 (N6 2002), allow you to link memos to specific text and then to print them together; doing so makes separating your interpretations from observations and other field data easier.

NOTING QUALITY

As you continue to read, begin to focus on the quality of the transcripts or notes. How were data obtained? If you are reviewing a set of field observations, how soon after the field activity were notes recorded? How vivid and detailed is the description? If the data report an informal interaction in the field, how spontaneously was the conversation initiated, and can you determine this from the notes? Were interview questions asked in a neutral way, or did the researcher suggest that some responses would be more valuable than others? These methodological problems will affect the credibility of your data; you must determine whether responses appear plausible, and whether there is sufficient contextual detail to add to your understanding. By including bracketed or italicized notes about such problems in your texts or in linked memos, you will give greater consideration to responses obtained through open-ended questions and less to those obtained through leading questions. You will also begin to develop a system, or audit trail, by which others can review your analytical work. (See pp. 168–169 in this chapter for more on audit trails.) Ultimately, the researcher's skill will enhance or reduce the trustworthiness of study findings.

IDENTIFYING PATTERNS

Once you have field notes or transcripts from several different sources (that is, different kinds of participants or different methods of data collection), review them as a set to identify important themes. Then start to examine the patterns in these themes. Patterns may include those that occur in all or some of your data, possible relationships between themes, contradictory responses, or gaps in understanding. Gaps suggest new questions for more exploration. As you collect additional data, repeat and formalize the process as we discuss later in this chapter. It may lead you to adapt your study design, seek different sources or types of information, or modify your interview or discussion guides to explore new topics.

Coding: Identifying the Emerging Themes

After you have read and become familiar with your first texts, you can begin to code the themes. Codes are like street signs, inserted into the margins of your handwritten notes or typed after segments of text to remind you where you are and what you see. In qualitative analysis using words or parts of words to flag ideas you discover in the transcript can make analysis of a large data file easier and more accurate. With key themes coded in this way, you can later search and retrieve interesting segments and look at them as a separate file. Having all the pieces of the text that relate to a common theme together in one place also enables you to discover new subthemes and explore them in greater depth. Though most qualitative researchers use some process of coding, there are no standard rules about how to do it. Researchers differ on how to derive codes, when to start and stop coding, and what level of detail they want. When more than one person is involved in coding, develop a process to negotiate or reconcile coding decisions. Be guided by what is most useful to you as you organize and make sense of the text, and remember to document coding decisions as you make them.

WHAT ASPECTS OF THE TEXT DO YOU LABEL?

Some researchers develop codes that closely match the ideas or language found in the textual data. They want to avoid imposing words or concepts that might prevent them from seeing their data in a new way. Others borrow terms from the social science literature that represent more abstract concepts important to their field. These have the advantage of being clear to a wider audience. Whether borrowed or emergent, labels allow you to assemble under one concept many seemingly disparate pieces of text and search for connections among them.

Common pitfalls include: (1) coding too finely (too many distinctions) so that important unifying concepts are missed; and (2) forcing new findings into existing codes instead of adding codes that could extend analysis in new directions.

Consider the text in Box 6.3, excerpted from an interview with a thirty-two-year-old woman from India with two children. She has been married for ten years to a man who is now HIV positive. She began working as a maid after marriage. She participated in a study to examine the relationship between women's work and their ability to make decisions about their health.

Several important themes emerge from this excerpt and help us understand the relationship between women's work and health-related decision making. They include the following:

- A description of financial decision making
- Attitudes toward women's work
- The role of the extended family
- HIV risk reduction behaviors

How do we code our text to enable investigation of these various themes? More specifically, how many codes should we use, and what words should we choose as labels?

There are no real guidelines on how finely to code your data. It may depend as much on personal style as on your research aims or professional field. We suggest coding your first several texts using fairly broad labels that correspond to the study's main research questions. For example, the categories we listed may be sufficient initially to label the texts. However, as you continue to read and code texts, you may find that such broad headings give you little sense of the main ideas emerging from your data. You will need to develop new codes that divide these themes into smaller components or subthemes.

BOX 6.3

Text with Codes in Margins

ID#RX234
32-year-old married woman
12/11/04
Interviewer: QRM

Text	Codes
Interviewer: Do you have to account for the money you spend?	
Respondent: No, we both . . . when he brings his salary, he tells me that	Financial decision making
[it] is this much; and I also tell him like this. If we have borrowed [money]	Borrowing money
from anybody, we decide together whom to repay. . . . And after all this,	
only one hundred rupees remain from both of our salaries. . . . *(Laughs)*	
Interviewer: In your family, who makes decisions?	
Respondent: We both decide together. He says, "No, we will not do this.	Financial decision making
We will do that instead." Since marriage, I have not bought any new saris.	Control
My brother gives me; my mother-in-law gives me. They also give clothes	Extended family assistance
to my children. We do buy one or two new clothes from our salary, but if	
we do not buy them clothing, my parents or my in-laws give us. My father	Burden on extended family
has four sons and one daughter. He has lots of responsibility. Still, he asks us	Material support
[if we need] food or looks after our needs. If I go to work, they look after	Child care
my children and give [them] food.	
My mother encourages me a lot to do a job. But my husband tells me not	Attitudes toward women
to work, not to work with other men. My husband says, "Whatever will be,	working
will be. You can work after I die. While I am alive, do not work. I do not	Emotional support
like it when you go to work. Now, you are working with other men. . . .	External control
[and] I am not there. If they ask you to go somewhere for a meeting,	
then you will have to go there." So my husband does not like me	Sexual faithfulness
working. He has doubts about me.	
Interviewer: "He has doubts" means . . .	
Respondent: Doubts means . . . I look beautiful. I must be having a	Sexual faithfulness
relationship outside. He wonders why I do not allow him to touch me.	Sexual power
It was written in my fate that I have to work outside and also inside	External control
the house. After all this, I get tired at night. . . . I feel scared that he	HIV risk perception
has this [HIV] and I do not, and during sexual relations, and if the	
condom breaks, then the virus will go inside of me and I will also	Condom use
get this disease. I have two children. All this comes in my mind.	
So I tell him, "I do not want to do [sexual intercourse]. Let me sleep."	Sexual communication
I tell him that I have to go to work in the morning. Then he also says,	
"Even I have to go to work. It is just two minutes' work. What has	Sexual pleasure
happened to you? You must be getting this [sexual pleasure] outside.	
That is why you are acting like this." He will talk like this.	

In our example in Box 6.3, we linked the code "Financial decision making" to the first two paragraphs. However, even within this short textual excerpt, several subthemes appear. For example, two potential subthemes emerge in the first paragraph. They have to do with <Communication about financial matters> and <Ways to cope with financial matters>. A third aspect of financial decision making might include information related to who controls decisions, touched upon in paragraph two. And suppose that additional data from the field suggest that both who makes financial decisions and ways of coping with financial problems depend on the type of decision and potential size of the spending required. Should you incorporate all these subthemes into your coding scheme? Not necessarily. It depends on how often such themes appear across your data and how rich or complex the ideas related to that theme. Comparing the process to a road map, you will create a "map" of your data that allows you to see the layout of the territory, where the main roads (main codes) intersect. Navigation becomes difficult when you use a map with too much detail. That is not to suggest that we will not explore the side roads (or less common subthemes). But we will wait to do so during the data display phase of analysis. (See the discussion of displaying data in this chapter on p. 157.)

Another coding decision is to determine which words to use when labeling your text. If theory has informed your study's design, it may suggest some of the important codes. For example, one theory applicable to women's work and health decisions is health locus of control (Wallston 1978). This theory relates to whether people believe that they or others have control over their health behaviors and outcomes (DeVellis and DeVellis 2000). In the example in Box 6.3, we labeled two sections of text as <External control>, reflected in the husband's reported words "Whatever will be, will be" and the participant's own views that having to work is "written in my fate." Self-efficacy theory has to do with an individual's performance of a particular health measure (for example, modifying what a person eats), as well as his or her perception of the ability to do so (DeVellis and DeVellis 2000). On first reading our sample text, we might be tempted to code text related to abstaining from sex as <Self-efficacy>. However, self-efficacy carries with it the notion that individuals can and should be independent decision makers, a Western notion that may obscure our ability to understand and explain women's decision making in India. Rather than impose deductive codes derived from theory on a piece of text, you may decide to develop labels that emerge from the data or merely describe them. (Codes that emerge from the data are often referred to as inductive codes.) For example, rather than <External control>, you might have used the emergent label <Fate>. The descriptive label <Sexual communication> would allow you to examine all communications between husbands and wives related to whether or not to have sex.

Whether you develop codes deductively, inductively, or in combination, it is helpful to define them. The definition should include information about the code's central meaning and may also provide examples of text considered within and outside the code's parameters. For example, in our study we might define *<Sexual communication>* as including any verbal communication between a couple related to whether or not to have sex, the timing of sex, and sexual behaviors that are accepted or rejected. It would include discussions about condom use. It would not include nonverbal communications. Software programs like N6 (N6 2002), NVivo (NVivo 2002), and AnSWR (McLellan and others 2004) provide templates for recording this kind of information.

The previous paragraphs relate to coding for content, but you may also want to note quality. For example, the participant's description of the couple's financial decision-making process is contradictory. On the one hand, she states that they decide together how to spend household income. Yet she also describes her husband as ultimately controlling decisions and further suggests that she does not purchase things for herself. In what specific ways does this participant take part in decision making? Does she initiate requests or only react to her husband's? Can she make autonomous decisions, and if so, in what circumstances? Why has she not purchased a sari in the last ten years? Has she chosen to forgo her own needs, or have others denied those needs? It is a good idea to capture such questions by inserting or linking memos to the text when data are ambiguous, contradictory, or missing, so that you can attempt to clarify information in continued fieldwork or account for it during the analysis.

THE EVOLVING CODING SCHEME

As additional texts are coded, the researcher will notice that certain labels begin to cluster and others separate out. For example, one might discover that participants report that many different kinds of people (husbands, in-laws, or others) have negative attitudes about women working outside the home and that a widespread concern is that women will succumb to outside sexual enticement if they work beside men. The sheer volume of discussion about sexual infidelity might lead the researcher to develop a new code to capture this idea. On the other hand, the researcher might find that a code that seemed relevant initially rarely emerges in later texts. A qualitative investigator should always be on the alert for new and surprising ideas and be ready to code them accordingly. For this reason a coding scheme is never rigid but evolves over time. (See Buston 1999 for more examples of the evolution of coding.)

It is a good idea to track changes in your coding scheme. One way is to keep a notebook or computer file in which you list each code, its definition, and an example of how it is used, and record any revisions of codes and the dates on which the coder made these revisions. When multiple coders are involved in a study, it is important to involve them as a group in coding decisions so that they understand how to apply codes to text. Be sure that everyone is clear on who has authority to alter the master file with the most updated version of the coding scheme. (See p. 120 in Chapter Five for more on training staff for data analysis.)

Choosing and Using Computer Software

It is possible to conduct qualitative analysis without a computer. For many decades qualitative researchers have used handwritten notes or transcribed verbatim interviews by hand. They have underlined text, written codes into page margins, or otherwise highlighted segments of print to distinguish ideas and messages. They have cut and pasted, sorted, and piled—organizing data around central themes. In fact, some researchers still worry that relying too much on computer shortcuts will impede the process by distancing them from the text.

However, modern computer software programs can ease the burden of cutting and pasting by hand while at the same time producing a vastly more powerful analysis by performing a number of basic data manipulation procedures. Such procedures include creation and insertion of codes into text files, indexing, construction of hyperlinks, and selective retrieval of text segments (Kelle 1997).

Some software packages make the coding process quicker and more consistent. For example, instead of typing every code into computer-stored text files, N6 keeps a record of codes as you create them and allows you to select already created codes from drop-down menus. This feature protects you from inadvertently altering your coding scheme and helps you later to assemble related text segments for further analysis. It also enables you to revise automatically a particular coding label across all previously coded text. One change in the master list changes all occurrences of the code. Other programs with this capability include AnSWR, EZ-Text, and QSR Nvivo.

Another function that most software packages provide is the construction of indexes. An electronic index lists all the substantive words in the text and their locations in terms of specific text, line number, or word position in a line. Once texts have been indexed, you can more easily search and find a specific word or combinations of words or move to the next occurrence of the word or phrase.

Most word processing software enables you to conduct simple word searches. Packages like EZ-Text facilitate such searches by allowing you to do the following:

- Find all words with a similar root: (decide, decision) (deci*)
- Specify a range of synonyms: (money, salary, or rupees)
- Join two concepts together: (deci* or choice) and health
- Restrict the search of one word or phrase to another located within a specified number of words: (deci* or choice) w/5 health

Hyperlinks enable you to cross-reference or link a piece of text in one file with another in the same or a different file. For example, you can write memos about a text segment or identify text from another source that relates to your original segment and then link them. If in separate interviews, for example, a husband and wife talk about how household decisions are made, you can link text segments from the two interviews for comparison. Hyperlinks also are used to link codes and their related text segments to one another. A number of software programs permit hierarchical ordering of codes. That is, you can identify a general code <Decision making> and link subcategories of codes <Joint, husband-controlled, wife-controlled> under the main heading. Depending on what your data say, you may find that each of these three approaches to decision making occurs in your data; no visible pattern exists in the different approaches. Or you may find that women in the study tend to describe decision making as husband-controlled, whereas husbands were more likely to describe joint or wife-controlled patterns. Some packages allow text segments to be linked to each other without using codes, or they enable you to build nonhierarchical networks of codes or text segments (Kelle 1997).

ADVANTAGES OF CONTINUOUS CODING

Continuous coding as data collection proceeds has many advantages. First, it imposes a systematic approach, assisting the analyst to identify gaps or questions while it is still possible to return to the field for more data. Continuously reviewing the coding structure in light of new texts may also reveal early biases and help you move beyond them, allowing you to redefine concepts without imposing unnecessary structure. As MacQueen notes in a field perspective at the end of this chapter, some software packages make it easier to code texts and revise coding schemes as you go.

For practical reasons researchers sometimes wait until all the data have been collected before starting to code. A transcription service may require you to submit all transcripts at one time rather than sequentially. However, coding cannot begin until you have text, whether handwritten or typed into a computer. Waiting too long to type your notes could cost you the opportunity to revise and refine your questions and thereby gain richer information on your research topic. In this situation good field notes and regular reviews of notes as a team are critically important.

CODING SORTS: BUILDING THEME-RELATED FILES

As you read, reread, and code text, begin to formulate ideas about what the data are telling you. You are then ready to start a more formal analysis, examining separately and fully each important theme as it emerges from the data. The first step is to conduct a coding sort, which is a collection of similarly coded blocks of text entered into new data files. Coding sorts can be done manually, using highlighting or cut-and-paste techniques; with simple word processing; or with qualitative text analysis software. In fact, most qualitative software packages enable you to generate different kinds of coding reports, from a report on an individual code that includes all relevant text segments (what we are calling a coding sort) to reports with summary information about the frequency with which codes appear in your data set.

Tip: Concentrate on one coding sort at a time—selecting the most central themes to begin with and then working your way out to related themes as they appear important. If you work in this fashion, you will begin to see how certain themes connect.

Box 6.4 shows an example from the microbicide trial, in which a coding sort has been developed to label text concerning whether a woman can use a vaginal gel without her partner's knowledge. We name this theme <Secret Use>. The transcribed and translated conversation is adapted from a multicountry focus group study that examined the acceptability of this new microbicide product to married couples in two African and two Asian countries (Bentley and others 2000).

We constructed this coding sort by blocking and copying computer text segments from original transcript files into a new computer file. If you do this work manually, you will need to enter identifiers that indicate the original source files for each block of text in the new, sorted file. However, many qualitative analysis software programs track this information for you. In Box 6.4 note that each block of text is identified by country, sex of group, and a group identification number. Letters or numbers typed into the original transcripts identify participants while ensuring confidentiality. When the speaker's identity is unknown, we have used a question mark.

BOX 6.4

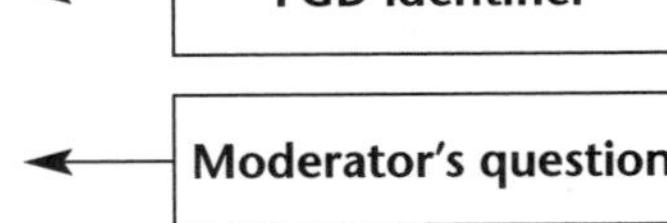

Coding Sort to Label Text by Theme

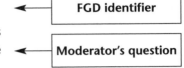

Segment 1. Country 1: Male Focus Group Discussion (FGD) 1 (Eight Participants) ← **FGD identifier**

Let us imagine the study is completed, and one day your wife secretly inserts this gel. Will you be able to tell that she has applied the gel when you have sex with her? ← **Moderator's question**

E: There will be no difference. The pleasure will be the same.

J: I will not be able to notice the difference.

?: We cannot know, since women are usually wet during sex. We can't tell if it is because of the gel or not.

H: I think it is possible to notice, because there is a difference in the sexual feeling when the gel is applied and without the gel. I will feel some changes because of the gel.

Participant ID (→ *J:*, *H:*)

Segment 2. Country 1: Female FGD 1 (Eight Participants)

In the future this product may be available for use without [having to use] condoms. So we would like to know whether you would be able to use this product without your partner's knowledge.

S: It would not be good for me to use the product without my partner knowing, because we are one body. And I would be in trouble if he discovers that I am using a product that he doesn't know about. But if I tell him, everything will be fine, and he will be aware of whatever is happening.

V: If this product was on the market and I used it without my partner wearing a condom, can't he develop sores on his penis?

Segment 3. Country 2: Male FGD 1 (Seven Participants)

Do you think that it is possible for a woman to use the product without her husband's or partner's knowledge?

No. 5: It is not possible, because if you find out later on . . . you might start suspecting that there is something wrong in her body. So she should tell you, "We are doing this." And then you agree. If she has a disease, she should tell me that she has a disease. Then we go together and seek treatment.

No. 6: For a woman to use [it] without your knowledge, aaah, I don't think that is fair. As a couple, we are one when we are in this house. If there is something you have to do, don't do it without telling your partner. . . . I don't want to find out about it accidentally. That is not good.

There are some who are not married but have girlfriends. Do you think that such a girl can use it without her partner's knowledge?

No. 5: Aaah, it depends on the girlfriend—whether she is a genuine girlfriend or she just does what girls do nowadays. Because if she is your real girlfriend, a man and woman who love each other, she should tell her partner about what she wants to do. But if she is like these prostitutes . . .

Let's say your wife just uses it, but you have sex. You, as a man, would you be able to tell that something has been used?

No. 6: You can feel it. Because with someone you have known for a while, you know what she is like.

No. 2: I would add that the sexual pleasure changes and the wetness.

Who has the power to decide whether the product should be used or not?

No. 3: The man has the power. He has the power because the woman cannot say that she wants to use it. What does she want to prevent? Because it is for preventing the virus.

In most qualitative studies, coding sorts consist of numerous text segments for each theme. The three segments in our example have been selected to illustrate how comments on one theme, clandestine microbicide use, can be identified in different transcripts and clustered in a single file.

SELECTING THE RIGHT SOFTWARE

Box 6.5 summarizes characteristics of four commonly used qualitative software packages: EZ-Text, Ethnograph, N6, and NVivo. Among the numerous computer text-analysis tools available to the qualitative researcher, these four are widely available and represent a range of data analysis needs from the relatively simple to the more complex. At one end of the spectrum, CDC EZ-Text is a good choice when the analysis plan is relatively simple and straightforward. This program works well for data that have been collected using a tightly structured guide in the same sequence and format for all interviews or focus groups in the study. Transcripts therefore should be focused, with clear links between questions and participants' answers or between codes and specific questions. Given these criteria, EZ-Text will allow you to organize data, search files, and retrieve information. Users, in fact, have referred to this software as "an electronic file cabinet," suggesting that although limited in application, EZ-Text has proven its usefulness in certain types of research.

In a file of moderate size (see field perspective in this chapter titled What to Look for in Qualitative Data Analysis on p. 172), the Ethnograph (Seidel 1998) can take the analysis farther. This software allows you to segment and sort data, focusing on small parts of the whole, noticing details and discovering relationships among different segments. As analysis progresses, you will begin to identify patterns and sequences that may lead to new coding schemes, new iterations, and new discoveries. The Ethnograph was one of the first programs to enable the analyst to identify overlapping themes and subthemes. A simple pencil-and-paper analysis can reveal broad thematic issues, but to look into and beneath an issue for closely related or overlapping ideas (subthemes) requires the precision of computer text analysis. The Ethnograph is more appropriately used by a single analyst than a research team, and intercoder reliability is more difficult to assess.

N6, formerly Nud*ist, is capable of handling not only a simple analysis but more complex data sets as well, including those with relatively little structure. Interviews or group discussions may have been free-flowing exchanges, ranging across many aspects of the topics presented, not necessarily in a predictable order. Themes and subthemes may appear in different parts of a file, scattered throughout the transcript. In qualitative research this apparent inconsistency is, in reality, an indication of richness and depth of expression in the data. However, the text-analysis program must have the power to disentangle the natural flow of the discussion and reassemble segments in a thematic scheme. N6 has this capacity for large, complex data sets, along with other useful features summarized in Box 6.6.

NVivo (2002) is similar to QSR N6 software and produced by the same company. NVivo has additional features, such as the ability to create models based on analysis, create matrices of data according to codes, and display all the codes that have been assigned to text documents while working in the document. Like QSR N6, because coded segments point directly to the full text document from which they derive, the

BOX 6.5

Comparison of Four Text Analysis Software Packages

Program characteristics	CDC EZ-Text	Ethnograph	QSR N6 (Formerly Nud*ist)	NVivo
Cost and availability*	Free download at http://www.cdc.gov/hiv/software/ez-text.htm.	Single user: $295; five pack: $1,180.	Single user: $340; five-user site license: $1,200.	Single user: $445; five-user site license: $1,565. (does not include maintenance and merge tool).
Text	Direct entry.	ASCII plus special formatting rules, can be done semiautomatically in the built-in editor or using cut and paste.	ASCII (.txt) plus special formatting rules to preformat text units.	Rich text format (RTF) plus special formatting rules to preformat sections.
Text units	Each answer is a single unit.	One line (forty-two characters).	Preselected before you start coding. Can be paragraph, line, or sentence.	Select as you code
Coding	Enter by selecting from a precreated list of alphabetically sorted codes.	Mark text with the mouse or enter start and stop lines.	Mark text with the mouse or enter start and stop lines.	Mark text with the mouse.
Analysis	Single code searches. Boolean operators can be used.	Single or multiple code searches.	Single or multiple code searches, with seventeen available operators.	Single or multiple codes, with Boolean and proximity operators. Modeling possible.
Sociodemographic data	Separate data entry for each file.	Demographic data can be added for each document or speaker within a document. Searches can be done using this data as filter.	No separate data entry for demographic data. Coding for demographic data can be automated.	Attributes can be assigned to documents and nodes.
Reports	Reports are generated by code, question, or ID.	Report shows complete information on text and displays coding stripes. Reports can be saved as ASCII (.txt) files.	Search results are saved as a node. These nodes can be browsed or saved as ASCII (.txt) files.	Search results are saved as a node. These nodes can be browsed or saved as rich text files.
Working in teams	Within specified limits, data files generated by different interviewers can be merged for multisite analysis.	Very limited.	Project merging is possible, and intercoder agreement can be assessed.	Project merging is possible, and intercoder agreement can be assessed. Different levels of responsibility and access can be assigned to different users.
Support	Help file, manual.	Help file, manual.	Help file, manual, tutorial, user listserv.	Help file, manual, tutorial, user listserv.

* Prices listed are from March 2004.

Source: Adapted from QDA software overview, March 2004. Available at http://www.quarc.de/body_overview.html.

BOX 6.6

Example of a Matrix Summarizing Data on Secret Use

Country 2	Not Possible	Possibility Not Ruled Out
Women		
Group 1	He will feel it.	Consensus unclear. (1/23/99, p. 24)
Group 2	Dangerous to do w/o your partner's knowledge. He may ask you to leave the house! He will catch you using [it]; he will divorce you [b/c assuming female promiscuity]. Better to be honest with him. (4/24/99 pp. 39–40)	If he feels that, it may cause problems. (p. 27) If a small amount, he may not notice.
Men		
Group 1	It cannot be done.	If she uses gel without my knowledge, she is not my real wife. (4/25/99 p. 23)
Group 2	I will feel something. . . . why did it get wet so quickly? You can feel the difference. Sexual pleasure changes.	It is not possible b/c if you find out later on, you might suspect something wrong with her body . . . I don't think that is fair.

full document is immediately available when clicking on a coded text segment. This approach also facilitates an iterative coding process, because reports on coded data can be further coded for finer levels of analysis. NVivo and QSR N6 both include mechanisms for developing and maintaining a comprehensive codebook and are an appropriate choice for qualitative computer modeling.

AnSWR (McLellan and others 2004) is a qualitative data analysis software package that is designed specifically for large, complex projects. Developed at the U.S. Centers for Disease Control and Prevention (CDC), AnSWR includes components that facilitate team-based research at multiple sites. In addition to a coding editor that allows flexible segmenting and coding of ASCII text (.txt) files, rich text format (.rtf) files, HTML documents, Microsoft Word or Excel documents, AnSWR has fully integrated quantitative data components, including the ability to build data entry screens.

A structured codebook format facilitates team-based codebook development and intercoder comparisons. Reporting options are flexible, with multiple selection criteria (files, codes, coders, and quantitative variables). Many of the reports include summary graphs. A unique feature of AnSWR is the Sensitive Phrase Substitution option that allows coding of sensitive data with user-designated substitution on reports. AnSWR is not for the novice computer user or faint of heart, however; there is minimal documentation and user support. But it is free for downloading from the CDC Web site at http://www.cdc.gov/hiv/software/answr.htm.

Displaying Data: Distinguishing Nuances of a Topic

Having extracted and combined all the information on a theme in a coding sort, you are ready to examine the theme more closely. Displaying data means laying out or taking an inventory of what you know related to a theme; capturing the variation, or richness, of each theme; separating qualitative and quantitative aspects; and noting differences between individuals or among subgroups. One way to approach the data-display phase is to develop detailed memos related to each main code in your coding scheme. Similar to the coding phase, the first step of data display is to identify the principal subthemes that emerge from the data, only this time you are working within a single coding sort rather than across all your textual data. In our illustration of the coding sort in Box 6.4, participants are expressing opinions on whether it is possible or feasible for a woman to use the microbicide gel in secret. Because most participants have taken a clear stand on this issue, their responses could initially be classified as supporting or rejecting clandestine use. As analysis continues, you will identify subthemes that reflect finer distinctions, for example, reasons for support or rejection of gel use.

Once you have identified a code's principal subthemes, return to the data and examine the evidence that supports each subtheme, both quantitatively and qualitatively. Quantitative aspects of a theme might include information about frequency or duration, size or quantity of a phenomenon. A qualitative examination of each would include attention to specific vocabulary that participants use to discuss the topic. Consider differences in the intensity or emphasis with which participants express an idea. Notice whether they relate an attitude or experience first- or secondhand. Examine the text for nuance, identifying different contexts in which the phenomenon occurs and consider what was not said. An example of how a researcher might flesh out details on the theme of secret use follows.

QUANTITATIVE EXAMINATION OF SECRET USE

Although treatment of quantitative data is beyond the scope of this book, in the example here it might include a variety of analysis techniques including frequency distributions of important codes, cluster analysis of themes, and multidimensional scaling. Whether or not more sophisticated approaches are used, it is important to determine how commonly themes occur in the data and whether they tend to emerge in specific subgroups, through particular data collection methods, or more generally across groups and methods.

Secret Use Might Be Possible At first glance it appears that most participants believed that the product could not be used without a partner's knowledge. Only three participants from one group, the men's group from Country 1, directly stated that "we cannot know" when a woman uses the microbicide.

Secret Use Not Possible At least some participants in all the groups believed that the product could not be used secretly. Though the majority remained silent on the subject, about one-third said they were fairly certain that a partner would discover secret use.

QUALITATIVE ANALYSIS OF SECRET USE

Secret Use Not Possible Two reasons emerged to explain why most participants believed clandestine use would not be possible. One concerned physical signs of microbicide use, namely that the male partner would feel "something different"—particularly if he were not wearing a condom. (Most participants in this conversation were somewhat vague about what exactly the man would feel.) One woman was worried that he might develop sores from direct contact with the gel. The same woman felt that some of the gel might leak out, and a man suggested that the amount of wetness would change. All discussions of this idea were short, emotionally detached—even rather clinical.

The second reason that participants considered secret use of the product impossible related to betrayal of the emotional bond between a man and woman and expectations about that relationship. In fact, participants offered such concerns more as an objection to secret use than belief that it would be impossible. They relate to the subtheme of partner bonding, which both men and women raised with comments such as these: "It is better for us to know as a family." "Our partners are part of our body." "As a couple, we are one when we are in this house." "If she is your real girlfriend. . . ." "If you have known (her) for a while, you know what she is like."

Included in the concept of partner bonding is the idea of obligation and an element of fear if that obligation is breached. For example, women remarked, "I would be in trouble if he discovers," and "He should not be disappointed." Men also implied that such a breach could have negative consequences for a woman. They commented, "You might start suspecting," and "I don't want to find out about it accidentally. That is not good." Such comments also hinted at the importance to men of control in the relationship, another subtheme that invites further exploration.

Secret Use Might Be Possible Several men indicated that they might not be able to detect microbicide use: "The pleasure will be the same," "Women are usually wet during sex." There was also some suggestion that secret use of microbicides might be acceptable in certain relationships but not without risk. One man suggested that "a woman who doesn't love you"—a prostitute—might not inform you that she is using it. Without explicitly stating it, he seemed to suggest that a man might be unable to detect a prostitute's use of microbicide.

Others implied that a wife who does not consult her husband about such matters might succeed in hiding it for a while but not in the long term and that the consequences of detection could be serious. It would break the bond between husband and wife. "If you find she uses the gel without my knowledge, she is not my real wife. Your real wife would not fail to tell you what she is doing." For a woman, it would risk her security: "He will catch you using [it], and he will divorce you." "It is dangerous to do something without your partner's knowledge."

Alternative Responses Some women and men redefined the question. Instead of focusing on secret use, several women talked about women's need for protection when their partners are unfaithful. A woman in one group and a man in another both suggested that changing risky behavior is better than using a microbicide, clandestine or not. Other participants said that a partner's unfaithful behavior is reason enough for a woman to use a microbicide. (Whether it can be used secretly is unclear.) For some men a woman's infidelity is reason to deny her use of the gel, because it would only reinforce her assumed promiscuity.

Developing Hypotheses, Questioning, and Verifying

We have shown how, by clustering segments around a theme, <Secret use>, you can extract meaning from data. As you continue organizing information associated with each theme, you will start to form hypotheses—hunches about the data that you want to investigate further. In fact, throughout the entire process of collecting, reading, coding, and displaying data, the qualitative researcher is formulating questions, interpreting responses, developing theoretical explanations, and trying to validate or reject emerging conclusions.

- Do the categories that I have developed make sense?
- What pieces of information contradict my emerging ideas?
- What pieces of information are missing or underdeveloped?
- What other opinions should I take into account?
- How do my own biases influence the data collection and analysis process?

ATTENTION TO DATA CREDIBILITY

How do you determine whether a research participant is giving you a credible response to a question? How do you make sense from the jumble of responses from different groups or individuals? Not all responses should be treated equally. It is important to examine how information was elicited and how it was delivered. Information is likely to be more credible when the following apply:

- The participant is responding to open-ended questions rather than highly suggestive ones.
- He is talking about his own beliefs, motivations, or experiences rather than someone else's.
- She does not contradict herself in subsequent dialogue.
- He speaks in detail rather than generalities.

The microbicide study contained contradictions in the data regarding whether physical signs of product use would be visible to a partner. A minority indicated that they would not be visible, but some said that condom use (advised to all participants in this clinical trial for ethical reasons) would mask the wetness of the gel. Data collectors could have probed more fully, comparing the perceptions of couples who failed to use condoms consistently with those who said they always used condoms. Another potential biasing factor could have been the selection requirement that women obtain their partner's approval to participate in the trial. It is not surprising, therefore, that many women in this sample rejected the possibility of secret microbicide use. Would women outside the clinical trial see more potential in secret use? Would women in the trial answer differently if they were interviewed individually rather than in focus group discussions or if their partners were not also participating in the trial?

It is important to weigh the credibility of your data as you interpret what you hear and attempt to confirm early conclusions. From a tactical perspective, it is helpful to question your data at every stage of the analysis. Some researchers enter questions, uncertainties, and misgivings directly into their transcripts, distinguishing commentary from raw data with brackets or parentheses, setting them in italic or bold type. Others link interpretive information as separate memos. As you review transcripts, if you are still collecting data, you can integrate new or revised questions into the interview or discussion process. On the other hand, if data collection is complete and you are now working from the coding sorts, you may want to enter separate memos about emerging conclusions, reminding yourself to return to your raw data for evidence to validate or reject your ideas.

Data Reduction: Getting the Big Picture

Data reduction is the process of distilling the information to make visible the most essential concepts and relationships. Along the way you have read through transcripts, identified important themes and developed a coding system to mark these themes. You have sorted data from your original transcripts into new files organized by theme. You have explored the rich variation of each thematic file, identifying key concepts and discovering the perspectives of different subgroups in your study.

It is time to step back from the data. The reduction process usually happens once all the data are in and you have become familiar with their content. The goal now is to get an overall sense of the data and distinguish central and secondary themes. This is also a process of separating the essential from the nonessential. To get this wider perspective on the data, using visual devices is often helpful (Ryan and Bernard 2000).

One such visual approach to data reduction is to develop matrices, diagrams, or taxonomies for each thematic file that has remained central to the study. We return to the microbicide example. Box 6.6 is an illustration of one approach to data reduction: a matrix constructed for the code <Secret use>. For one country (Country 2), it identifies key phrases that relate to the theme's two main components: (1) secret use not possible or feasible under certain conditions and (2) possibility of secret use not ruled out. Page references identify the comment's source in the text file. If more than one focus group participant has expressed essentially the same idea, it is noted after the phrase. By including other countries or population segments in this matrix, the researcher is able to visualize and compare responses across different groups and subgroups.

A matrix enables the researcher to assemble a lot of related text fragments in one place, abbreviating comments from the coding sorts to reduce a complicated data set to a manageable size. Other matrices that we developed for this study included acceptability of the gel and intentions about using it if available, experiences with actual use, effect of product use on sexual experience, and one-word descriptors that participants used to describe the product. Some software makes it easy to develop such matrices, although they can also be developed by hand. Although the process can be time-consuming, data reduction helps the researcher establish the boundaries of important themes. In fact, when multiple researchers are involved in the analysis process, each can pursue different themes and present findings to the group. Lively discussion may ensue as the group explores how themes connect, overlap, or contradict each other.

Although it makes sense to develop matrices to capture the essence of some themes, different mechanisms may be more appropriate for other themes. For example, the code <Financial decision making> emerged from the earlier study on women's work and health care decision making. Further analysis of that code identified several approaches to financial decision making, including one in which husband and wife confer beforehand on purchases and have the ability to veto a partner's wishes (<Joint>), one in which the husband controls all decisions (<Husband controlled>), and one in which the wife controls decisions (<Wife controlled>). The diagram in Box 6.7 helps us clarify the relationships among these three different decision-making approaches. It suggests that husbands maintain a central role in most household financial decisions. In households with a joint decision-making process, women may have some influence over the purchase of expensive items like televisions, vehicles, or land. It also suggests that some women are able to exercise complete control over some household decisions, but these tend to be the day-to-day purchase of food and household items or school supplies. Finally, some husbands relegated day-to-day household decision making to their wives, while controlling the amount of funds they could spend and expecting a regular accounting of spending.

Data reduction may not be necessary for all codes; some may be discrete enough that further refinement is not needed. The code <One-word descriptors> used in the microbicide study would be one such example. Other codes may contain multiple ideas and necessitate development of several different matrices, diagrams, or taxonomies in order to reduce complex constructs to main themes and subthemes.

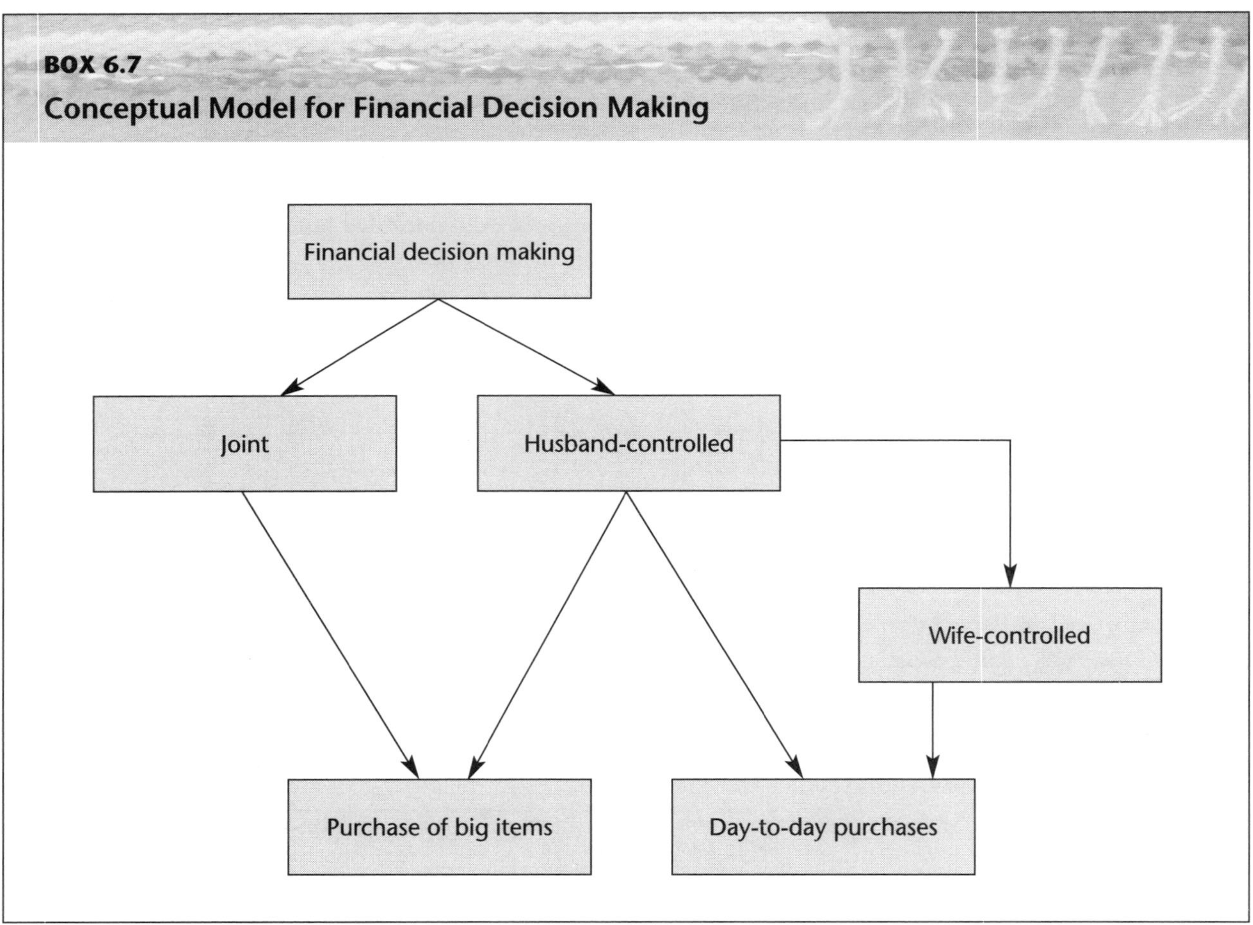

Interpretation

In this last section, on interpretation, we focus on three issues: how to arrive at the essential meanings of qualitative data, how to ensure that the interpretation you offer is trustworthy, and how to interpret data when your study has used both qualitative and quantitative methods.

Interpretation is the act of identifying and explaining the data's core meaning. It involves communicating the study's essential ideas to a wider audience, remaining faithful to your participants' perspectives. The purpose of interpretation is not simply to list a handful (or pages full) of interesting themes and their examples, leaving readers to draw their own conclusions. Rather, it is to identify ways that the many different pieces of the research puzzle (emerging themes and subthemes, connections, and contradictions) fit and what it all means. Although the meaning that you extract from your analysis should reflect the intent of your study participants' responses, it must also have relevance to a larger population and provide answers to questions of social and theoretical significance.

Developing credible or trustworthy interpretations of qualitative research includes arriving at understandings that would make sense to the men and women who have agreed to be observed, answer questions, or participate in other ways in the study. Of course, some comments may reveal that some or all study participants do not want certain information acknowledged and will publicly deny or suppress it. Such might be the case, for example, if release of findings could undermine the relatively more powerful or privileged positions that certain individuals hold over others. Conversely, participants might deny or want to suppress information if they fear it will put less-advantaged individuals or groups at greater physical or social risk. In such situations checking the trustworthiness of your interpretations against community understandings may be difficult. In addition, credibility of qualitative results does not necessarily mean that the findings are reproducible. Other researchers might examine the same data and interpret them differently. Contradiction in this case is similar to arriving at different quantitative conclusions when researchers have used different statistical analysis techniques. In both qualitative and quantitative scenarios, the researcher must reevaluate the first analysis, looking for factors that contribute to the different results, use his or her best judgment in deciding which procedure to favor, and present the process for external scrutiny. This convention is inherent to scientific method and the generation of knowledge.

When both qualitative and quantitative data have been collected and analyzed, the interpretive process must include integration of the two types of data. Qualitative and quantitative researchers working together identify where different approaches produce similar or complementary findings and where they are contradictory. When findings are contradictory, the researchers must decide how or whether to reconcile or prioritize them to arrive at an overall interpretation of study findings.

SYNTHESIZING FINDINGS: GAPS AND CONNECTIONS

Following the steps recommended in this chapter, you have read and reread your texts and developed and refined codes, noting the detail of each coded theme and extracting the central ideas. Novice researchers are often tempted to conclude their qualitative analysis at this stage, presenting a list of themes and examples with little thought as to how the elements of the analysis fit together as a whole. But as experienced qualitative researchers know, the main task now is to search for relationships among themes or concepts identified from the analysis. Doing so can be difficult because of the large number of themes and subthemes that often emerge in qualitative research. One way to accomplish this step is to develop diagrams or other visual representations that map out relationships in the data.

In qualitative research on adolescent abortion, teams from two West African countries conducted a study to identify social, economic, and cultural factors that led to unwanted pregnancy and resulted in illegal abortion for some unmarried adolescents (Tolley and others 1998). A number of themes emerged, including the following:

- Adult and adolescent perceptions of current sexual mores
- Boys' and girls' expectations about relationships with the opposite sex
- The role of economic pressures and how they influence decisions about sexual partnerships, contraception, and pregnancy outcomes
- Communication patterns between adolescents, teachers, and parents about sexual and other issues

- Adolescent and adult knowledge about reproduction and contraception, as well as abortion techniques
- Reported contraceptive behavior
- Providers' attitudes and behaviors related to reproductive health services for adolescents
- Adolescents' experiences with clandestine abortions

The researchers struggled to make sense of so many different themes, wondering how to present them in a way that a larger audience could understand them and find them useful. Through the process of coding and sorting data and developing thematic matrices and diagrams, they found that three contextual factors seemed to explain differences in adolescent sexual behavior and reproductive decision making: differences in how boys and girls are socialized, economic differences, and the influence of adults and peers. Teachers, parents, and youth differed in their opinions on why or under what circumstances adolescent couples had sexual relations, how they made (or avoided making) decisions that might lead to pregnancy, and how they eventually made the choice to keep or abort the pregnancy. However, their different perspectives could be explained by examining sexual relations, contraceptive use, and pregnancy-related decisions through the lens of three broad areas: economic roles, gender roles, and social norms.

After several attempts at creating a visual representation of the pattern they found in the themes, the research teams developed the diagram in Box 6.8. The centrality of contraceptive use (or its lack of use) as a pathway to pregnancy enabled the researchers to focus on their findings' policy implications. This diagram gave them a central organizational structure for presenting all their data. The final report then summarized in greater detail how each of the three sets of factors influenced sexual and contraceptive behavior and decisions related to pregnancy outcome.

INTERPRETATION OF QUALITATIVE DATA IN A MIXED-METHOD DESIGN

Before linking the findings from qualitative and quantitative data analysis in a mixed-method study, it makes sense first to analyze each data set separately according to procedures associated with its paradigm (see Chapter Two). How you then integrate these findings is guided by the purpose of each component in the study design. Their respective purposes influence whether qualitative and quantitative components will have equal weight in the study design, whether one is primary and the other secondary, and whether qualitative and quantitative components are conducted sequentially or at the same time (see Mixing Methods section on pp. 45–49 in Chapter Three).

Often the two components of a mixed-method design are conducted sequentially, but one is considered the main study (see Box 3.6, p. 48). If, for example, qualitative data were first collected to inform development of structured data collection instruments for a quantitative survey on teenage drug use, analysis would focus on identifying those issues that lead young people to consider, try, continue using, or reject drugs. It would investigate the ways adolescents obtain drugs, as well as the language they use

BOX 6.8

Using a Diagram to Organize Findings

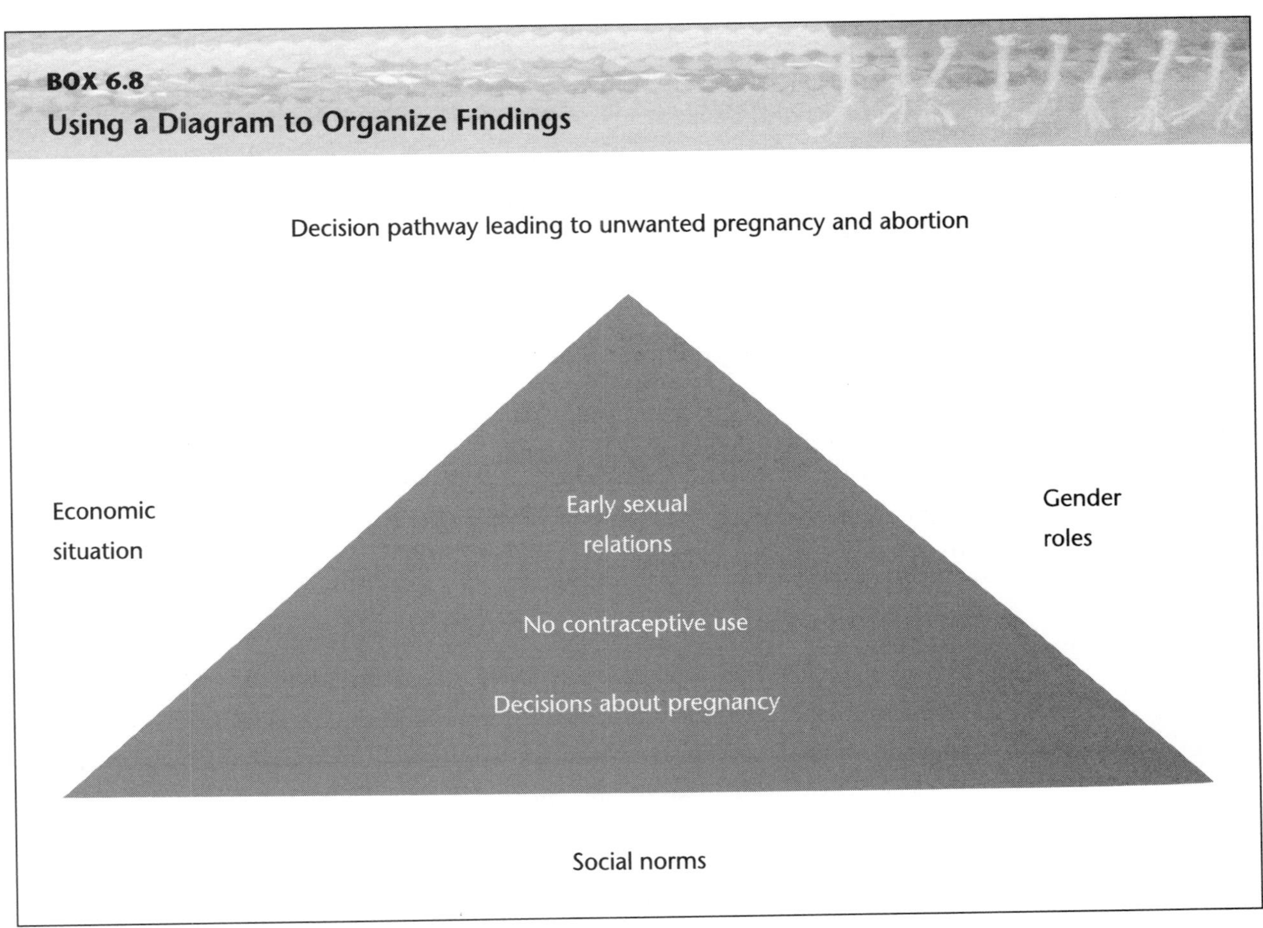

to talk about such issues. Qualitative analysis would then be completed first, resulting in a list of topics, perhaps even specific questions with a range of structured responses—words or phrases, examples, or metaphors that the intended audience could easily understand. On the other hand, if the results of a regional stratified random sample survey among middle and high school students suggested that drug use were particularly high within several school districts, qualitative research might be conducted after the survey to help explain district-level differences in drug use, focusing on school and community-based drug policies; the availability of extracurricular activities for adolescents; the characteristics of adolescent peer networks; and other emergent issues.

When qualitative and quantitative analyses are conducted sequentially, or when one set of analyses clearly dominates the study design, linking the findings from the two research approaches can be fairly straightforward. However, linking qualitative and quantitative findings may prove more challenging when both methods in the study design have equal status (Tashakkori and Teddlie 1998) or when they are conducted in parallel. In these more truly integrated studies, a combination of methods may be used to confirm research findings or to increase their explanatory power.

Difficulty arises when qualitative and quantitative methods uncover dissimilar or even contradictory conclusions. What should a researcher do when the data do not agree? A first step is to look for explanations that reconcile initially contradictory explanations. Reconciling the findings may require additional analyses of either or both types of data. In the field perspective on rapid analysis in South Africa at the end of this chapter, qualitative findings on women's feelings of vulnerability and the difficulty of negotiating condom use conflicted with the quantitative finding that protection from STIs was within most respondents' control. After returning to the qualitative data and examining the language that women used to express their understanding of control, the researcher concluded that most women were giving hypothetical answers to the structured (quantitative) questions on control of STI prevention methods. They also appeared to have answered these questions from the standpoint of desired rather than actual decision-making responsibility. Another way to resolve contradictions is to stratify or regroup quantitative data for further analysis on the basis of the qualitative results. Or you can stratify the qualitative results by significant predictive variables in the quantitative analysis.

But despite all attempts to reconcile contradiction, different findings are sometimes irreconcilable. In such cases we advise the researcher to present the divergent interpretations and allow readers to draw their own conclusions. It is especially important in this situation to provide sufficient information on the data collection and analysis strategies to allow readers to evaluate for themselves the credibility of your interpretations and perhaps to arrive at different conclusions. Following are ways to maximize the credibility of your qualitative findings.

ESTABLISHING TRUSTWORTHINESS

Analyzing qualitative data is intense. Having immersed yourself in a process of reading and rereading, labeling, dissecting, questioning, and synthesizing, you may find it difficult to step far enough back from your emerging interpretations to determine their ultimate trustworthiness.

In Chapter Two we introduced four criteria—credibility, dependability, confirmability, and transferability—by which to assess the truth value of qualitative findings. We now return to these four criteria and show how to incorporate them into the analysis.

Credibility Credible interpretations of qualitative data offer explanations that are consistent with the data collected and are understandable to people in the study population. Such interpretations are contextually rich. They are sensitive to differing perspectives in the study sample, perspectives that sometimes diverge or even clash. Credible interpretations develop explanations that somehow reconcile or show how divergent findings relate to the context under study.

There are several techniques for ensuring that interpretation is credible: (1) looking for negative cases for emerging hypotheses; (2) testing rival explanations; and (3) seeking explanations for inconsistencies arising from triangulation of respondents, methods, theories, or researchers (Patton 1999; Kidder 1981; Krueger 1998).

In a study to assess the quality of Norplant services in Senegal, for example, one issue we examined was access to Norplant removal after fewer than five years of use

(Tolley and Nare 2001). (Norplant is a system of five capsules containing progesterone that are implanted just under the skin of the upper arm and provide contraceptive protection for five years.) The study included a group of women who currently were using the method, a second group who had discontinued Norplant after five years, and a third group who had used the method less than three years before stopping. It also included providers.

All providers recognized—in principle—that a woman has the right to have her implants removed whenever she wants. However, on further probing, fewer than a third of providers said they told their clients that they could request removals at any time for any reason. Interviews with current and past Norplant users confirmed that few providers gave them information on Norplant removal. In addition, reports from some past users that they had trouble convincing providers to remove their implants early led us to speculate that women were actively discouraged from using Norplant fewer than five years. However, our data showed that some early discontinuers had little or no problem getting their implants removed.

We delved further into the stories of early discontinuers who did and did not have problems. Most women who had problems said they requested removal because of increased bleeding. In contrast, most women who obtained removal easily did so for other reasons, either to improve their health or to get pregnant. Furthermore, almost all women who gave health-related reasons had stopped using the method on the physician's advice, not at their own request. Were there any exceptions? We returned to the transcripts to find that one woman had, in fact, requested removal of Norplant on her own volition because she could not tolerate changes to her menstrual cycle. Her situation seemed different from other women in the study. She herself was in the medical profession, and her colleague had removed the implants.

By looking for cases of women who got their implants removed early without objections from providers, we arrived at three interwoven notions related to Norplant removal. One was that providers often held different views from users about acceptable and unacceptable reasons to discontinue the method. The second was that women differed in their ability to negotiate removal for reasons that providers might not view as important. The third was that users often resorted to strategic explanations for their desire to have it removed. Thus, closer analysis revealed that these seemingly contradictory results did, in fact, reflect real issues for users.

Showing that you have moved beyond your initial understanding of a research question to gain a more in-depth perspective also builds credibility. One way to show this progression is to consciously compare your final interpretation with what you first expected to find. By identifying and documenting your motivations, interests, and perspectives initially and throughout the research process, you will be better able to navigate around those biases to represent the study respondents more fully and credibly. Some researchers write down what they expect to find before implementing the study. If you find no surprises in the data, no contradictions or revisions to theories, then you may not have dug deeply enough but instead discovered only what you originally set out to discover (Lincoln and Guba 1999).

Dependability In quantitative research an important test of reliability is the extent to which findings can be replicated. The goal is not only to replicate the results of a study (which, given intervening time and change, may not be perfectly possible) but to be able to replicate the processes used to obtain these results (King and others 1994).

To increase the dependability of qualitative findings, on the other hand, you might incorporate a team approach or use multiple independent coders or analysts. This tactic will help to offset the subjective bias of any one researcher. The process of resolving differences in interpretation can be a check against individual bias to some degree, but differences in individual power or status might still influence process. Or you may have a second independent investigator analyze data. This allows you to reduce the potential for individual influence over interpretation, but there is no way to rectify differences in independent interpretations. If two significantly different interpretations of the data emerge, you might need to resort to a third independent investigator or present both interpretations of the results, allowing the reader to draw conclusions from both perspectives.

Qualitative researchers should also address issues of process dependability—other scientists' ability to replicate the study procedures. Because qualitative data collection is often more fluid and researcher-dependent than quantitative interviewing, such documentation should include information about the researcher's background and professional and project-specific training. Other important information includes field decisions to change methods, revise questions, and so forth. For example, in the Norplant study cited earlier, we originally intended to use the same technique (focus group discussion) to gather information from current method users—those who had completed four or five years of use—as well as from early discontinuers. During pretesting, however, we discovered that women who had stopped using the method early were not showing up for group discussions. In follow-up visits to these women, we discovered that many were anxious about sharing personal opinions and experiences in a larger group. Most, however, were willing to talk to us privately in their homes.

Confirmability By definition qualitative research recognizes the researcher's central role in defining issues for study, interpreting information, and guiding the research process. Qualitative researchers do not claim to be detached and neutral scientists, unencumbered by their own experiences and values. They do believe, however, that by being conscious of their own subjectivity, they can better understand and limit its effects on their research activities (from data collection to analysis), thereby allowing participants to express their experiences, values, and expectations without constraint. Qualitative researchers can check whether they have sufficiently maintained the distinction between their own and their subjects' ideas by opening the study process to outside inspection and verification.

One such approach is the audit trail (Lincoln and Guba 1985). An *audit trail* is a record that enables you and others to track the process that has led to your conclusions. It is created from notes and other field materials collected and stored along the way. Six categories of information contribute to a good audit trail:

- Raw data—uncoded transcripts, tape recordings, field observation notes
- Data reduction and analysis products—list of codes, theoretical notes about working hypotheses, matrices
- Data reconstruction and synthesis products—diagrams and notes showing how different themes relate, a final report
- Process notes—methodological notes, notes about trustworthiness, audit notes
- Materials relating to intentions and dispositions—study protocol, personal notes about motives and expectations of the study
- Instrument development information—interview guides, data collection protocols

An audit trail also enables other researchers who review analysis decisions to decide for themselves if interpretations are well grounded in the data.

Transferability Because qualitative analyses are so firmly rooted in specific contexts, some researchers believe it is not possible to make inferences to other populations. Others appear to draw general conclusions from their research too casually. Although the first approach limits the usefulness of qualitative research, the second limits its potency or effectiveness. The middle ground is to apply lessons learned in one context to similar contexts. But how can we do this?

First, as qualitative researchers, we should draw our conclusions carefully, ensuring that the data support them. Second, we can describe enough of the research context, the characteristics of the study participants, the nature of their interactions with the researcher, and the physical environment so that others can decide how transferable the findings are to other contexts. Finally, the results are more likely to be transferable if one objective of the original research design was to test a model or build a theory. Such designs will have identified theoretical constructs or components of a conceptual model to be tested in or adapted to a new study population. We can then expect that the study outcome will lead to support or refinement of a model, clearer limits on generalizability, or an alternative model or theory. Thus, the analysis process will have moved discrete fragments (segments) of data to a credible conclusion, based on evidence and capable of advancing our understanding of a complex behavioral health phenomenon.

Field Perspective

Rapid Analysis of Qualitative Findings: A Case from South Africa

Theresa Hatzell, Ph.D.

Family Health International

Ministries of health battling public health crises often cannot wait for evidence from the published literature to make decisions. That reality became apparent when a director of a unit focusing on sexually transmitted infection (STI) and HIV unit for the Department of Health (DOH) of South Africa requested immediate guidance from a public health research unit. The DOH was making decisions regarding resource allocations for condoms as part of the national HIV/AIDS prevention strategy. Working in collaboration with Family Health International, the public research unit had recently conducted a survey with women who had participated in a pilot launch of the female condom. The director of the STI/HIV unit asked our team for research findings indicating how well the national male condom–promotion program was responding to women's needs to protect themselves and whether there was any justification for spending money on the female condom as well. Pressed by budget-cycle deadlines, the director asked that we report preliminary conclusions from our survey results as soon as possible.*

We were able to provide the director with the information he needed. With analysis of a combined quantitative-qualitative structured survey instrument, our findings enabled him to justify allocating at least a small portion of the condom budget to female condom procurement. Here's how we did it.

We had collected data through face-to-face interviews during which we administered a structured survey instrument that included fixed-response questions linked to more open-ended questions. For example, we followed the fixed-response question "Have you ever tried using a male condom?" with several open-ended questions, including, "If not, why have you never used them before?" and "Is there anything in particular that has prevented you from trying them?" Therefore, the instrument yielded both quantitative and qualitative data that we were able to subject to an integrated statistical and content analysis. The design of our instrument proved crucial to understanding South African women's limited ability to control consistent male condom use, in spite of their own good intentions.

To respond to the priority concern of the STI/HIV unit director, we explored study participants' perception of their risk of STIs. All of these people had been exposed to the nation's intensive male condom–promotion initiative. We first used a statistical software package for quantitative analysis of the data derived from our survey's closed-ended questions. This exercise provided us with results such as the percentage of women responding that they are worried about becoming infected with an STI; who say that protection from STI is completely within their control, somewhat within their control, or not at all within their control; and who say their risk of becoming infected with HIV is none, slight, moderate, or great.

We asked open-ended qualitative questions, such as "Can you tell me why are you worried about becoming infected with an STI? What makes you feel that protection is completely within your control? Why would you say that you have no/slight/moderate/great chance of becoming infected with HIV?"

Verbatim written responses were entered into a single text document using a standard word processing software package. The three questions served as headings; and each survey participant's response, marked by a unique identifier, was listed beneath the corresponding question.

Other team members read through all the responses to note both commonly repeated themes and rare points of view. Following this review of the data, we named and defined a set of codes that represented commonly cited ideas and unique but intriguing concepts that were relevant to the issue of risk perception. These included the following:

Code	Definition
NOTRUST	Cannot trust partners to remain faithful.
FORCE	Partner uses threat of physical force to have unprotected sex.
PLEASURE	Male condoms are associated with reduced sexual pleasure.
YOUCHEAT	Asking for condom use implies suspicion of the partner's infidelity.
MECHEAT	Asking for condom use implies an admission of infidelity on one's own part.
MCBREAK	Male condoms are unreliable because they break.
TAMPER	Male condoms cannot be trusted because partners can tamper with them.
REFUSEMC	Partner refuses to use the male condom.
ALWAYS	I use a condom for every sexual act.
INCONSIST	Male condom use is irregular.
PASTSTI	Had an STI in the past.

Next, we copied the text into a file compatible with a computer software program for qualitative data analysis. We read through the data a second time and classified text by marking responses or segments of responses with the codes we had defined.

Once the text was coded, we used the program's computer-assisted search procedures to tally the frequency of selected concepts, as indicated by the codes. These simple frequencies helped us to identify major themes expressed by the participants, for example:

- Feeling vulnerable to infection because women suspected their partner's infidelity but could do nothing about it
- Doubts about the protection offered by male condoms because they are allegedly prone to breakage
- Difficulty getting partners to use male condoms all the time

At that point we took another look at the quantitative data. We saw that 85 percent of the respondents said that protection from STIs was completely within their control. This finding really puzzled us, given that only 47 percent of the respondents said they were current users of male condoms. We ran a cross tabulation and found that the women who were completely in control were no more apt to report current condom use than those who admitted less than complete control.

Once again we returned to the qualitative data. We used the capacity of the Ethnograph software to stratify searches and were able to tally code frequencies and retrieve coded text for a selected subset of respondents. In this case we were especially interested in the qualitative responses of women who indicated that they were completely in control of protection from STIs. Once we took a closer look at those women's verbatim responses, we surmised that many survey participants were probably responding hypothetically to the question about being in control.

Women were essentially saying, "In theory the ability to protect myself from STIs is completely within my control." They supported this assertion with normative statements such as "It is my responsibility to protect myself"; "It is my body. Only I can protect it"; and "If I don't take care of my health, who will?"

Meanwhile, this subset of in-control women commonly reported they are at risk of infection due to their partner's suspected infidelity or the alleged unreliability of male condoms. With the insight gained from our qualitative data, we were able to make an important clarification of the initial quantitative finding indicating that most women felt they were in control of protection. We reported to the STI/HIV unit director that there was substantial evidence that many women continued to feel vulnerable to infection, despite their ready access to male condoms. This information, combined with evidence of women's ability to use the female condom in situations in which they could not manage to use the male condom, helped to convince the director that he was justified in using some funds for female condom purchase and distribution.

**A limitation in conducting a rapid analysis based on combined qualitative and quantitative data is that the process tends to be purposeful and narrow in scope. It provides less opportunity for iterative open-minded exploration of data than is normally advised in qualitative analysis.*

Field Perspective

What to Look for in Software for Qualitative Data Analysis

Kathleen M. MacQueen, Ph.D.

Family Health International

Software options available for qualitative data analysis (QDA) have been steadily increasing in recent years. This is both good news and bad news. Good, because it means it is getting easier to match the best tool to the task. Bad, because it means there are more opportunities to choose a tool that works poorly or not at all for the task at hand. How to make the best choice?

Concerns in choosing QDA software include the following:

- How complex are the data?
- How complex is the analysis?
- What resources—staff, time, and technology—are available?

As these questions suggest, QDA software decisions are an important part of the research design process. When researchers put aside those decisions until after collecting the data, they often find that they have collected more data than they can manage or analyze in a systematic way.

How Complex Are the Data?

Qualitative data present organization and management challenges that are different from those of quantitative data. Data such as field notes, recorded and transcribed interviews, video recordings, written responses to questions, and photographs can contain many layers of information that will need to be carefully peeled apart during analysis. The greater the amount of data, the greater will be the complexity of organizing and managing it.

Choose software that helps you organize the computer files containing your data. Particularly when working with large, complex qualitative data sets, you should look for software that lets you decide where to store your data files, rather than requiring you to place data files in a particular directory on your computer. For example, if you are conducting a two-stage multisite research project with three different data collection instruments per stage, data should be hierarchically organized in folders that reflect the underlying logic of the data collection design.

How Complex Is the Analysis?

The more complex the analysis goal, the more important it is to choose software that is up to the task. Analytic goals can range from simple summaries of responses to complex theoretical modeling or hypothesis testing.

- At the simpler end, the goal of summarizing responses about individual topics may be fully met using a word processor to insert topical codes in the text, conduct word searches on those codes, and copy text excerpts to summary tables. Depending on the volume of text, this goal could also be achieved using paper, highlighters, scissors, and tape.
- A somewhat more complex goal would be a description of the way different topics are related to each other. For example, you might want to code issues from discussions on multiple topics. Software that produces reports on the co-occurrence of codes would be helpful. If the data are rich with layers of information, the software should also let you organize your codes into hierarchical trees and networks so that you can easily go from a broad overview to a detailed view of content. Look for software that will generate summary tables that show which codes occur together and how often, as well as text sorted by the codes assigned to it.
- If complex modeling or hypothesis testing is the goal, then you may need several software programs so that you can go beyond text analysis to decisional analysis, cluster analysis, and multidimensional scaling. A key issue here is the ability to import and export data. Of course, such complex approaches also require equally sophisticated

research design and data collection strategies. Unless you already have at least some formal training in or experience with most of these methods, you probably should not choose this as your goal.

- Another issue is the amount of sociodemographic data that will be used as part of the qualitative analysis. For example, for a single analysis you may want to contrast responses for men and women, for different age groups, for different ethnic groups, and for different research locations. The more kinds of groupings you want in the analysis, the more important it will be to choose software that lets you link this type of information to the qualitative data so that it will automatically sort the data in different ways.

What Staff, Time, and Computer Resources Are Available?

The number of staff who will be working on an analysis will affect your choice of software. As staff increases, so does the need for organization. This includes tracking who is doing what, ensuring that everyone is using the same standards, and merging the results of each team member's analysis task. If there is a lot of data or the analysis goal is fairly complex, you should choose software that helps with these tasks.

Many QDA packages require a significant amount of time to learn, and the packages may cost hundreds of dollars. Therefore, if you are familiar with a particular software package, continuing to use that package may be worthwhile if it meets most of the needs for a new project. But if you are attempting a project that is more complicated than your previous work, you should make a detailed outline of the data management and analysis steps that it will require. Then test them out using the software you intend to use to make certain it will work and determine the requirements in terms of time and effort. Also, you will want to make certain that your computer(s) have enough memory to store the data and run the program without crashing (or straining your patience).

Software Needs Based on Study Complexity

SIMPLE QUALITATIVE STUDY

Such a study would have most of the following characteristics:

- A limited descriptive goal, for example, to summarize the range of responses on five or fewer major topics
- Limited data needed to achieve that goal, for example, less than 250 pages of text, no more than twenty in-depth interviews, or no more than ten focus group discussions
- Analysis to be done by one or two people
- Little or no sociodemographic data to be used during the analysis, for example, only sex and ethnicity differences to be noted

For example: in preparation for a larger community-based intervention trial to enhance access to prenatal care, a qualitative researcher conducts twelve in-depth interviews with women who gave birth at the local hospital without previously receiving care. The goal is to describe some of the experiences of women in this situation to enhance the training of the staff who will implement the intervention. The interviews elicit information on each woman's home environment, her access to transportation, the extent to which she relies on traditional healers, her perceptions of the value of prenatal care, and her experience with the hospital during her recent birth. Two focus groups are also held with hospital staff to determine what they perceive as the major barriers for women seeking prenatal care. The interviews are audiotaped and transcribed. A research assistant helps with data analysis. The software requirements are minimal; the objectives can be met by using a word processor with search, copy, and paste tools.

MODERATELY COMPLEX

This type of study would have two or more of the following characteristics:

- An explanatory goal, for example, why a particular outcome is observed
- A moderate amount of data, for example, 250 to one thousand pages of text, twenty to fifty in-depth interviews, or ten to twenty focus groups
- Analysis team to have two to four people
- More than five major topics to cover in the study, with overlapping issues within at least some of the topics

- Limited sociodemographic information to be used during the analysis, for example, no more than twenty variables

For example: once the intervention trial described here is under way, it becomes clear that first-time mothers are not being effectively targeted. The researchers implement a substudy to find out why. They begin by conducting five focus groups with a variety of women to find out how to locate and enroll women who are pregnant for the first time or are likely to become pregnant for the first time. They initially use the interview guide developed for the simple study; but after conducting eight such interviews, they identify a new set of issues that have not been previously addressed. They modify the interview guide accordingly. In addition, they note that income, education, employment, and housing appear to influence access; so they develop a set of standardized questions on these factors. They conduct another twenty interviews. All focus groups and interviews are audiotaped and transcribed. Another research assistant joins the analysis team. This type of study works best with the help of software specifically designed for QDA. Almost any QDA software package will work.

COMPLEX STUDY

This study would have two or more of the following characteristics:

- A major scientific goal, for example, theoretical modeling or hypothesis testing
- Data collection on a large set of topics organized into hierarchies or networks of information
- Very large volumes of text, for example, more than one thousand pages or more than one hundred text files
- Detailed quantitative measures or descriptors that will be linked to the qualitative results
- Coordination of one large analysis team (five or more people) or multiple small teams with discrete analytic tasks

For example: the community intervention trial to enhance access to prenatal care is successful, but a follow-up study two years later shows a subsequent decline in access, especially for first-time mothers. The researchers hypothesize that this is related to a combination of local cultural values that tend to isolate childless women, in combination with economic factors that increase the dependency of young women. They suspect that long-term, sustainable improvements in first-time mothers' accessing prenatal care will require greater involvement of their spouses or partners. They design an ethnographic study that will collect information on all of these issues (gender roles, age roles, family roles, socioeconomic status, pregnancy, motherhood) through a series of interviews with men and women aged fifteen to forty-five. Data collection strategies include structured interviews that are audiotaped and transcribed, informal interviews for which notes are taken and then compiled, and field notes describing observed interactions in a variety of settings. Two senior researchers and four research assistants conduct data analysis in stages. Several structured interview guides are developed, based on interim data analysis.

A project of this magnitude requires systematic file and data management, the ability to link text and quantitative data, the ability to export summary data for use in other software programs, and the ability to track and replicate analysis decisions. Most QDA software packages will support some of these tasks but not all of them. In this situation it is important to carefully evaluate the options included in a software program to determine whether it will meet your needs.

Information on QDA software

The Centers for Disease Control and Prevention has developed two QDA software programs with a special emphasis on facilitating team-based analysis projects and the integration of qualitative and quantitative data. They are free and available online. EZ-Text is designed primarily for use with open-ended responses to structured questionnaires. It is available at http://www.cdc.gov/hiv/software/ez-text.htm. AnSWR is designed for more complex qualitative projects and is available at http://www.cdc.gov/hiv/software/answr.htm.

The following Web sites offer a variety of additional resources for software selection: Software for Qualitative Data Analysis at http://www.car.ua.edu; and the Computer Assisted Qualitative Data Analysis Software Networking Project at http://caqdas.soc.surrey.ac.uk/.

CHAPTER SEVEN

Putting It into Words

Reporting Qualitative Research Results

Writing up qualitative research "convert[s] private problems into public issues, thereby making collective identity and collective solutions possible."
(Richardson 1990, p. 28)

APPLIED REPRODUCTIVE HEALTH RESEARCH frequently has as its goal to influence policy, strengthen programs, or change health provider practices. The main product of qualitative research, however, is text—papers, reports, articles, books, and data archives.

As researchers, what can we do to make our writing matter, have an impact? What influence do we have over how people will interpret or use the text we have generated? How can we present results convincingly, especially to people who may be more accustomed to understanding issues in quantitative terms?

Writing up qualitative data is a process that includes determining whom to address and why, revealing one's point of view in relation to the data, and dealing with special issues of trustworthiness. This chapter discusses publication of qualitative data in reports and scientific publications, including how to organize methods and results sections; the importance of distinguishing between presentation and interpretation of findings; treatment of quotes; appropriate length; and techniques for combining quantitative and qualitative findings. Much of this dicussion is also applicable to the preparation of proposals for research or new programs in public health. Even if the work is yet to be done, your written proposal should take into account many of the same principles for creating a credible and persuasive argument.

Ethical Norms in Writing

The very nature of qualitative research—the active generation of insights and meaning by study participants sharing their stories—has important practical and ethical implications for how researchers report study findings. Be aware of qualitative reporting conventions even before you begin your study, and use them to guide your work.

In general, the ethical norms that govern how we write about people's lives include "the four non-negotiable journalistic norms of accuracy, nonmaleficence, the right to know, and making one's moral position public" (Denzin 2000, pp. 902–903). When you write up sensitive information on human sexuality, contraceptive decision making, and client-provider interaction, keep four basic principles in mind:

- *Aim for balance and accuracy, not neutrality.* Qualitative writing aims for balance and accuracy in reporting findings, not neutrality. It presents multiple sides of the particular reproductive health issue being studied. It aims to elicit the knowledge, understandings, and insights of the research participants and to present their insights in context.
- *Assure that no harm comes to participants.* You must not only assure that no harm comes to those interviewed as a result of their participation in a study, but also assure that no harm comes to them as a result of the publication, presentation, or dissemination of their views or experiences. Even when the published work does not give names, information could reveal the identity of some participants.
- *Give public voice to findings by sharing participants' own words.* The aim of most social scientific inquiry is to generate knowledge and insights for the scientific community and ultimately to benefit society. The tradition in qualitative research of presenting study participants' insights in their own words is both a philosophical commitment and a qualitative writing norm. Try to include quotes or even brief phrases (if possible, in the participants' original language, along with translation). By presenting participants' perspectives in their own words, you both empower them and convey important contextual information to readers, such as depth, detail, emotionality, and nuance (Denzin 2000).
- *Describe the context of your interactions and disclose your role.* Generally, qualitative researchers learn about other people through interaction in specific roles such as interviewer/interviewee or participant-observer/persons observed (Richardson 1990). In order to be able to judge the quality of the research, readers must have adequate information on when and how you gathered information, awareness of the nature of your relationship with those studied (your conversational partners), and knowledge of your standpoint and motivation in carrying out the study. At some point in your report, clearly state all sources of funding for your work.

  The concepts of voice and reflexivity are of central importance in qualitative writing. Reflexivity in writing means letting readers see our individual insights as historically, culturally, and personally situated. Because qualitative research always explores the context in which phenomena occur, qualitative writing involves presenting relevant aspects of the larger historical, political, cultural, or scientific context of the issues we study and the findings we generate.

Getting Ready to Write

Many investigators new to qualitative methods ask when they should begin writing up research for publication. Because qualitative research generates rich information, determining where to focus one's attention, getting organized, and deciding on the level of detail to be shared is often difficult. How do you know when research is ready for writing? Do you have other considerations—time, money, donor interest, and so on—that may necessitate ending the study and beginning to write?

RECOGNIZING WHEN TO WRITE

When you have come as close as possible to the point of saturation in your analysis, where additional data are not yielding new insights, you are ready to write. At this point, if you have followed a systematic research process, you should have a full set of files that document your reflections on what you learned. You will also have the following:

- A final list of codes
- Tables, matrices, or other summary devices that identify aspects of the reproductive health concepts you have studied
- A clear understanding of the thematic structure: how your themes fit together and how they relate to your conceptual framework

In conducting your study, you have generated information in the form of text, photos or images, and sometimes numbers. As you interpreted and analyzed the information you gathered, you also began to write up your thinking. You may have made notes in the margins of your transcripts (for example, "most married women are reluctant to ask husbands to use condoms") or determined text headings to depict sort categories (for example, "fear of pregnancy" or "fear of sterility"). Now your task is to put what you have learned from the study into a narrative: to produce text that weaves everything together and will make sense to your intended readers, text that members of the group you have studied would also consider accurate and complete.

CHRONICLE WHAT YOU HAVE LEARNED

There is an intermediate step between data analysis and compiling a report, writing for scientific publication, or preparing a presentation: writing a chronicle of your personal discovery. Some people call this phase "writing it out of your head" (and onto paper). In this intermediate step, you take the insights you have gathered and start writing the story of what you have learned. Your task is to take all you know and make it concrete for yourself in a relatively concise summary—typically about three to four pages.

To do this, begin by clustering the fragments of thematic ideas and integrating them into a meaningful account of what is going on. Talk about linkages and interrelationships you see among ideas or themes. You may take different vantage points on the findings—a gender or economic perspective, for instance—but focusing on a clearly defined aspect of the material will help you organize your account. Often there is more than one analysis for a study, and you will need to focus on a particular set of findings.

As you write, keep asking yourself, *What is this (really) a study of?* Having a clear understanding of how your concepts are linked is the most important signal that your analysis is finished. If you are getting ready to write and do not yet have a clear understanding of how key themes fit together, go back to your data before proceeding. As described in Chapter Six (see pp. 164–165), some qualitative researchers develop a visual or graphic diagram of how their key themes or concepts fit together, making sure this relates back to their conceptual framework. In writing they then touch on each aspect of the diagram, describing how the concepts are related. Another approach to sorting out the links between study themes is to convene a meeting of key informants and the research team, break into small groups to discuss how the themes fit, then reconvene as a larger group to work toward consensus on the meaning of the data and relationships among key ideas.

One of the greatest challenges that qualitative researchers have in writing up findings is to remain focused on the research questions and objectives while linking the questions to the findings. In qualitative research the study findings—which are the product of analysis—are the researcher's insights from sorting the data, identifying a small handful of key themes, describing how they fit together, and understanding how they fit in the larger sociocultural context. Quotes from participants, the raw data, should not be considered or presented as results but rather as illustrations of insights arrived at through your analysis. Just as a quantitative researcher would not provide raw line listings in the results section of a paper, a qualitative researcher must do more than present strings of quotes. The results or findings represent a synthesis. The quotes provide richness and detail.

Choosing a Format, Audience, and Voice

Qualitative research is primarily about text, although in some research, images, body maps, and photos are considered and analyzed as forms of visual language. Like modern scientific writing, which reflects conventions first developed in the late nineteenth century, qualitative research writing has its own traditions and conventions regarding presentation of data and the visibility or invisibility of the author-researcher in the writing itself. However, these conventions are still evolving as qualitative research expands in its use and application.

An array of stylistic conventions can be used for presentation of qualitative data on public health. Not all qualitative researchers choose conventional scientific formats for presenting findings; many experiment with form, format, voice, shape, and style. Reporting people's insights can be accomplished through genres such as fiction, poetry, performance, graphic arts, photographs, videotapes, and multimedia presentations (Gergen and Gergen 2000). Other approaches range from testimonials, such as first-person accounts by hospital obstetric patients regarding the quality of labor and delivery services, to scientific papers, which might include selected quotes from study respondents on contraceptive acceptability. The range includes such familiar formats as research reports, scientific journal articles, reports for donors, field reports, evaluation reports, operations research reports, oral presentations, fact sheets, and slide presentations. Even when using familiar formats, however, certain conventions differ from quantitative research reporting and writing, including use of quotes and the sequencing of certain information.

Determining how to write—which presentation style to choose—requires first determining your purpose. Are you writing to influence community opinion leaders, to inform policymakers, or to promote changes in health provider practices? Is your purpose to further academic discussion with scientific colleagues, to satisfy your faculty tenure committee, or to fulfill an obligation to share findings with study participants? Being clear about your purpose and identifying secondary objectives will help you determine what audiences to write for. At the same time, balance your aims with available resources by undertaking a frank assessment of your time and resource constraints.

In general, those writing for academic audiences commonly write papers for presentation at conferences or publication in social science, health, or medical journals. Such papers typically articulate conceptual frameworks or theories, describe methodologies used, and present and interpret data. Qualitative research journals usually allow longer length for articles than journals with a quantitative orientation, whereas scientific monographs provide space for the fullest exposition of results.

Papers published in journals for less-academic audiences, including some health practitioners, may also provide theoretical frameworks for better understanding an issue, such as the gender dimensions of risk behavior and sexually transmitted infection (STI). Writing that targets an audience of health providers often includes concrete suggestions for better practices, as well as broad policy recommendations. It is important to include appropriate scientific references or citations in materials written for health professionals.

Writing intended for lay readers or the public typically presents the human face of a persistent public health problem, for example, abortion-related morbidity and mortality. Such writing should either suggest reform of current practices or policies or give guidelines for how to alleviate a problem or improve practices (Denzin 2000).

Determine what is the basic story you are going to tell, who is to do the telling, and what type of narrative format you plan to use to weave your data. Your choice of presentation style will depend on your audience, purpose, and obligation to the study participants. The format you select may also depend on your study's characteristics. For example, a narrowly focused ethnographic study of commercial sex workers in one establishment may lend itself to a narrative style, but a more widely focused study may not. Your selection of a format may be influenced by various other factors as well, including availability of staff time or financial resources for writing, upcoming opportunities for presentation at conferences, or a tradition in your organization to write reports instead of publishing in journals. Once you have ascertained which primary and secondary audiences you intend to reach with your report, you will be able to assess which writing practices would be appropriate for a presentation of methods and findings.

One way to get an audience of health professionals to pay attention to your findings is to imitate conventional scientific-writing styles but modify them to suit the presentation of qualitative findings (Miller and Crabtree 2000). If you are writing for clinicians, for example, you might use certain biomedical writing conventions in your report—such as visual presentation of findings through tables, charts, diagrams, and data matrices—or present case reports, a narrative approach familiar to clinicians. A case study approach typically includes a detailed description of the cultural context; assumes the researcher will seek rather than test hypotheses; and relies on the author to integrate and interpret the findings in a historical, cultural, organizational, and political

Tip: For examples of scientific journals, university presses, and commercial publishers that accept articles that report on qualitative studies, see Appendix Ten.

context (Cernada 1982). Selected use of such scientific-writing conventions may increase the likelihood that readers more familiar with quantitative science will pay attention to what you report.

VARIATIONS IN THE STANDARD REPORT FORMAT

Depending on your study, purposes, and audience, you may need to modify the standard scientific report outline to fit your material. Your outline should reflect your audience's information needs and other factors, such as the importance you assign to discussion of theory. Other widely used approaches to organizing qualitative writing include much of the same material as presented in a standard scientific report but with certain variations in the ordering of contents.

Problem-Solving Approach State the problem and describe the importance of the research topic and its implications for health policies or practices or its impact on theory. Briefly describe your methods. State what you have learned about individual reproductive health themes or concepts. Offer your conclusions.

Narrative Approach Tell your story by way of a chronological narrative, illustrating a problem or process—such as barriers to contraceptive services—step-by-step or from multiple perspectives. (A narrative approach can be very dramatic. See an example in Ronai 1995.) In your conclusion explain why and how the process occurs. For example, if your study examines community perspectives on female genital cutting and adherence to the practice varies from village to village, you might organize your findings site by site.

Policy Approach Present a conclusion as to why a process or behavior occurs or fails. Walk through the evidence to show how you reached this conclusion. Journalistic and policy-oriented reports typically follow this pattern for busy readers who have little time for reading a lengthy article until they have grasped the relevance of the material. (See an example in Appendix Eleven.)

Analytic Approach Organize your findings in terms of the theoretical or conceptual framework you used to develop your study. Describe what you have learned and how it fits in the larger framework. (For an example, see Kaler 2001.) If you use a locus of control model to examine domestic violence, for example, explain how your findings support or differ from the model and related thinking.

No matter what format you choose, be sure to follow the basic principles that hold for all scientific writing: demonstrate a knowledge of available scientific literature, and get your facts right (Rubin and Rubin 1995).

Once you have determined your audience and the basic format you will follow, find and read samples of excellent writing that address similar audiences. Analyzing styles and formats by other researchers in your field can help you organize your data and insights effectively.

For example, if you are writing about a series of focus group discussions on health decision making, try to find articles that describe research that uses comparable methodologies:

- How is the material organized?
- Does your material lend itself to this kind of format?
- How does the author describe his or her methods and analysis strategy?
- Where is the author in the text? How has the author dealt with reflexivity; that is, how has the author revealed his or her standpoint vis-à-vis the topic? (Richardson 1990)

You will need to anticipate the approximate length of your manuscript, so that you can balance detail with space considerations. Aim to provide enough description to convey meaning, but do not overwhelm the reader with length. The level of detail you will provide about your study and the length of your writing will depend to a large extent on the audience you choose to address. Choosing a specific journal for submission or determining a specific format to emulate will also help you identify an appropriate length for your material. (See Appendix Ten for information on where to publish qualitative studies on reproductive health.)

Finally, if you are writing as a research team, determine from the outset who will be an author and agree on roles before you begin (see Appendix Twelve).

How to Begin Writing

Write a statement of purpose. This helps you find and maintain a focus (Wolcott 1990). Here are some examples:

> This paper examines the dynamics of condom use among female commercial sex workers (CSWs) in Durban, a large coastal city in KwaZulu-Natal province. Our objectives were to explore the socio-behavioral determinants of condom use between CSWs and their partners, both in professional sexual relations with clients and in personal relationships with domestic partners. We also sought to examine the extent to which HIV/AIDS influences CSWs' condom use in these situations (Varga 1997, p. 75).

> In this article, we describe our methodology for exploring conjugal physical and sexual violence. In addition, we present some of our initial findings concerning informants' perceptions regarding the nature of this violence, its antecedent causes, its consequences, and the strategies employed to deal with it. It is our hope that this research will not only contribute to academic knowledge but will help to resolve people's problems by means of the application of the results in education, health, political and other fields (Glanz 1998, pp. 377–378).

Do not continue writing until you are satisfied that your brief statement of purpose captures the essential components of your study: what you looked at and where, how, and why you studied it.

Next, put together a detailed written outline, a sequence, or an expanded table of contents (Wolcott 1990). In addition, decide first how you are going to present your

BOX 7.1

How to Organize a Standard Scientific Report

If you want to publish in a prominent academic journal or prepare a report for ministry of health officials, you may choose to follow a fairly standard scientific format. Most journals limit articles to twelve typed pages (2,500 words) plus references and two to three tables, following a general outline:

I. Introduction
   - A. Literature review
      1. Relevant facts from previous studies
      2. Questions unanswered by previous studies
   - B. Purpose of the study
      1. Main question and summary of basic approach used to answer it
      2. Anticipated contribution of study results
   - C. Brief description of the study
      1. Who did the study, where, and when
      2. Brief description of the methods and participants
      3. Description of relevant cultural or contextual information (for example, religion or religiosity, socioeconomic context)

II. Methods
   - A. Study design
   - B. Sampling methods
   - C. Data collection methods
   - D. Data analysis methods

III. Results
   - A. Presentation of the results
   - B. Interpretation of the findings
   - C. How the results relate to earlier studies and your conceptual framework
   - D. How methodological difficulties could have affected results

IV. Conclusion
   - A. Importance of the results to others thinking about the problem
   - B. Logical next steps for research
   - C. Implications of findings for the specific purpose of the study

V. Recommendations
   - A. Policy or service delivery recommendations
   - B. Community action recommendations (if applicable)

VI. Acknowledgments

VII. Bibliographic references and citations

authorial voice (Wolcott 1990). To use a dramaturgical metaphor, will you be offstage but clearly directing the performance, or will you be the narrator interpreting meaning between scenes? Your stance or voice should reflect the basic processes of data collection used in your study. Rubin and Rubin (1995, p. 268) recommend that "if the interviews were deeply interactional, with the parties exploring ideas together and coming up with a joint conclusion, then the researcher's voice and role should be apparent in the report."

Once you have written a clear statement of purpose, identified your audience, chosen a presentation format, and written an outline, you should be ready to begin your report or article. We discuss next what is typically included in the main report sections—introduction, methods, results, and conclusion—and where that differs from scientific writing on quantitative studies.

INTRODUCTION

Begin by describing how your topic and design fit within the existing body of literature. If you studied maternal mortality by interviewing husbands of women who died in childbirth, be sure to cite both epidemiologic and ethnographic literature on maternal mortality, as well as literature that would cast light on the use of family members as key respondents for reporting reproductive health events. Some investigators find it useful to write both their statement of purpose and this section on the study's relationship to existing literature even before they begin the study.

METHODS SECTION

Describe how you went about your study in as much detail as space allows, presenting those aspects that most affected collection and analysis of data. Explain how you identified whom to interview, how you gained access to the interviewees, and why they were willing to talk to you (Rubin and Rubin 1995). When did you conduct the fieldwork? How extensive was your involvement? How long did you stay, and what was your role? Present a straightforward description of the setting and events and invite the reader to see through your eyes. Make sure to describe your sample, including sociodemographic characteristics such as age, marital status, religion, sex, education, and other descriptive information related to the research problem. Presenting this information in a table format is often reassuring to audiences more familiar with quantitative methods.

Also, describe important aspects of the local context or culture. For example, if abortion is among the topics investigated in the research, provide background on the legal status of abortion in the country, and describe prevailing cultural or religious beliefs and whether the study population's beliefs differ from these. Studies in sexual and reproductive health often include reproductive history as well as, for example, number of pregnancies, age at first birth, and contraceptive use.

As you write, be sure to detail how you "navigated" while in the field, including how closely you interacted with the interviewees (Golden-Biddle and Locke 1999), how you involved others at the research site, and how you created a friendly and trusting climate for the research. You will need to discuss the ways in which you collected and analyzed the field data. How did you modify your design? Did you use more than one

BOX 7.2

Content Checklist: What to Include in Study Write-ups

Whether you write up your data as an oral history, final report, or a social science journal article, your manuscript will need to answer the following questions:

- What was the research question, and in what context does the problem exist?
- How was the research designed?
- What techniques or methodologies did you use for data collection and analysis? What types of data were collected?
- Why were the research design, sampling strategies, data collection approaches, and analysis techniques appropriate to the question you posed, in the particular context of your research?
- Was the research process iterative?
- Is the interpretive process used in the analysis clearly described?
- What did you find out, and what do you think it means?
- What was your relationship with informants, and how did you and they influence each other during the research process?
- Have you demonstrated an understanding of the world portrayed in your text in a way that readers will feel accurately represents the local perspective?
- Have you conveyed adequate levels of detail about the people and context you studied, including specialized or commonly used language regarding the aspect of public health you examined?
- Have you grounded your findings by systematically integrating negative cases and contrasting them with cases that are very different? (Flick 1998)
- Have you explicitly shared with readers your own personal biases, perspectives, and motivations and how these might affect your research?
- What were the limitations in your study?

Sources: Adapted from Miller and Crabtree 2000; Golden-Biddle and Locke 1999.

data collection technique? Under what circumstances was information cross-checked? What were the limitations of the study? What aspects of your decision making had the greatest impact on your research? Answers to these questions will help your readers understand how to evaluate the merits of your findings.

RESULTS SECTION

Make a clear distinction between presentation and interpretation in writing up your results. Virtually every stage of your work will reflect simultaneous analysis and interpretation: your study findings are interpreted data. When you present findings, define them as such. When you discuss what you believe the findings mean in relation to other data or concepts, let the reader know you are interpreting those findings.

A typical way to write qualitative research is to move through themes sequentially as you follow the evolution of some issue. With this approach you first present study findings, then share your insights on what they mean. How you order your presentation of themes is like constructing an argument. "Qualitative theory is developed by elaborating and interpreting the unexpected and the apparently contradictory. If you have evidence for both sides of an argument, then present it and explain it" (Rubin and Rubin 1995, p. 263).

In a qualitative study in Haiti of women's roles in sexual decision making, the authors led the reader through five themes to illustrate how Haitian women's capacity to negotiate safe sexual behavior, including the use of condoms, may be related less to their knowledge of the disease than to their customary role in sexual relationships (Ulin and others 1995). Expanding on key thematic ideas, they present a range of study participant perceptions, descriptive information about participants who offer comments and quotes that illustrate both themes (for example, beliefs about vulnerability to and consequences of AIDS) and subthemes (for example, social rejection, destruction of family, uncertainty about a spouse's fidelity) that they determine to be important. Following this presentation of results, which includes some explanatory interpretation, the authors offer a conclusion, which contains their analysis of the findings with regard to the eight specific study objectives posed at the outset of their investigation. They present the conclusion section much like a series of distinct discussion sections for a scientific journal article, each about a page long. Finally, the authors end with a recommendations section, presenting their viewpoint on the study's implications for intervention.

You can choose the approach you take to organize your presentation and discussion of findings to reflect aspects of your research design, whether you have conducted in-depth interviews, focus group discussions, or participant observation. Instead of separating the presentation of data from interpretation, some authors choose to weave the presentation of results into their analysis in a way that parallels their conversations with study participants over time. This kind of writing is similar to storytelling, with the researcher-author serving as narrator.

For example, in a study of adolescents in Detroit, Michigan, who intentionally infect themselves with HIV (Tourigny 1998), the author presents key themes in a series of case studies. Interview transcripts from a larger study had revealed that a subgroup of teenagers infected themselves with HIV in order to feel visible and important, others to access care and social services, and still others to elicit community or family support. The author decided to focus on this phenomenon through case studies of six self-infected young people she knew well and to present her interpretations by way of personal commentary woven throughout the six case studies.

If your presentation of findings is logical and coherent, you increase the probability that the audiences for whom you are writing will accept your work. This principle is valid even when dealing with multiple sources of data and presenting highly complex issues. Having a consistent structure for presentation of results helps you organize the material more efficiently and helps those who read your report make sense of the information.

BOX 7.3

How to Organize and Report Findings from Mixed-Method Studies

A structure that works particularly well for studies using more than one methodological approach is to organize the presentation of all findings by key themes. You will need to be selective in your choice of themes—with so much data it will be essential to leave some material out. As you write, guide the reader through findings from one methodological approach, present the findings from a different approach, and then tell the reader what you think the combined findings mean regarding that theme. After treating all your key themes sequentially in this way, write a conclusion that explains the linkages between themes, explains the findings in light of your theoretical framework, examines how applicable the findings would be in other contexts or with other groups, and discusses whether the findings are consistent with other studies.

Sometimes a study that uses both quantitative and qualitative methods gives different results when examining the same phenomenon. Reaching a unifying conclusion regarding discrepant findings is not your responsibility, but you should present these contradictions and offer supporting data for the reader to assess.

In his combined-methods study of sexual cultures and sexual health among young people in Lima, Peru, one author (Cáceres 1999) begins by presenting his study objectives and discussing the social theories or philosophies he employs. Second, he outlines the qualitative and quantitative phases of his study, describing the tools and processes used in data collection and analysis, stating ethical considerations, and providing sociodemographic information on the study population. Next, he leads the reader through each thematic topic, alternately presenting qualitative and quantitative findings, as available. He organizes the findings by thematic areas: gender images and norms, factors in sexual socialization, sexual experience, the process of sexual initiation, the structure of sexual risks, and special contexts for sexual experience (paid sex, coercive sex, and concomitant use of alcohol or drugs).

Like Cáceres, you can successfully alternate between presentation of qualitative and quantitative data on specific points—even where themes break into subthemes—and still retain your focus. In writing on sexual risk, Cáceres presents quantitative data on the proportion of young women who report having experienced undesired pregnancy and on cofactors for undesired pregnancy. Without interrupting the narrative flow of his elaboration on this phenomenon, he shifts into qualitative findings regarding young people's thoughts on factors that lead to undesired pregnancy, factors such as the relative stability of the couple or the use of tricks by one partner to achieve pregnancy as a way of trapping the other in the relationship. In his analysis he provides selected quotes by adolescent study participants to illustrate key insights. Finally, once all relevant findings are presented on a given theme, he provides a unifying conclusion: his interpretation of what the findings mean, how variations in the findings can be understood, and what is important about what he learned.

However you structure the presentation of your findings, offer your interpretation and use your field notes to provide concrete illustrations and examples. Sharing the process allows readers to arrive at their own conclusions as to the data's meaning.

Make use of numerical tables and other quantification where you can. It can help your readers, for example, to learn that "Individuals in all but one of the six focus groups believed in some way that oral polio vaccine spreads AIDS." Using numbers gives readers an indication of the relative importance of an idea and allows them to weigh the evidence you present. But be careful: one of the most common mistakes in reporting qualitative research is to treat data from qualitative samples as if they were quantitative data. For example, because the sampling for qualitative studies is not representative, overemphasizing numbers and distributions is erroneous and misleading. This is why providing appropriate examples would be helpful.

As you write, get your facts and references right the first time; and if you make generalizations, use specific instances to support your conclusions (Wolcott 1990). Write about whether you feel the findings from your study would make sense to a study participant and why. Tell the reader what steps you took in the study to ensure that the study question and the results were consistent with participants' views of their world.

Like the choreographer, the researcher must find the most effective way to tell the story and to convince the audience of the meaning of the study. Staying close to the data is the most powerful means of telling the story, just as in dance the story is told through the body itself.
(Janesick 2000, p. 389)

CONCLUSION SECTION

In the conclusion section of your paper or report, tell the reader whether the research has generated information that you didn't expect. Relate your themes to your statement of purpose and original question(s), and describe how your data support your explanation of the question or your conceptual framework if you used one. If you have created a visual diagram showing how your themes fit together, reflect on your original framework and whether it was borne out or not. What do your findings, the cluster of ideas, mean in a broader context? How might these findings apply beyond the original study population? Be careful not to suggest that your findings can be generalized, but rather state or show why you believe they are extensible (meaningful to a wider public health community) or not.

Describe findings that indicate controversy or polarization. If these relate to gender, say so. For example, if you conducted a series of focus group discussions on the influence of religious beliefs on family planning, note where women say one thing and men say another. Likewise, if you find that contraceptive discontinuation is associated with changes in menstrual bleeding patterns, be sure to discuss whether the results fit with findings from similar studies conducted elsewhere. If not, can you explain why they do not? Make clear the multiple and sometimes contradictory perspectives reflected in your data.

State the policy or programmatic implications of your findings, if applicable. Some writers place these in a separate section of recommendations that follows the conclusion section.

How to Use Transcript Quotes in Narrative

Your use of quotes in your writing depends on what you are trying to accomplish. Also, as you select and present quotes, take care to represent participants' viewpoints fairly and respectfully.

Remember to choose quotes that illustrate significant findings, manage the marking of quotes in transcripts efficiently, and present them in ways that preserve the contextual information necessary for readers to understand them accurately.

HOW TO SELECT APPROPRIATE QUOTES

Use representative quotes to illustrate norms or shared perceptions. These quotes should succinctly represent concepts that interviewees would recognize as their ideas. For example, in one West African study of service delivery for the contraceptive implant Norplant, the majority of respondents independently mentioned the phrase *va-et-vient* ("coming and going" or "being given the runaround"). Hearing so many women say that to get Norplant removed, they had to endure being given the runaround by service delivery personnel alerted the researcher that this service delivery phenomenon was entrenched. The women's shared phrase pointed to this phenomenon as a key theme to explore in future research.

Use provocative quotes to highlight insights not generally held but perhaps innovative or pioneering. For example, if a focus group participant mentions that women like the female condom "because they can insert it before they leave work," you might explore whether potential users in that area perceive themselves to be at high risk of rape when commuting and whether they feel the female condom would offer disease protection. Be careful not to give undue importance to quotes that may reflect atypical positions.

Draw on different people's voices, not just the most articulate. Be sure to check whether the range of people you quote reflects the range of people interviewed. One way to illustrate a range of perspectives and variations in language is to list short phrases related to your theme:

> *My wife and I decide together how many children we'll have.*
>
> *It's up to the man to decide how many children he can afford, because he's the one who earns the money.*

Use quotes to show the importance not only of what people say but how. Language use or tone can indicate decision making, discord, ambivalence, underlying emotion, or social expectations. Things said with great emotion or powerful word choices may indicate provocative issues below the surface.

HOW TO PREPARE TRANSCRIPTS AND MANAGE FOREIGN LANGUAGE TRANSLATIONS

Mark key quotes to use in writing as you read through your transcripts. Have a good system for flagging possibly useful quotes as you read through the text, for example, writing participant or group ID code and line numbers on the transcript. As you write or make notes on your interpretation of the data, you can use the code as a temporary shortcut for the illustrative segment, for example, FG2-UM, 75–120, where the reference is to lines 75 to 120 in the transcript from your second focus group of urban males. Otherwise, trying to relocate a memorable quote when you need it can be a frustrating search. If you are using software to do your analysis, you can designate a code to retrieve salient quotes (see Chapter Six, p. XXX).

As a general rule, use verbatim quotes. However, minor changes may be needed to make a quote clearer—especially if it is a translation. Do not let clarification change some subtle meaning. If you need to shorten a quote or change some words, the convention is to put your substituted words in square brackets [ ] and replace omitted words with a space and then three dots, called ellipses. For example: "My boyfriend and I want to protect ourselves from these [sexually transmitted] diseases, but . . . we don't always have condoms when we need them."

Many words or expressions in other languages have no literal translation, or if translated, lose the subtlety of the original statement. The best way to handle these is to use the word that the translator believes comes closest to the original but also to include the original word or phrase in italics within parentheses. For example: "An [informally] married *(placé)* woman agreed that 'life on the streets is hard. . . . a woman without employment can't stand up to her partner.'"

Include key foreign words or phrases to enable readers who do know the language to judge the validity of the translated data. For example:

Moderator: What kind of people can contract the AIDS disease?

First Haitian respondent: People who are fooling around *(viv deyo),* living promiscuously *(nan epav),* but if both people are not living like that, you will not get it.

Second Haitian respondent: What she says is right, [but] some women who live with men are not involved with other men *(li pa nan anyen),* while their men may be involved in everything *(nan tout afel).*

Weave explanatory quotes into your interpretation. The usual approach is to make the point in your narrative and follow it with an illustrative statement from a participant. You can wrap the quote into the narrative: "Most women seemed to believe that men expect to make the decisions about family size. As this thirty-two-year-old woman lamented, 'I really wanted only two kids, but my husband—you know how men are—insisted on a big family.'"

Or you can set longer quotes off as indented paragraphs, usually with a slightly smaller font. Use quotation marks when the quote is embodied in the narrative but not when it is set off in its own indented paragraph:

> A forty-two-year-old nonliterate mother of six volunteered the following illustration to explain how friends help each other:
>
> > *When two women meet, they talk about the disease. I will say, "My dear, the AIDS disease is out there. Are you being careful?" And my friend might say, "I have this man I've been sleeping with, but I don't know if he has other women. Do you think I should break off this relationship?" And I say, "You can use a condom."*

Note that quotes become more alive if they are labeled with descriptive information, for example, "a sixteen-year-old woman pregnant for the first time," or "a forty-year-old unemployed factory worker." Remember never to put the respondent's name in your report or quotation. You may have descriptive information in background data sheets (see Chapter Five). Your choice of descriptors will depend on the information you consider most relevant to the point you are making in your narrative. These descriptors can also follow the quote, for example:

> *I hide the pill packet in my clothes when my husband is home. I don't want him to find it, because he does not know I'm going to the family planning clinic.*
>
> —Market woman, primary schooling, twenty-seven years old

You can also link several short, related quotes, indicating clearly that they are different speakers, for example:

> *I hide the pills in my clothes when my husband is home.*
>
> —Twenty-seven-year-old market woman

> *I take my pills before he comes to bed—I go to bed before he does.*
>
> —Thirty-three-year-old teacher

> *When my husband asks, I just say I'm not using them.*
>
> —Thirty-year-old farmer

Keep quotes down to short segments of text—enough to suggest the context and not so long that the reader loses the thread. Ask yourself whether the segment is a good reflection of the point you want to make. Because very long quotes tend to distract the

BOX 7.4

Does Your Study Matter?

- Have you identified gaps in the literature and suggested ways [in which] your work offers new thinking in an area of importance?
- Are the results consistent with other studies? How applicable are the findings in other contexts or with other groups?
- Does your study rebut accepted thinking on the public health topic you addressed, at least to some extent?
- Does your writing provoke readers to reexamine their assumptions underlying prevailing theories or lines of thought?

Sources: Adapted from Golden-Biddle and Locke 1999; Lincoln and Guba 1999.

reader from the narrative's flow, make them just long enough to give some life to the text. The narrative should speak for itself; that is, it should make the point or show how the quote illustrates something you have written. You can also provide interpretation after the quoted remarks, for example, pointing out that the clandestine users quoted earlier have different strategies for keeping their contraceptive use secret.

When using quotes in oral presentations of your research, keep them short. Just as presentations of quantitative studies are usually accompanied by slides or transparencies that summarize the data in statistical tables, qualitative researchers use words, or brief excerpts from transcripts, to illustrate the points they are making. You can prepare these displays exactly as you would for a written report, except that you should avoid presenting long passages on the screen. Short quotes, using some of the conventions we have discussed for abbreviating verbatim statements, can help an audience visualize the data or hear the participants speaking through you, the researcher. Presenting verbatim expression of your study participants enables the listener to share in the excitement of discovering life from the perspectives of the people living it.

Your report will be more credible if it is organized around a conceptual framework, if the framework is elaborated throughout the report, and if it is supported with adequate qualitative evidence (Lofland 1974).

External Review: Assessing the Product

As a qualitative researcher, your obligation is "to gather the most highly credible information possible within the constraints of your situation and to present your conclusions in a form that makes them . . . understandable and useful" (Morris and others 1987, p. 8). Whether or not you communicate effectively with specific audiences will influence whether those groups will consider your study credible. Policymakers, fellow researchers, and community members will determine their confidence in your study by examining both what you say and the manner in which you say it.

You can use three basic strategies to enhance the credibility and communicability of your study report:

- Make sure the study question and results matter to your intended readers (relevance)
- Understand your audience's needs (length, level of complexity, conventions regarding credibility)
- Attend to the basics of good writing (clarity, accuracy, logical development of ideas)

Individuals and agencies that use qualitative results to achieve their objectives are likely to have developed their own frameworks to help them evaluate what they receive from investigators. Similarly, publishers, professional societies, thesis committees, conference committees, evaluators, and government monitors all have their criteria for establishing the quality of proposals or written accounts of research. Donors and journal editors provide their reviewers with checklists and guidelines that reflect their priorities. The essential points for ensuring quality range from stating the problem through design decisions and analysis, and finally putting the whole process and outcome in writing. The checklists on page 184 and in Appendix Nine provide useful reviews of these steps.

No matter whom you communicate with, your readers will consider your text in light of their own needs and interests—both personal and professional. For example, if you report on in-depth interviews with married women who discontinue use of an intrauterine device, your intended readers will interpret and act on the text by relating what you present to their own views on the subject. These may relate to client-provider interaction, spousal decision making, or even the value they assign to qualitative as opposed to quantitative approaches to studying contraceptive use. In order to convince readers that your findings hold merit, you will need to achieve a balance between challenging their assumptions and reiterating the familiar—in terms of the format, style, and content of your report.

Take care that what you say and the evidence you marshal to support your insights will seem realistic to your intended audiences, as well as to those you interviewed or observed in your study. Does your writing convey to readers "a sense of familiarity and relevance as well as a sense of distinction and innovation" (Golden-Biddle and Locke 1999, p. 374)? Most readers will judge your written presentation as a direct reflection of the quality of your research. To convince the reader that you have accurately recorded and understood the meaning of what study participants said, present detailed descriptions and key quotations, and back up your argument with evidence (Rubin and Rubin 1995). Then check your work by reviewing the content checklist in Box 7.2 (p. 184). If you follow these steps, you will go a long way toward convincing your readers of your report's credibility.

An important related issue is effective communication—writing that engages your readers intellectually and emotionally. The goal of qualitative writing is "to represent the world of your interviewees accurately, vividly and convincingly" (Rubin and Rubin 1995, p. 261). Your results will be important "if your report is read and its vividness influences decision-makers" (p. 53). Writing has the potential to motivate readers to change practices, to explore new avenues of research, to inform health advocacy efforts, or to spur communities into action. Your responsibility is to make your study report as accessible, credible, and engaging as possible. Vivid stories can provide convincing descriptions of health conditions or issues, touching your readers more profoundly than abstract discussions alone. Hearing reproductive experiences in people's own words is gripping and powerful. Individual stories convey excitement, fear, drama, and realism. Do not be afraid to share emotion in bringing the interviewees' insights to life for your readers (Rubin and Rubin 1995).

The ultimate interpreter of the quality and usefulness of your work is the reader, who interacts with what you have communicated and decides whether to integrate it into his or her work and worldview or to dismiss it. Your report's credibility and communicability will determine to a large extent whether readers will use your findings and whether the findings will have an impact on health policies, practices, and behaviors.

Field Perspective

What One Editor Looks for in Qualitative Research Papers

Marge Berer, M.A., Editor

Reproductive Health Matters

Reproductive Health Matters (RHM) is an interdisciplinary journal in the sexual and reproductive health field with a diverse international audience. It commonly publishes papers that report on qualitative research, for example, social science research or users' perspectives in conjunction with clinical trials in the field. What follows is what I, as an editor, look for in a qualitative research paper and what it needs to include in order to be publishable.

RHM's editorial policy states that it is looking for papers that identify and help us to understand women's reproductive and sexual health needs and to evaluate and improve upon existing policy and practice for women's benefit. Qualitative papers can raise fundamental concerns and dilemmas and expose the multifaceted nature of problems and their solutions. RHM looks mostly for papers that have a women-centered perspective and that foster new thinking and action in the field, whether at the local, national, or international level. Findings need to be relevant cross-culturally and able to be put to good use by others, no matter where they happen to live.

Good qualitative research requires as rigorous a process of research implementation and reporting, within accepted and broad guidelines, as does quantitative research. It is at least as difficult to do and to write about well. Much has been written about how to do this sort of research. For those who have no training, it is worth reading about how to do it before starting out. A paper is only as good as the research on which it is based, with good writing skills added in. If the research itself is flawed, there is nothing an editor can do to help, except to point this out.

Describing the Research

A paper needs to start off by stating what problem or situation led to the research; followed by what the aim of the research was; where, when and how it was carried out; and by whom. If the study was an integral part of a larger research project to collect quantitative clinical or other data, then the larger research study must be described as well, in order to place the findings in the context in which they were gathered. If these wider aspects of the study are described in detail in one or more other papers or reports, whether published or unpublished, these should be summarized briefly and referenced.

Study Participants and Methodology

Qualitative research by its very nature takes time and cannot easily include large numbers of participants because it involves in-depth, field-based methods. Even so, to be relevant to others, especially at the international level, the findings must have sufficient value to be worth knowing about and publishing. For example, they must be important enough to affect future work on a new contraceptive method or to alter some aspect of health education, counseling, service delivery, or policy. This means that the research methodology must be carefully thought out and implemented, as with quantitative research, and reported in enough detail so that the process is clear. For example, the participants must in some way be representative of the group from whom they are drawn, such as young, unmarried women attending family planning clinics in a particular city. (This does not mean representative in a statistical sense; see the discussion of sampling in qualitative research in Chapter Three.) The way in which participants are chosen must be described. If they do not make up a random sample, how were they found? Why them and not others? If key informants were consulted, how and why were they chosen and not someone else? Describe what participants were asked to provide. Procedures for obtaining consent to participate in the study should be detailed in the paper.

The methodology for obtaining the information also needs to be described, that is, what questions participants were asked, who interviewed them, how the data were recorded and analyzed, and so on. Qualitative research may be on a sensitive subject, for example, sexual relationships and behavior or illegal abortion. It isn't always easy for participants to tell the whole truth, especially in one possibly short interview with a stranger. Hence, in order to judge the quality of the information being reported, the reader needs to know the means that were used to elicit the information. For example, sometimes researchers go back to talk to all the participants two or three times or have tested and found successful sensitive ways of probing for details. If efforts were made to get in-depth responses and not superficial or normative responses, such as holding focus groups to find out social norms and then in-depth interviews to find out actual behavior or practice, this should be explained.

Findings

The paper needs to be about who the participants are, what was learned from them, and why their perceptions or views were important, but not about the process of finding the information out. Hence, the presentation of the findings does not need to follow the order in which the questions were originally asked. It makes a difference whether all the participants, half of them, or only a few of them have experienced a problem or believe something that is described.

Possibly the most common mistake authors can make is to think that because their research is not quantitative, it need not contain any quantitative data or follow any accepted process of reporting. Although too many numbers can clutter up a paper of this kind, no sense of numbers in participants' responses means it is difficult to know the significance of what is reported. Nuances and distinctions are worth teasing out as well.

Quotes from participants should illustrate points being made better than the text, but they should not repeat what is in the text or vice versa. It isn't necessary to include more than one quote to illustrate a point but rather to make it clear that a certain number of participants said something similar. Sometimes when a striking comment, a point of view, or an experience is uncommon but important and relevant, it is worth quoting as an exception.

Translation of quotes into English, where required, does not need to make people sound stupid or foreign. It should be in correct English (current usage) appropriate to the participants' style (colloquial, formal) in their own language.

Discussion and Recommendations

The discussion should not summarize or repeat the findings but interpret them and discuss their significance. What potential effect will they have? The author(s) should make recommendations about any changes that should be made as a consequence of the findings. If the study had limitations in this regard, these also should be discussed. Further research would provide work for the researchers, but recommendations of further research should be restricted to taking knowledge or practice forward more broadly.

If the research team disseminated its findings to others, this process should be described. If team members went back to the study site and consulted the participants for their input into the report or provided information to them about the findings or the subject of the research for their own benefit, this also should be reported.

RHM's editorial policy is to appreciate research that is linked to action, that is, in which the results of the study are used to benefit the participants and others in similar circumstances and not research done only for its own sake or to benefit mainly the researchers. A research team may not be in a position itself to carry out an action component, but it can work with others who can.

If I were permitted to make only one recommendation to authors about how to proceed, I would recommend that they read the papers of researchers and authors in the field whose work is valued and study those papers well before designing a study, going out to do fieldwork, and writing their papers. Worthy goals in the pursuit of knowledge, the ability to hear and understand the significance of women's and men's experiences, creativity and sensitivity in the research process, using proven research methodology—together these will result in excellent research reports that are well worth publishing. Good writing and editing skills help too!

CHAPTER EIGHT

Disseminating Qualitative Research

The ultimate goal of qualitative research is to transform data into information that can be used.

(Rossman and Rallis 1998, p. 11)

WHEN WE WRITE about people's notions of health risk or quality of care, we are fulfilling a practical and social mandate common to applied research: to create information for use by programs to improve services or by decision makers to inform policies. The end product of applied qualitative research on public health should be to give public voice or visibility to private or hidden issues, cast new light on puzzling questions, make invisible problems clear (allowing solutions), and make health problems more understandable (allowing better solutions) (Rubin and Rubin 1995).

Because applied research aims to generate information that can be used, the dissemination of study findings—what, why, by whom, to whom, and how—needs to be considered from the beginning. If you want your results to be used, start planning for dissemination even when you are designing the study and developing a budget. Your specific purposes for dissemination can vary and may include the following processes or products:

- Strengthening and increasing the frequency of communication between the researcher and study participants
- Providing tools or materials for researchers and health advocates to communicate in support of policy change
- Helping other researchers, scientists, or decision makers understand the social, cultural, political, or economic factors that influence reproductive health
- Empowering marginalized, silenced groups (such as victims of sexual violence)
- Providing practical information to solve programmatic problems
- Keeping health issues alive in the media, donor, and public health communities

Dissemination activities may include individual or group discussions before, during, or after study completion; professional meetings and conferences; publication in peer-reviewed journals; distribution of fact sheets; use of traditional media (for example, songs, posters, puppet theater); coverage by news media; audiovisual presentations; or training workshops.

Contrary to the popular notion that dissemination implies only end-of-study activities, such as a seminar to brief senior health administrators, *research dissemination is a process, not a one-time event.* You do not have to wait until you have analytic saturation before you start to disseminate. From the first day you introduce your study to ministry of health officials or community leaders, you are actively disseminating information on the purpose, scope, and potential impact of the study. When you return to key informants to say, "This is what I'm hearing. Does it make sense to you? Why or why not?" you are sharing preliminary findings and opening a collaborative dialogue on their meaning.

In short, dissemination is an ongoing part of the dialogue with stakeholders that characterizes applied qualitative research. The methods used in qualitative research bring you into repeated contact with opinion leaders, community members, and other stakeholders; these interactions serve both to gather and to share information. Having unearthed in-depth, often deeply personal information on what people think about health issues, you must share study insights as widely as possible—whether such dissemination is formal or informal, direct or indirect.

As you develop a research dissemination strategy appropriate to your study, you will likely encounter obstacles. These can range from resource constraints or skepticism about the validity of findings on the part of policymakers and scientists unfamiliar with qualitative methods to personal reservations regarding your interpretive role or resistance on the part of health bureaucracies to information suggesting new practices. Many researchers believe either that research dissemination is outside their professional capacity or simply not their responsibility. Others think they are responsible for dissemination only to the research community. It is important to consider from the outset where your research responsibilities will end and whom to involve in order to promote effective use of results.

Although many of the strategies and activities used to disseminate qualitative research are identical to those used to disseminate other types of studies, a few issues are specific to qualitative work. For example, a frequent complaint among both scientists and policymakers who have previous experience with qualitative studies that were poorly designed and implemented is this: "Why should we believe that these results mean anything? This information is anecdotal!"

To accomplish the ultimate purpose of applied research, to produce new and useful information, you will need a strategy for presenting your results effectively and persuading audiences that your findings are credible. We recommend at the very least disseminating your findings to study participants, health advocates, and the local or international research community. Incorporating participatory dissemination from the beginning, a process to which qualitative methods lend themselves, will generate better data and give your research results a better chance of being used.

Research Ethics Require Dissemination

The obligation to disseminate information back to study participants has been part of the professional code of applied sociologists, anthropologists, and other social scientists for decades, as has been the public disclosure of findings. The Association of Social Anthropologists of the Commonwealth (1999), for example, states that a researcher's "obligations to the participants or the host community may not end (indeed should not end, many would argue) with the completion of their fieldwork or research project. . . . [Researchers should] communicate their findings, for the benefit of the widest possible community."

Qualitative researchers are ethically bound to disseminate findings for several reasons. First, we share the fruits of research—namely, information on study findings—to ensure that community members will continue to cooperate in future studies. Second, the use of qualitative research methods—whether focus group discussions with commercial sex workers or structured interviews with health educators—is based on creating trust. We reciprocate that trust by sharing information, returning the benefits of research to the individuals and communities that have contributed their insights. This ethical commitment to reciprocity has been formalized in guidelines for the informed consent process for international research involving human subjects, including qualitative research. In large part because community members in countries where AIDS research is being conducted have demanded that the benefits of research accrue to them more directly, international guidance documents are increasingly recommending that communities as well as study participants be informed of study findings after research is finished (Heise and others 1998; UNAIDS 2000b).

There are other reasons to take seriously your role in dissemination. For example, effective dissemination of findings is a cornerstone of the research partnership and a proxy indicator of research impact (Harris and Tanner 2000).

An Inclusive Dissemination Process Promotes Use

Ideally, qualitative study designs include a component in which study participants are contacted and asked whether the preliminary findings appear valid to them. For logistical and financial reasons, this phase is not always possible. Nevertheless, do what you can to check that your findings would make sense to your conversational partners. You might, for example, conduct exit interviews with stakeholders before leaving the study site. Every time you ask your participants how they understand the meaning of the data you are generating, you are inviting them to contribute to shaping the messages that will emerge from the research, while at the same time disseminating information on the study. Such interactive dissemination leads to more grounded and therefore more credible study findings.

Experts in diffusion of information agree that an inclusive and ongoing approach to research dissemination also leads to a greater likelihood that findings will be used (Rogers and Storey 1987; Havelock 1969; Cernada 1982). To foster a climate in which research is seen as relevant, involve stakeholders in as many research dissemination activities as possible. Stakeholder participation can mean very straightforward, simple activities. Maintaining frequent communication with key groups through visits, telephone calls, e-mail correspondence, or technical support is a powerful way to promote interest in and use of study findings. A recent study on the dissemination of research-based HIV prevention models to community service providers in the United States found that dissemination efforts are more successful when they "occur in the context of ongoing relationships between researchers and service providers, and when staff-training technical assistance is followed by opportunities to plan and problem-solve how to implement the research-based intervention" (Kelly and others 2000, p. 1087). The authors of this randomized control trial concluded that the frequency of outside contact reinforcing and supporting initial dissemination messages to health administrators and providers had a significant impact on adoption of new research-based HIV service delivery approaches.

How to Develop and Implement Dissemination

To develop a strategy for disseminating study findings and promoting their use, you will need to make decisions on what to say, to whom, and through which means—and make sure you have the staff and financial resources to conduct your plan. In practical terms a modest but effective package of dissemination activities might include facilitating the development of an information resource center in the study community (for example, a minilibrary containing the study report and relevant materials), publishing a newsletter with research results, collaborating on research reports, publishing journal articles, defining messages of importance to stakeholders, determining appropriate dissemination vehicles, or translating results for policy audiences.

Communication and participation are actually two words sharing the same concept. Etymologically the Latin communio *relates to participation and sharing.*
(Dagron 2001, p. 33)

At a minimum aim to do the following:

- Write a report and discuss it one-on-one with key decision makers
- Plan a half- to one-day presentation meeting for health professionals and advocacy organizations
- Return information to the community through community discussions, a brochure on findings (see Appendix Thirteen, which shows a brochure designed to share study findings with the communities that participated in the research), or other means
- Distribute copies of your report to local universities, libraries, and key local and international organizations

To increase the likelihood that your study results will be used, keep in mind that the information must be communicated to the appropriate potential users (primary and secondary users). Study findings must address issues that users perceive to be important, and reports must be presented in a form that users will understand and consider credible. Information must be delivered to each audience in time to be useful, such as during revision of national guidelines on health service delivery practices (Morris and others 1987). Special events such as World AIDS Day or International

BOX 8.1

Ways to Foster Two-Way Communication in Research

Research stakeholders are more likely to use study findings if they feel they have participated in creating the results and are consulted and kept informed throughout the research process (Rothman 1980). To promote use of study findings, plan to include two-way communication steps such as the following:

- Collaborative development of subprojects
- Regular two-way communication and consultation with stakeholders
- Regular written feedback to stakeholders on study purposes, progress, and findings
- Substantial face-to-face dialogue about progress, preliminary study results, implications of results for programs or policies
- Field trips with managers and stakeholders to view activities in order to create understanding, enthusiasm, and ownership of study results
- Collaborative seminars to interpret findings
- Joint development of a family of related print materials written at appropriate levels for different audiences
- Follow-up visits to ministry of health officials or other key parties to personally deliver and review the study report
- One-on-one discussions with stakeholders for informal discussion of results, with written communication regarding next steps

Source: Adapted from Population Council, 1994.

Women's Day may offer an opportunity to focus attention on your study. Also, try to make your communications as pleasant as possible—consider serving lunch at your dissemination seminar or combining tea and an informal talk with government officials to whom you hand the report.

No matter how modest or ambitious your dissemination goals are, develop a written strategy based on audience needs, your needs and resources, current and emerging opportunities, timing, and the power of your study findings (Rogers and Storey 1987).

A strategy should include the following twelve general steps and considerations:

- *Conduct a needs assessment to help shape the dissemination of findings.* One of the most important elements in dissemination to promote use of research findings is adequate understanding of what users need (Havelock 1969). Determine the degree of interest among researchers, health professionals, stakeholders, women's groups, and others who work to improve the public's health.
- *Make a list of what people want to know* and why they want to know it (Morris and others 1987). Consider the decision-making process and the most influential people working on this issue in the setting you are studying. Your stakeholders can also help create this list. Do not assume you know all the groups that could benefit from

BOX 8.2
Dissemination Factors That Promote Utilization

- The information needs of specific audiences are considered when designing the study.
- The credibility and reliability of the research findings are accepted by users of the study.
- Findings are disseminated to multiple audiences using a variety of channels and formats.
- Presentation of findings emphasizes the important lessons learned, especially from the point of view of the intended audience, rather than the need for more research.

Source: Adapted from Sharma 1996.

the information. Also, be aware that sometimes stakeholders may not want to disseminate information to certain groups; try to ascertain whom they do not want you to talk to and why. Remember that different groups of people need different kinds of information in different forms and at different times (Morris and others 1987). Ask who might be influential in action to improve health conditions, attitudes, programs, or policies suggested by research findings or recommendations and whether such individuals or groups have an explicit advocacy agenda.

Audiences that may be appropriate to involve in dissemination, either as creators or recipients of information related to your study findings, may include other researchers, health program directors, planning ministries, donor agencies, news media, or nongovernmental organizations (NGOs) that focus on women's health, human rights, adolescent health, or civil society.

- *Ask yourself if your findings will or should matter to your audiences.* Be realistic. Ask whether the information in your report is

  Relevant to the user's real and compelling problems

  Practical from the user's perspective

  Useful and applicable to their situation

  Understandable to potential users

  Timely (Morris and others 1987)

- *Ask if the findings will have a negative impact or be controversial.* When you originally designed your study, you should have considered the potentially disadvantageous uses of the data you planned to collect. In planning your dissemination strategy, be sure to revisit these issues. Anticipate whether your study results might be embarrassing to program administrators, parliamentarians, or other community leaders accountable for decisions and oversight of health programs and policies (Hess 1989). Consider whether news media or citizen groups may take the findings out of context. Be aware that "the study will be used, one way or another, and sometimes those uses are different from the ones [the researcher] intends" (Rossman and Rallis 1998, p. 11).

Sometimes study findings lend themselves to misinterpretation and therefore need special consideration in dissemination planning. For example, in a combined qualitative and quantitative study of the social and economic consequences of family planning use in the southern Philippines, researchers found that one-fourth of all women, rural and urban, reported ever having been physically harmed by a spouse (Cabaraban and Morales 1998). The study found that among the significant correlates of violence were the wife working for pay and the husband sharing household chores. When initially presenting these results in the community, some audiences mistakenly concluded that male involvement in cleaning and washing leads to violence. One man commented, "Therefore, in order to avoid violence, we must not do household chores." To correct further misinterpretation of the results, the research team met with stakeholders to develop a dissemination strategy (personal communication from M. Cabaraban to E. T. Robinson, Aug. 2001, unreferenced). Jointly, they developed an approach to serve the community interest while avoiding potential distortion of the data. They recommended that churches use the research results in developing guidelines for marriage counseling, that local institutions be encouraged to provide safe haven and legal services for battered women, and that health providers—including traditional midwives and healers—be trained to provide assistance and referrals for women experiencing violence.

How your study results will be used may be outside your control, but you are responsible for anticipating the potential negative uses of the information. By planning ahead, you can assist stakeholders and members of your research team to prepare for findings that may be controversial or lend themselves to distortion.

- *Find out what criteria the audience uses to assess the information it gets.* To promote effective communication, determine which sources of information the group considers to be credible, useful, or timely (Goldstein and others 1998). Note the style of dissemination that best meets this group's needs. Some may prefer brief or graphically interesting materials, whereas others do better with a more comprehensive or academically oriented presentation. Sometimes written dissemination is not culturally appropriate, but a series of community discussions would be. Different groups need different information, in different languages, using different terminology, delivered in formats that respect cultural or other norms. Timing and opportunities will also differ by group.
- *Identify people to work with.* If you have determined that you have time to disseminate your findings only through written reports, consider working with local groups that could plan and implement broader dissemination of the findings. These might include professional associations, librarians, broadcast journalists, NGOs, or folk media committed to disseminating health messages.
- *Find as many ways as possible to report results back to key groups* interested in the findings. Ask yourself who could best deliver the information. The knowledge dissem-

BOX 8.3

Working with the Media

The media play a key role in conveying health information to researchers, clinicians, and the general public (Grimes 1999).

Mass communication using news media, advertising, and marketing channels works particularly well to publicize new information and influence social norms. Media coverage of public health issues can demonstrate the benefits of particular policies, articulate obstacles to health services, or model behaviors such as responsible parenthood (Smith WA 1995). If your study purpose involves communicating results to a wide group of people and you have sufficient resources to do so, seek out a media professional or health advocate who can help you plan effective activities, keeping these guidelines in mind:

- Establish your message.
- Consider your audiences and direct your messages to them. Your audiences are mostly interested in how they are affected by what you say.
- Know your facts.
- Use human language. Everyone relates best to human experiences, so use stories drawn from your research to make your key points easier to absorb. Try to avoid technical terms. Use quotes from research participants to illustrate your message.
- State your conclusions clearly, from the beginning (Seidel 1993). For example, you might say, "This study showed that prophylactic provision of emergency contraception prevents abortion, and let me tell you why."
- When interviewed, stick to a couple of key points; practice articulating a very brief message that broadcast journalists can use as a sound bite.

ination and use literature shows that information produced internally—in contrast to information imported from outside an organization or a country—is often more acceptable and more credible. Consider various options, including copresenting the information with a health program manager who intends to use the findings. Find out if existing consortia, such as a national health task force, can either integrate their dissemination efforts with yours or reinforce your efforts with supporting messages. Offer a local health Web site the opportunity to post your study report's executive summary.

- *Identify opportunities for dissemination* and consider the possibility of controversy. Identify other relevant activities going on in the setting (for example, conferences, events, or media coverage of a related issue) that could either support or conflict with your dissemination plan.

  Community organizations can sometimes use research summaries or fact sheets as supporting information in their proposals to donors for funding service delivery projects.

  In short, plan specific ways to reach out to each important audience through channels that have appropriate "reach, frequency, and cultural impact" (Seidel 1993,

p. 2). If time and financial resources allow you to collaborate with a communications consultant or a local NGO skilled in dissemination, ask them to develop and pretest materials and messages for various intended audiences.

- *Identify dissemination priorities using a collaborative process* as you develop your strategy. Perhaps you work at a major university and have conducted in-depth interviews on the use of emergency contraceptive pills in collaboration with research partners in several locations. You might decide—and your study participants might tell you—that health professionals, women's advocates, and policymakers all could benefit from the findings. In this case your strategic priorities, developed with appropriate input, might be to do the following:

  Widely disseminate technical data on emergency contraception and the specific study results (locally, nationally, internationally).

  Help local experts or other partners understand that how they translate findings and technical information into political or programmatic terms is key to gaining support for policy or program changes.

  Build local capacity for ongoing dissemination and policy reform related to provision of emergency contraceptive services (Porter and Hicks 1995).

If you intend to influence an audience, know its motivations and its idiosyncrasies.

(Morris and others 1987, p. 15)

As a researcher, you likely will not implement a comprehensive dissemination strategy without assistance. You may be too busy, may not consider it appropriate, or may not have the needed resources or skills. But your role in identifying dissemination priorities is crucial: you have sifted through the data and articulated what they mean.

- *Begin disseminating from the outset.* From the first day of your contact with stakeholders, inform them of your study's purpose, its limitations, and its potential outcomes. A participatory approach increases the likelihood that the eventual results will be discussed and used. Where feasible, inviting policymakers to contribute questions of importance to them encourages interest among leaders in a position to initiate change.
- *Help study participants play an active role in informing others.* Simple dissemination activities, such as handing out a short letter describing your study's goals, may help to create a climate conducive to research and empower research stakeholders to support your work. Be cautious to present such material in a way that avoids the appearance of a public announcement, being clear that it is an internal communication to the research team or participants. Consider also that once you have provided written materials to individuals or groups, your materials may be inappropriately used or printed in a local newspaper.
- *Help your readers identify the most important information.* If you are developing printed materials, use headings; write topic sentences; and pay attention to spacing, margins, and graphic design. In short, do what you can to improve the readability of your material (Morris and others 1987).

BOX 8.4
How to Make Study Findings Accessible

Obtain an International Standard Book Number (ISBN) number or other standard cataloging information for each substantial document you produce. It will help promote correct cataloging and easy retrieval by local and international library reference staff and users.

- Submit your citation to bibliographic indexing databases such as POPLINE, Asia-Pacific POPIN, and WorldCat to ensure that researchers will have worldwide access to your article or abstract through libraries, commercial information services, and the Internet.
- Post study reports for which you hold the copyright on the Internet—either on your institution's Web site or that of a sister agency interested in disseminating health information.
- Make your data set available to other researchers for additional secondary analysis through a major university archive in your country or region or to the Social Science Information Gateway or the Inter-University Consortium for Political and Social Research. Sharing your data set is one of the most cost-effective forms of research collaboration. Data set archives should include copies of data collection protocols, study reports, analyses, and computer files of the actual data, searchable by region, country, study population, date of study, and the variables covered by the study (Piotrow and others 1997).

See Appendix Fourteen for more details.

How to Reach Policy Audiences

Health policy reform is a process composed of three dynamic, interactive activities: defining a problem, generating solutions, and building political consensus (Porter and Hicks 1995). If shared effectively, your research findings can influence policy in defining health problems and shedding light on possible solutions. Translating research findings into terms that address the interests and concerns of decision makers and other groups active in public policy is not easy, but it is vital (Porter and Prysor-Jones 1997). As Rist (2000, p. 1005) notes, "Qualitative research can be highly influential . . . with respect to problem definition, understanding of prior initiatives, community and organizational receptivity to particular programmatic approaches, and the kinds of impacts (both anticipated and unanticipated) that might emerge from different intervention strategies." Make use of the power of your participants' words and stories to engage those who influence policy. Select the "face" or aspect of the problem that is most relevant to the interests of your particular audience: a simplified understanding of the problem is crucial in generating support for solutions (Porter and Hicks 1995).

If you want to capture the interest of busy policymakers, include an executive summary to accompany a more lengthy report. An executive summary should state the following: (1) what you studied; (2) why you conducted the study; and (3) what major findings, conclusions, and recommendations you have generated. Some readers may not have the time or expertise to read through your report, but they will want to know what you found and how it applies to them.

Identify locally credible champions—not necessarily experts but respected individuals able to convey research-based information—to make the case for change with those who can actually influence health policies and their implementation. Working to influence policy is a form of behavior change intervention, a field in which both theory and data point to the importance of participative decision making and face-to-face interactions that lead to commitments to change (Stevens and Tornatzky 1980). Never underestimate the importance of personal contact in your policy dissemination efforts.

Oral Presentation of Qualitative Findings

Oral presentation of qualitative findings is very similar to presentation of quantitative study results, with the distinction that treatment of quotes from participants usually replaces statistical summaries of the data. As with all dissemination formats, be sensitive to audience needs and expectations (for example, by determining the time your audience has to listen and speaking less than the maximum time allotted); know whether overhead slides or projection images will be better received and what contextual information will be important to provide; and focus on the main question, paying attention to the quality of what you say. When structuring your oral presentation, include the following sections:

All information is subject to misuse; and no information is devoid of possible harm to one interest or another. Researchers are usually not in a position to prevent action based on their findings; but they should, however, attempt to pre-empt any likely misinterpretations and to counteract them when they occur.
(Association of Social Anthropologists of the Commonwealth 1999)

Opening. Set the scene by telling a story that will interest your audience.

Introduction. Tell your listeners what your presentation will cover:

- What health issue did you study?
- Why did you conduct the study (objectives) and why was it important?
- What questions did you ask, and how did they evolve as you analyzed initial responses?
- What methods did you use, and how close did you get to the participants in the study setting?
- Which results will you discuss?

Body of the talk. Discuss your results sequentially, and relate them to your theoretical framework. Clarify each point by using examples and presenting selected short quotes from study participants to illustrate major findings. Offer your interpretation of how applicable the findings may be to other settings, and describe the limitations of your work.

Summary. Summarize for the audience the important points in your talk. Articulate any unanswered questions, and identify areas that need further study.

Two of the most important elements of successful presentations are (1) to keep overheads, slides, or other visuals short and simple; and (2) to practice giving your

BOX 8.5
Policy Dissemination Tips

- Keep reports brief.
- Provide talking points to policy stakeholders who may either use or disseminate your study results.
- Recognize that research results may have larger political implications, requiring consensus of many stakeholders before action can occur.
- Encourage policymakers to weigh data from different sources.
- In planning for use of information for policy purposes, consider the availability of resources, the institutional capacity to change practices, and political risk (Rist 2000, pp. 1013–4).

talk beforehand. To hold your audience's interest and to share ownership of the findings, consider inviting a key informant or other stakeholder to copresent the findings. Remember that you are sharing the words and experiences of people who entrusted their stories to you. Do not be afraid to try presentation formats that convey the drama and emotion of their lives.

Outcome Indicators for Dissemination

Because you do not know precisely where the research will lead or to whom the findings will be important, you cannot define outcome indicators for effective dissemination at the outset of your qualitative study. Nevertheless, as you proceed with the study, do your best to identify appropriate indicators for use of the results. Defining possible ways to measure the effects of dissemination will help focus your efforts on activities with greater impact.

To develop indicators, make use of existing theoretical frameworks developed by scientists who study knowledge dissemination and use. For example, Havelock's classic review (1969) of four thousand studies on knowledge dissemination and use framed how individuals and groups use knowledge in terms of three categories: (1) problem solving; (2) social interaction; and (3) research, development, and diffusion. Try to visualize how different groups might use your study to address health care or service delivery problems; how the findings might influence relationships among individuals or groups concerned with your topic; and how your study findings might affect future research, public awareness, or community empowerment to improve health. These possible outcomes may become your dissemination indicators. They may include changes in the information resources available to stakeholders or changes in their knowledge base, information-seeking behavior, or decision-making processes (Menou 1993, 1999; Thorngate 1995).

Process indicators for dissemination of study findings are data and indicators compiled at the program level. What might the application of your findings mean to program planning, allocation of resources, procedures, or functions (Buckner and others 1995)? Process indicators for the short-term or intermediate outcomes (or effects) of public health research dissemination may include the following:

- Publication of study findings in-country as well as internationally
- Presence of study reports in local, national, and international libraries
- News media coverage of study findings
- Number of individuals or groups who need the information reached with summaries of results
- Locally initiated translation of study findings into local languages or easier-to-read formats
- Increase in the number of ongoing opportunities for and instances of communication between community stakeholders and health researchers or policymakers
- Number of short courses or conferences at which study results are disseminated
- Funds allocated for additional communication of results
- Adoption by sister research agencies of future research priorities suggested by your study

The long-term or ultimate outcomes (or impacts) of qualitative research dissemination are harder to measure but nevertheless important (Beck and Stelcner 1996a, 1996b). They may include the following:

- The number, variety, and mutuality of relationships between those interested in the health issues you studied and those who are in a position to help them (Cernada 1982; Havelock 1969; Human Interaction Research Institute 1976)
- Enhanced mutual understanding of terminology or language used by different groups (researchers, politicians, community members) to describe health concepts
- Increased accuracy in the information that stakeholders share in dialogue or debate (Communications Initiative Partners Meeting 2000)
- Growing respect among research stakeholders for each other's perspectives, manifested in greater degree or regularity of consensus on action steps favoring improved health care delivery
- The number, variety, frequency, and persistence of forces that can be mobilized to use the knowledge generated (Havelock 1969)
- Changes in health services or policies attributable to your research
- A high level of citations of your report in scientific papers and international bibliographic indexing databases
- Increased long-term news media coverage of the topic you studied (as measured through content analyses over time)

- Allocation of funds or government support for further research on aspects of the topic you studied
- Systematic use of study findings in public health, educational, and training institution curricula
- The percentage of organizations that subsequently offered an evidence-based model of services in line with your research findings

Common sense tells us that if we know where we want to go, we are more likely to get there. Identifying outcome indicators for dissemination is one way to keep your sights on the potential use of your study findings by people who need them.

Conclusion

The biggest challenge to disseminating qualitative research may lie within ourselves and our conceptions of our roles as researchers. If we do not perceive communication as an explicit research responsibility or are uncomfortable in the role of dissemination, our work and the insights it generates are unlikely to make a difference to people's well-being or to the health programs and policies that serve them.

Neither academic nor medical and health research institutions . . . regard it as their responsibility to communicate their research findings to local policymakers, practicing health professionals, or the public.
(Kitua and others 2000, p. 821)

Even if your orientation, interests, and resources allow you to develop ambitious research dissemination objectives and plans, you will likely face challenges and frustrations as you proceed. A participatory approach to collaboration with stakeholders in the iterative process of dissemination or materials development takes more time than implementing dissemination unilaterally or limiting dissemination to publication of a scientific paper. Community members or health service delivery staff may not be convinced that change is desirable or possible. Recommendations suggested by the findings may be considered too innovative for the current political climate. Or research findings may not be focused enough to provide guidelines for action, and you may need to confer again with stakeholders able to create and take responsibility for disseminating action-oriented recommendations.

For qualitative researchers research dissemination is both an ethical obligation and a practical necessity. It is most effective when planned and implemented from the outset with significant involvement of research stakeholders. We urge qualitative researchers to question prevailing notions of their role in dissemination; incorporate ideas into dissemination plans as they surface in the research process; and take active steps to bridge the information gap between the research community, health practitioners, health advocates, and policymakers.

Field Perspective

Involving Librarians, Researchers, and the Media in Dissemination Planning

Edmond Bagdé Dingamhoudou

Population Council, Senegal

In 1997–1998 the Centre d'Études et de Recherche sur la Population pour le Développement (CERPOD) and Family Health International conducted a qualitative study in Mali of women's experience with contraception—what they expect from it, why many are reluctant to try it, and why some start but do not continue (Castle and others 1999). Researchers followed fifty-six new contraceptive users in Bamako, the capital, over an eighteen-month period to see how family pressures encourage or discourage contraceptive use, focusing on communication, support, and strategies women use to control their fertility. Women were recruited during their initial visit to the Association Malienne pour la Protection et la Promotion de la Famille clinic and interviewed three times at eight- to nine-month intervals. Eleven focus group discussions were held with approximately one hundred experienced users, married men, and older women with daughters-in-law. Thirty-two women who had never used contraception also were interviewed.

The study yielded a number of findings that the research team thought were useful for family planning program staff and others. What good are findings that are shared only among the people who have conducted the study, without further dissemination? This question is becoming increasingly relevant to research endeavors on the African continent. It follows that no dissemination process can achieve its desired results as long as the messages that it seeks to convey do not address issues of public concern.

While CERPOD was finalizing a written report on the study (CERPOD 1999), our documentation center was also organizing a regional workshop on disseminating population and reproductive health research findings. We hoped to set up a regional reproductive health network of librarians and documentation specialists who could work with both journalists and researchers. The program included a training session on dissemination concepts in which participants developed practical ways of disseminating research findings using drafts of unpublished brochures.

The workshop participants were split into four groups. Each group was asked to list the elements of a dissemination campaign and to present its ideas on how to distribute the family planning study brochure. All possible means of dissemination were recorded. An introductory session on the Internet was even offered to the many participants who were not yet familiar with this tool. During the plenary session, all the ideas were synthesized and discussed to see which ones converged. At the end of the workshop, each participant went home with a written dissemination plan for the CERPOD materials.

Direct contact with journalists, documentation specialists, librarians, and researchers made it possible to examine closely the barriers to an effective dissemination process. The researchers, documentation specialists, and librarians were very open about their fear of working with journalists. They considered them to be too hurried and motivated by sensationalism. Importantly, they believed that journalists tend not to credit the source of the information (the researcher) or the contribution of the documentation specialist or librarian. In turn, the journalists criticized the others for being suspicious and overly cautious about distributing information.

Eventually, participants discovered the complementary roles of the different groups involved in the dissemination process. The journalists showed the researchers, documentation specialists, and librarians how to write a press release for the media, announcing the availability of the new publication. The journalists then learned from the others how to conduct documentation searches.

Any dissemination process must pay special attention to the support materials; the message itself; and areas of technical, professional, and even artistic design. My advice to qualitative researchers planning study dissemination is to use any opportunity to reach those who could use the information in their work or lives. Also, I recommend involving other relevant groups, such as librarians and journalists, as we did in the CERPOD workshop.

Field Perspective

Transforming Research Findings into a *Telenovela*

Patricia Bailey, Dr.P.H.

Family Health International

Toward the end of Family Health International's five-year multinational Women's Studies Project, those of us who had worked on the project's studies and dissemination planning in Bolivia discussed how to share project findings with groups outside traditional academic and public health circles. As the research projects in Bolivia were ending, we planned a final dissemination conference for ministry officials, nongovernmental organizations (NGOs), and women's health advocates. The conference format, which included panels on specific themes that emerged across the studies and activities, allowed participants to synthesize findings and articulate practical recommendations. We also contracted with a local video producer, Fundación Solón, to take these themes, write a script, and produce a video, which was transformed into a four-chapter miniseries produced for television. This short *telenovela* fictionalized the lives and voices that were revealed to us and became an instrument of entertainment, education, reflection, and controversy. As a co-investigator on several of the Bolivia studies, I found the popularization of scientific findings to be a unique and exciting experience.

The five studies used a range of qualitative and quantitative methodologies, including a case study of women-centered health care services; a cross-sectional survey of couples; in-depth interviews with men and women; a longitudinal survey of women; and a situational analysis of services that included interviews with clinic staff, clinic users, and nonusers. In different ways each generated rich insights into our research question: how the use and nonuse of family planning services affected women's lives.

We met several times with the video producer, who was convinced that the qualitative nature of the findings translated well into a drama with great human interest. The producer intertwined several subplots to reflect the complexities of urban life in El Alto, a fast-growing city filled with immigrants who arrive from rural areas with their cultural traditions and customs intact. The producer chose to depict the tensions of everyday life through a character who loses his job and, humiliated, must turn to his wife for financial support; discrimination between social classes and ethnic subgroups; a young woman seeking to ensure a better life and her partner who is threatened by her independent behavior and desire to delay childbearing; an adolescent who is faced with an unwanted pregnancy and in desperation seeks an abortion; and an unhappy physician who finds neither his personal nor his professional life satisfying. All these themes came directly from the findings of the five studies. In the *telenovela* these difficulties and challenges are mediated by images of the rising sun in the *altiplano* (the highlands), the poignant hilarity of a tuba-playing drunk, a coy flirtation between two elderly clinic workers, and the compassion that individuals express when faced with the suffering of others.

Subplots in the *telenovela* illustrated perceptions and conditions that study participants shared with us:

- An adolescent discovers her unwanted pregnancy and resorts to an unsafe abortion with severe complications. She almost loses her life, but the young physician intervenes and saves her, restoring his faith in himself and his professional calling to help others.
- A middle-aged man loses his job and drinks excessively; his wife becomes the sole support for the family. In order to cope with this new responsibility, she wants to use a contraceptive method to avoid future pregnancies. Together they attend the physician's clinic, are counseled, and leave with condoms.

- A young woman, a university student, seeks an intrauterine device without telling her partner. She wants to delay childbearing in order to finish her degree; but when her partner finds out, he attacks her and goes to the clinic and assaults the physician.
- An elderly cleaning woman at the clinic and the clinic gardener begin a relationship, but she has misgivings about sex after menopause. The physician assures her that sex at her age is fine.
- The physician suffers a personal and a professional crisis. His wife throws him out when she discovers he has visited a prostitute. His car is stolen, and he decides to quit his work to take a job as a car salesman, like his friend.

Reflecting tensions revealed in the research, the physician character stands for the superiority of Western medicine whereas the older indigenous clinic cleaning woman, a traditional herbalist, represents traditional medicine. When the irate young husband beats up the physician, the cleaning woman successfully treats the physician, who gains new respect for traditional medicine. Class, social, and ethnic tensions are exhibited between the indigenous older woman at the clinic and the young doctor who treats her poorly—for example, he won't give her a ride in his car because she might be dirty.

Besides being shown on television, the video will be used in preservice training for medical and nursing students in Bolivia and elsewhere in the region. It is to be used also among health care professionals at NGOs and in the public sector to promote discussion of the many factors that influence health. Differences in gender, ethnicity, culture, and social class all translate into an imbalance of power and lack of recognition of human rights within civil society as well as among health care professionals. Meanwhile, we await the public's reaction to this human, powerful, and accessible teaching medium. (The telenovela is entitled *Fueguitos del Alma,* or *Fireworks of the Soul,* and is available by contacting Patricia Bailey at Family Health International, P.O. Box 13950, Research Triangle Park, NC 27709.)

Field Perspective

What We Learned from Conducting Qualitative Research on Reproductive Health in China

Baochang Gu, Ph.D.

China Population Information and Research Center

A study on the impact of family planning on women's lives in China (Xie and others 2000), conducted as part of the Women's Studies Project of Family Health International,* was the first study conducted through international collaboration in China with the explicit goal of investigating directly how family planning has affected women, both positively and negatively. The study employed both focus group discussion (FGD) and a questionnaire survey. The FGDs, which allowed hearing the voices of both women and men whose lives are immediately affected by family planning, turned out to be a novel study methodology that provided valuable information for program implementation.

A number of studies have been conducted since the mid-1980s using quantitative data to assess the abnormally high ratio of male to female births in China. However, the FGD approach used in this study revealed how people rationalize sex preference in children and why people in rural China so desperately want to have a son. Some women in North Anhui said: "To have high status in the community you need a son. Otherwise you are looked down upon in the family and community." "Without sons, your husband will dislike you; you will be very much discriminated against by the mother-in-law and the family." "These women live miserable lives, especially if they are sterilized. Then there is no more hope. You terminated your family line."

In fact, our fieldwork suggests that the methodology greatly altered the relationship between the researcher and the researched. With a questionnaire survey, people tend to act as information providers, seeing the study as unrelated to their own interests and well-being. Sometimes respondents are unmotivated or even become bored and uncooperative in responding to a long list of questions. But participants in an FGD tend to use it as an opportunity for their voices to be heard. They feel respected and heard.

At the beginning of the project, the research staff were worried about whether women would be willing to talk openly, especially on sensitive topics related to their personal reproductive lives. During the sessions, once the purpose and subject of the session were explained, there was an initial silence, and then women would start to speak one after another. Sometimes several women were vying for the chance to speak out; they did not want to miss the chance to talk. In all of the study areas, participants often had so much to tell that the session had to go beyond the scheduled time.

Such a situation made the note taker's work difficult and the recorded tapes difficult to transcribe. However, getting women and men to talk from their hearts was something that was unusual in China and something that a quantitative survey could never achieve. The human touch of the qualitative approach requires the investigators to place themselves in an equal position with the participants. A key lesson that we learned is that FGD sessions could not be successful unless participants were convinced that they could trust the investigators and that the study would bring some improvement to their lives.

Successful fieldwork requires the support and cooperation of local government, particularly because management of the highly sensitive subject of family planning is devolved to local government leaders in China. Acutely aware of the implications, the field team met first with local program leaders and managers to explain the purpose of the study and detail procedures, including how participants would be selected and their desired characteristics. We emphasized that the study would not assess the performance of the local program but that the people interviewed would provide information to make general improvements in the China family planning program. Local assistance is necessary not only to gain the cooperation of the local government but also to recruit local field assistants for the FGDs.

A questionnaire survey that complemented the FGDs was carried out in the same project areas. The combined quantitative and qualitative methods provided rich, complementary information and helped us to interpret our findings in a more convincing way than we might have in using either methodology alone. This triangulation of data strongly helped the leaders and managers of the family planning programs to understand the need to hear women's own views of the relationship between family planning and other aspects of their lives.

This research was conducted at a time when China is considering how to shift away from its long-time emphasis on demographic goals. Our study provided a context to understand the need for a client-centered orientation in family planning and helped pave the way for an innovative quality of care experiment that China's State Family Planning Commission has conducted since 1995. This study took the rare step of listening to individuals' voices, a departure for China's family planning program in the mid-1990s. Since our work was implemented, understanding and meeting clients' needs for quality reproductive health care has increasingly become the central theme of the family planning program in China. The voices of women and men from south Jiangsu, north Anhui, and central Yunnan were heard clearly by family planning leaders not only in their own provinces but also by national leaders in Beijing.

**The Women's Studies Project was funded primarily by the U.S. Agency for International Development. This study in China was funded by the Rockefeller Foundation and the Ford Foundation.*

APPENDIX ONE

Samples of Behavioral Frameworks

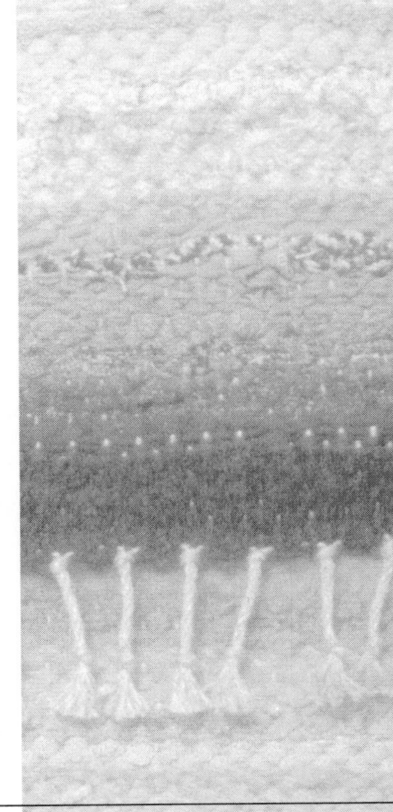

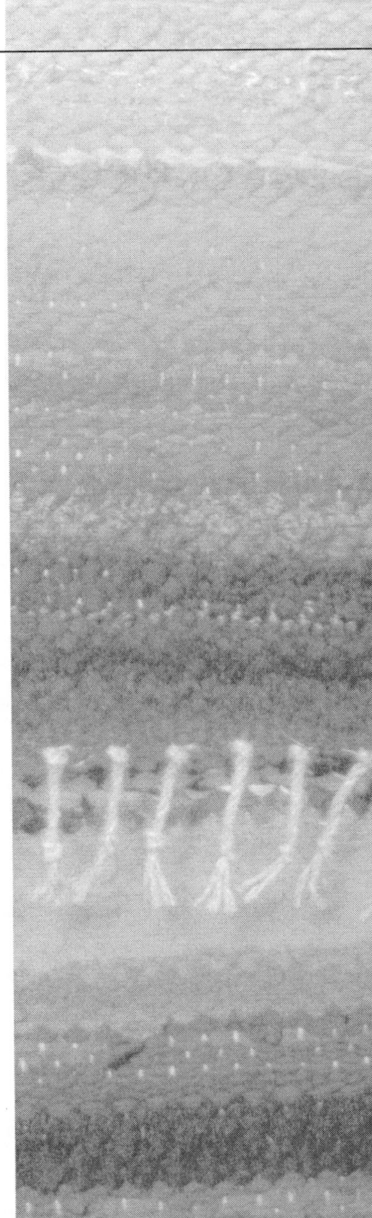

THEORETICAL FRAMEWORKS from the behavioral sciences can be a valuable source of ideas for developing a research problem and a way of linking one's research to a wider theoretical context. In qualitative research, however, the investigator must take care not to impose structure at the expense of spontaneity and new insight into the problem. Nevertheless, frameworks that have been developed, tested, and refined in numerous studies of a common behavioral phenomenon, such as taking action to reduce health risk, contain useful concepts and relationships that can add clarity to a research problem without putting constraints on the methodology.

Qualitative researchers should also note a common limitation of most behavioral frameworks, namely their focus on individual behavior. For instance, many women feel at risk of HIV, not due to their own behavior but because of their sexual partners' behavior. Qualitative designs that use concepts drawn from behavioral models must also encompass the wider social and cultural context—economic constraints, normative influences, and as always, gender and power differences that could explain or contradict the findings of a study limited by a predetermined model.

Following are summaries of five frameworks that have been useful to researchers in sexual and reproductive health.

Health Belief Model

One of the most commonly used frameworks in health behavior research, the health belief model, offers useful guidance for understanding sexual risk behaviors (Rosenstock and others 1994). Basic premises of the model are that individuals differ in two ways:

(1) how they perceive the personal benefits or value of avoiding illness or getting well and (2) their expectations that a specific action can prevent illness. People are more likely to take action to prevent or control an ill-health condition if the following apply:

- They believe it to have potentially serious consequences.
- They believe that a course of action available to them would be beneficial in reducing either their susceptibility to or the severity of the condition.
- They believe that the anticipated barriers to (or costs of) taking the action outweigh its benefits (Glanz 2002; VanLandringham and others 1995).

This model can address programmatic or practical questions, such as "Why are women discontinuing the use of intrauterine devices?" or "Why are commercial sex workers not using condoms with their steady partners?" Key concepts are the following:

Perceived susceptibility: people's perception of their chance of getting a condition such as pregnancy or HIV infection (Brown and others 1991)

Perceived severity: opinions of how serious are the medical, social, or financial consequences of a health condition

Perceived benefits: perceptions of the efficacy of the recommended action (for example, abstinence, condom use, contraception) to reduce health risks

Perceived barriers: perceptions of the psychological, social, or financial costs of adopting the new health behavior

Cues or triggers to action: events that increase the likelihood of action, including symptoms of infection or exposure to messages on the radio

Self-efficacy: the conviction that one can successfully carry out an action, such as consistent use of preventive measures required to produce certain outcomes (for example, prevention of pregnancy or disease) (Bandura 1977)

Other variables: especially sociodemographic factors such as educational attainment, as they influence an individual's perceptions and thus indirectly influence health-related behavior

Stages of Change Theory

In this framework behavior change occurs as a sequence of stages that vary by individual. It can be a useful tool for tailoring health interventions to the needs of target groups—segmented by behavioral stage—and for evaluating programs by measuring behavior change at different stages (Prochaska and others 2002).

Key concepts are the following:

Precontemplation: the stage in which an individual is at risk but with no intention to modify behavior (for example, sexually active adolescents who do not believe they can get pregnant, diabetic women who are uninformed about the dangers of repeated pregnancies, or smokers who ignore the consequences of nicotine and tar in tobacco).

Contemplation: the stage at which an individual recognizes the need for change but is ambivalent.

Preparation for action: individuals at this stage intend to take action and may have initiated limited behavior change (occasional attempts to stop smoking); they may be good candidates for behavior change programs that focus on action steps (smoking cessation programs).

Action: the individual has made specific modifications in behavior or lifestyles sufficient to reduce the risk (a decision not to purchase cigarettes).

Maintenance: sustained behavior change for more than six months.

Factors that influence movement through this sequence of changes may also come from other frameworks, for example, perceived severity of risk or sense of self-efficacy as in the health belief model.

AIDS Risk Reduction Model

The AIDS risk reduction model (ARRM) provides a framework for explaining behavior change in relation to the sexual transmission of HIV/AIDS (Catania and others 1990). It incorporates several variables from other behavior change frameworks, including several from the health belief model: self-efficacy and theoretical understanding of interpersonal processes. Like the stages of change framework, ARRM hypothesizes a sequence of three stages of change: (1) recognizing and labeling one's behavior as high risk, (2) making a commitment to reduce high-risk sexual contacts and to increase low-risk activities, and (3) taking action. The last stage is further classified as seeking information, obtaining remedies, and enacting solutions. Phases may occur concurrently or may be skipped, depending on the individual.

Variables that influence movement through these stages include the following:

- Knowledge of sexual activities associated with AIDS transmission, belief in personal susceptibility, believing that AIDS is undesirable
- Costs and benefits of action, self-efficacy, knowledge of the health utility and pleasure of a sexual practice
- Social networks and problem-solving help, prior experience with problems and solutions, self-esteem, verbal communication with sexual partner, partner's beliefs and behaviors

In addition to the influences listed here, ARRM postulates other motivators to change such as public education campaigns, informal support groups, or an image of a person dying from AIDS. In the past ten years, ARRM studies have examined a variety of populations, including people attending HIV-testing clinics, gay and bisexual men, unmarried heterosexuals, and adolescent women attending family planning centers. Results from a published study revealed how difficult it was for women in Zaire to label their high-risk behavior as problematic; only one-third of the study participants felt personally at risk for contracting HIV/AIDS (Bertrand and others 1992).

Locus of Control

This theoretical construct is derived from social learning theory. It has been used to conceptualize the distinction between the belief that events in one's life are the result of one's own action and the belief that such events are governed by forces independent of oneself (Wallston and others 1978; Lau 1982). Health locus of control has been measured by a scale composed of items that determine the relative strength of external or internal health beliefs about health and illness. Key concepts are the following:

External locus of control: belief that outcomes are under the control of powerful others or are determined by fate, luck, or chance

Internal locus of control: belief that outcomes are directly the result of one's behavior

Locus of control is relevant to research problems that focus on behavior change to reduce the risk of HIV. For example, a fatalistic attitude toward one's risk of acquiring the HIV virus (internal locus of control) is likely to be associated with inconsistent or incorrect use of condoms, in contrast to consistent use of condoms by individuals who believe they offer protection against disease (external locus of control). However, a woman who believes in the efficacy of condoms might also believe that she has no power to control the decision to use them. For her behavior change is limited by an external locus of control, in this case the perceived influence of "powerful others."

The Social-Ecological Model

The social-ecological model is not so much a theory with a characteristic conceptual framework as it is a general approach to designing health promotion research and programs. The basic premise of the model is that individuals are located in social, institutional, and physical environments and that interaction between the individual and forces in their environments influences health and well-being (Stokols and others 1996; McLeroy and others 1988; Sallis and Owen 2002). Research designed from a social-ecological perspective typically examines relationships between two or more of the following levels:

- Individual: knowledge, attitudes, skills, physiology directly attributable to a single individual
- Interpersonal: interactions between health providers and clients or between members of couples, families, networks of friends
- Organizational: formal and informal groupings of individuals around particular interests, including workplaces and social institutions
- Community: relationships among organizations, physical environment
- Policy: legislation at local, national, or international level

In health fields the primary research focus is often the individual, but this model draws attention to aggregate levels of influence on individual and group behavior. It suggests levels of investigation for study design, but specific constructs are more likely to come from other social and behavioral theories. We have summarized several theoretical frameworks with examples of individual-level constructs. For example, research designed from a social-ecological perspective with a focus on obesity among young adolescents might include the following:

- In-depth interviews with normal and overweight adolescents to explore issues related to self-esteem, perceptions concerning idealized and actual body size, knowledge and attitudes related to diet and exercise, perceptions of self-efficacy in adopting new dietary and exercise-related behaviors
- Group or individual interviews with parents of normal and overweight adolescents on food management decisions, including food budget, meal planning, food preparation, portion sizes, and interactions between parents and children about food
- Observations of physical environments of the households and communities of normal and overweight adolescents, including access to safe spaces for physical activity

Theories that relate to other levels of the social-ecological model include social support at the interpersonal level (Cohen and Wills 1995), organizational change at the organizational level (Emmons and others 2000), and both diffusion of innovations (Rogers 1983) and empowerment and social change (Freudenberg and others 1995) theories that address individual, organizational, and community as well as policy levels.

APPENDIX TWO

Examples of Oral Consent Forms

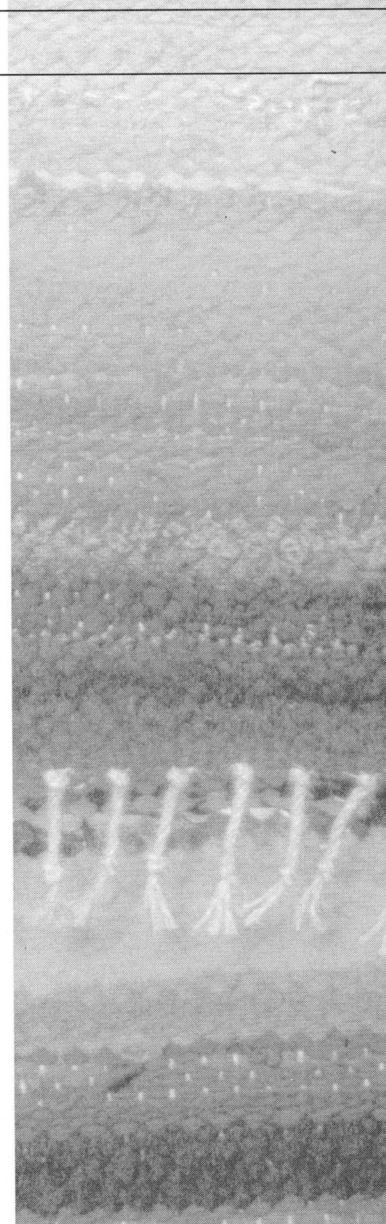

Example 1

FAMILY HEALTH INTERNATIONAL

ORAL INFORMED CONSENT FOR FOCUS GROUPS

(FOR MODERATOR TO READ TO FOCUS GROUP)

Name of research study:

Principal investigator:

Reason for the Research:______________________________

We would like to talk to you about taking part in discussion group(s) conducted by *(name of organization)* to *(objectives of the research study in easily understood words).*

You are being asked to take part in a group that will have a trained leader. The groups will talk about *(discussion topics).*

Your Part in the Research Study

About *(number of women/men/couples)* will take part in this research *(specify at this site and/or at number of sites).*

If you agree to take part in the research, you will be in _______ groups lasting _______ hours each.

Your participation is voluntary, and there is no penalty for refusing to take part. (If you do not take part, it will not affect any health care that you would normally receive.) Also, you may quit being in the groups at any time.

How You Were Identified

We are asking you to participate because we are talking to people who use the *(name of clinic).*

Possible Risks and Benefits

There is a small chance that what people talk about in the group will make you feel uncomfortable. There is also a small chance that others in the group may tell someone you were taking part or report what you said.

Confidentiality

No one except the group leaders and the other group members will know that you took part in the research. The groups will be tape recorded with voices only. *(To protect confidentiality of research participants, state what will be done with the audiotapes after being used for focus groups.)* Note takers will write down opinions and what group thinks during the sessions. We will not record your name or any other personal things about you during the groups. We ask that participants not reveal outside the group information they may have heard in the group. Even though we will ask people in the group not to reveal anything to others, we cannot guarantee this. We will protect information about you and your taking part in this research to the best of our ability. If the results of this research are published, your name will not be shown.

Compensation

You will be paid _______ or given gifts worth _______ per session for taking part in this research.

Contact for Questions

(Give separate list of contact numbers to subjects when oral consent is used.)

Consent Form for Moderator to Sign

1. Read and review the oral consent for focus groups with each participant in a private setting.
2. Ask the following: "Are you willing to be in a focus group to talk about _______________?"
3. Read the Oral Informed Consent for Focus Groups to the group before the first session begins. Whenever possible, (voice) tape record this reading before the group.

I have reviewed the Fact Sheet with the research participants, and they have fully agreed to be in this focus group research. I further agree to keep confidential anything that is said in the discussion group.

Please print clearly:

_______________________________ _______________________________

(Moderator's name) (Moderator's signature)

____

(Date)

Example 2

FAMILY HEALTH INTERNATIONAL

ORAL INFORMED CONSENT FOR SURVEYS AND INTERVIEWS

Name of research study *(may be simplified)*

This interview is for a research study that is being done by *(name of organization).*

This research will gather information on *(how people in this city think about AIDS and HIV).* We are talking to people who use the *(name of clinic).*

The interview will include questions on *(sexually transmitted diseases, AIDS, condom use).* It will take most people about _______ minutes/hours to answer the questions.

The names of people who agree to be interviewed *(will not be recorded without their permission).*

Your participation is voluntary, and there is no penalty for refusing to take part. (If you do not take part, it will not affect any health care that you would normally receive.) You may refuse to answer any question in the interview or stop the interview at any time.

(Give a separate list of contact numbers to subjects when oral consent is used.)

Every aspect of the research outlined above has been fully explained to the volunteer in his/her native language, *(specify).*

________________________________ ________________________________

(Signature of person obtaining consent) (Date)

APPENDIX THREE

Example of a Qualitative-Quantitative Research Design

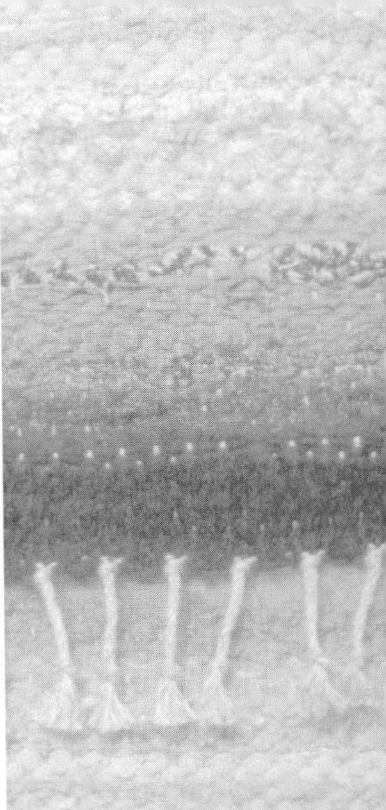

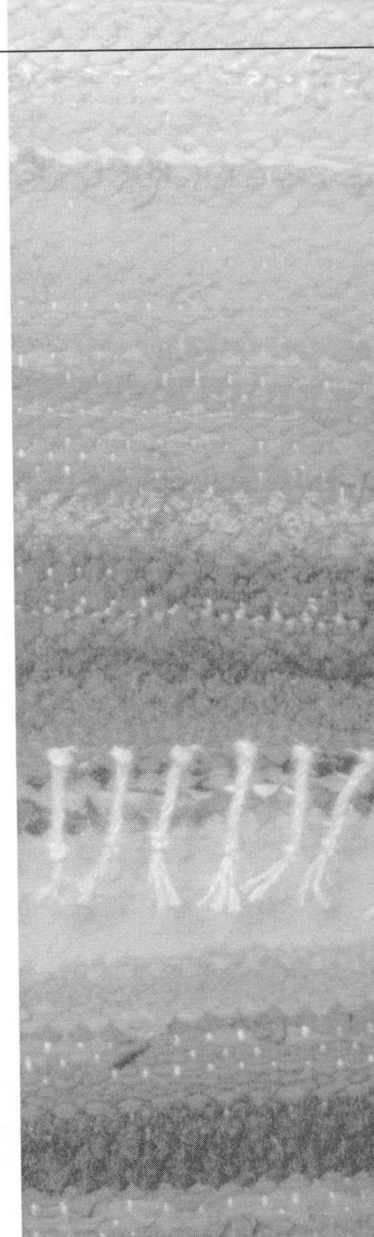

Unintended Pregnancy and School Dropout Among Women Students in an Urban Secondary School

This partial research design shows the progression from an area of research linked to a policy issue to development of research questions and selection of methods. Note that the full design would also include a conceptual framework and plans for data analysis and dissemination.

AREA OF RESEARCH

Unintended pregnancy and consequent discontinuation of studies among female adolescents attending secondary school.

POLICY ISSUE

Immediate punitive suspension of pregnant students for one year from date that pregnancy is discovered by school authorities.

RESEARCH PROBLEM

- To explore and compare the experiences of sexually active young adults with respect to (1) pregnancy prevention, (2) the effect of pregnancy on school achievement, (3) vocational goals, and (4) perceptions of personal control in their lives
- To explore attitudes of school authorities toward female students who become pregnant while still in school

STUDY OBJECTIVES

1. To identify patterns of sexual activity, contraceptive use, contraceptive help seeking, and pregnancy experience in a sample of adolescent women
2. To compare academic and vocational aspirations of four groups: (a) sexually inactive women students, (b) sexually active women students who have never been pregnant, (c) women students with histories of pregnancy, and (d) women (former students) who left school permanently because of pregnancy
3. To explore young women's sense of personal control in relation to pregnancy prevention, school achievement, and vocational goals
4. To identify the potential for policy change regarding suspension of pregnant students
5. To describe the experiences of adolescents who seek contraceptive information and service

EXAMPLES OF RESEARCH QUESTIONS

Objective 1: Patterns of Sexual Activity

- Quantitative: At what ages did women in the study population become sexually active?
- Quantitative: To what extent have sexually active young women used contraception (age, methods, consistency, continuity)?
- Quantitative: What have been the outcomes of pregnancy when it occurs (births, abortions, live children)?
- Quantitative/Qualitative: How and where have young women sought contraceptive methods and at what ages?
- Qualitative: To what extent do young women believe they have been successful in obtaining contraceptive information and methods? If not successful, why?
- Qualitative: What were young women told or advised to do when they sought contraceptive information and methods?

Objective 2: Academic and Vocational Aspirations

- Qualitative: In what ways do students and former students believe their academic and vocational goals have changed since they began secondary school?
- Qualitative: How do current academic and vocational goals differ among sexually active students who have never been pregnant, students who have ever been pregnant, and former students who dropped out due to pregnancy?
- Qualitative: How do students perceive the policies and attitudes of school authorities toward student pregnancy?

Objective 3: Personal Control

- Qualitative: How do sexually active and sexually inactive students, as well as women who have left school due to pregnancy, differ with respect to their beliefs that they can act on their own desires or decisions regarding having sex, becoming pregnant, pursuing education, and choosing a vocation?

- Qualitative: What influences or circumstances do women in each category perceive as encouraging and discouraging their ability to control their reproductive, academic, and vocational decisions?

Objective 4: Potential for Policy Change

- Qualitative: What are the opinions of schoolteachers and administrators concerning the suspension policy?
- Qualitative: In the views of school authorities, how should the school respond to a pregnant student?

Objective 5: Contraceptive Information and Service

- Qualitative: How do women students describe their experiences in pharmacies and clinics when they have sought help for pregnancy prevention?
- Qualitative: How do students' accounts compare with observed behavior of pharmacists and clinic personnel?

SOURCES OF INFORMATION

Quantitative: Phase I

School sample: eight hundred female students, fifteen to eighteen years of age, enrolled in a large urban secondary school; all eligible respondents

Community sample: seventy-five women factory workers, twenty-five years of age or less, who say they discontinued schooling because of pregnancy

Qualitative: Phase II

Subsamples of phase I respondents, purposively selected to represent four groups:

- Sexually inactive women students
- Sexually active women students who have never been pregnant
- Students who have dropped out of school during a pregnancy and returned
- Former students who dropped out of school due to pregnancy and did not return

Key informants, purposively selected:

- Four school administrators from a different but demographically similar school
- Four schoolteachers from a different but demographically similar school
- Four family planning providers from a reproductive health clinic in the study community
- Four pharmacists from the study community

Total: three family planning clinics and three pharmacies

METHODS

Quantitative: Phase I

Structured questionnaire, multiple-choice responses with skip patterns, administered to all phase I respondents in one session (n = 800)

Qualitative: Phase II

- Focus group discussions with two groups of participants from each of the phase II subsamples, repeated in a total of three discussions with each group, or twenty-four discussions
- In-depth interviews with key informants: school administrators, teachers, family planning providers, and pharmacists
- Mystery client observation in family planning clinics and pharmacies serving the study community

ANTICIPATED ETHICAL ISSUES

Sensitivity to Preference of Some Students Not to Participate

Prospective participants need full explanation of the nature and purpose of the research, possible risks (breach in confidentiality), and expectations on them as respondents to the phase I survey questionnaire, as well as in phase II if they are selected and agree to participate.

Parental Consent if Required by an Institutional Review Board

Informed consent of adolescent participants in social (nonclinical) research may be sufficient. If parental consent is required, the researcher must take great care not to suggest that any individual student is or is not sexually active. Emphasis should be on healthy reproductive decisions in relation to educational and vocational achievement. If possible, the request will come from the school as part of an ongoing health education program.

Protection of Confidentiality

Survey questionnaires will be administered by researchers, not school personnel. School personnel will not be present during any data collection. Only researchers will have access to data, which will be secured in a locked place. Participants in phase II will sign a pledge to respect the confidentiality of their peers. Focus group moderators will guide discussion toward normative aspects of the research problem by inviting participants to comment on common experiences and feelings of young women. They will not ask for disclosure of personal experience. Selecting key informants from schools other than the study site will minimize possible student anxiety about school officials being in the study.

Deceptive Nature of Mystery Client Observation

This technique will be used only if pharmacists and clinic personnel grant permission to conduct occasional anonymous and unannounced observation visits by simulated customers or clients over a six-month period.

APPENDIX FOUR

Procedural Guidelines for Managing Focus Group Discussions

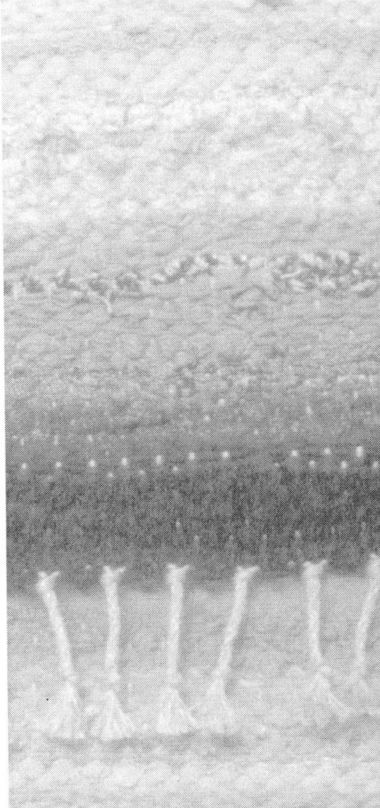

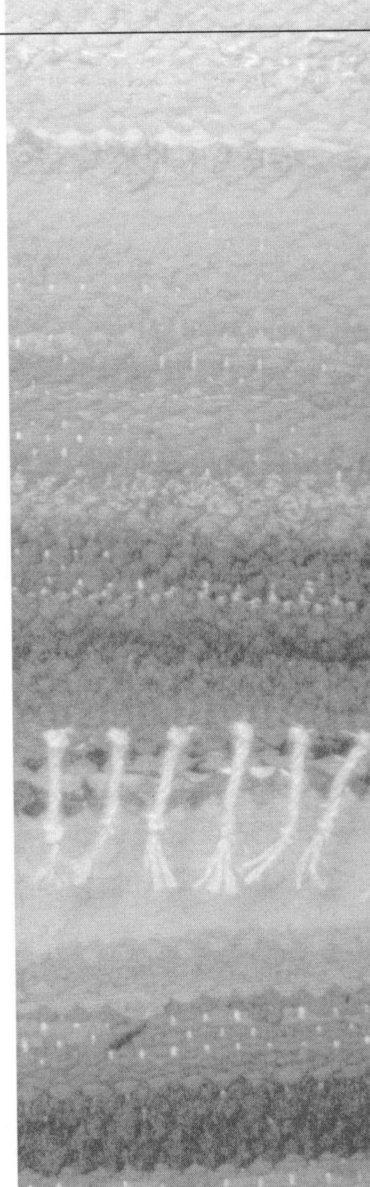

Before Leaving for the Site

Review notes. Include notes from focus group discussions conducted earlier for this study, including team debriefings if they were done.

Review study protocol and topic guide.

Gather materials.

Prepare tape recorder, extra tape recorder, sufficient cassettes, extra batteries, notepads, pens, labels, name tags, topic guides, gifts, snacks or travel reimbursements for participants, other materials.

Test tape recorder.

At the Site Before Discussion Begins

Set up the room. Refreshments should be available before focus group discussion begins. Ensure that participants help themselves or are served. Arrange mats or chairs in a circle. A table may or may not be present, depending on cultural norms of conversation.

Test the tape recorder.

Label the cassette with the date and group identification code; load and test it.

Greet the participants.

Collect sociodemographic data informally.

Make labels with numbers corresponding to data sheets if you are using them to identify individual speakers during recording and note taking.

Starting the Discussion

Introduce yourself and invite participants to introduce themselves.

If names are used, use the first name only.

Summarize the purpose of the study.

Describe the focus group discussion process. Emphasize that there are no right or wrong answers; all should participate; all should respect the opinions of others; help to keep the discussion on track; describe the use of the tape recorder; remind participants that notes will be taken. Advise the group that the discussion will last approximately 1½ hours. Invite questions.

Review the statement of informed consent. Make sure that everyone understands.

Encourage confidentiality. Ask participants to guard the confidentiality of others in the group.

Conducting the Discussion

Begin with warm-up questions.

Be aware of who is talking and who is not. Do not allow one or two individuals to dominate; bring silent participants into the discussion.

Use broad, open-ended questions. Avoid yes-or-no or short-answer questions in a questionnaire format. Frame the discussion with more general questions and encourage participants to raise issues that are important to them.

Always probe. On some occasions moderators may want to probe for additional information when a participant's initial answer appears incomplete. Probing does not mean suggesting a more interesting answer. Probes that suggest answers are leading probes and must be avoided.

Following are examples of leading probes *not* to use:

- Do you mean . . ?
- Are you saying that . . ?
- Is that the only thing you can think of?
- You do not mean that . . ?

Good non-leading probes are usually general inquiries such as the following:

- How do you mean?
- In what way?
- What other methods (means of) do you know?
- There is no hurry. Take a moment to think about it and tell me all that comes to your mind.

Do not hesitate to use silence (waiting expectantly while a speaker thinks through her idea) and nonverbal prompts (raising your eyebrows, nodding your head, saying "hmmm," and so on). They tell the respondent that you are listening and interested in whatever she has to say.

Note any questions that the group does not seem to understand, as well as questions that stimulate good discussion. Revise the topic guide after the session if necessary for future discussion.

Record body language and other nonverbal communications. The participant's tone of voice or physical movements may communicate more than she is actually voicing. An idea stated forcefully or even angrily might emphasize the strength of a participant's convictions. A hesitant manner might suggest the participant is not sure about the idea she is stating or that she anticipates disagreement from others in the group. Rivalries or one-upmanship between group members may also be communicated nonverbally. Such dynamics should be noted. Body language and nonverbal communications, just as verbal expression, should also be noted.

Use the guidelines flexibly; return to topics that were not fully discussed or that needed more thought.

End of the Discussion

Thank the participants.

Explain how the discussion information will be used.

Remunerate discreetly. Distribute travel reimbursement, small gifts, or honorarium if used.

Collect the tape recorder, tapes, and sociodemographic data sheets if used. Check that all cassettes are appropriately identified with coded information.

After the Discussion

Expand your notes in outline form. The note taker and moderator should do this together, immediately following the session if possible, or at least on the same day as the focus group discussion. Record in writing any nonverbal data.

Transcribe the tapes. This may take four to eight hours. The task may be shared or rotated from note taker to moderator. Develop a system to transcribe tapes as quickly as possible.

Review the transcribed notes. Add the researcher's comments in parentheses. These could include observations about the group, remarks to probe in later discussions, or methodological problems.

Translate.

APPENDIX FIVE

Sample Budget Categories for Planning Focus Group Discussions

Michele G. Shedlin, Ph.D.
National Development and Research Institute

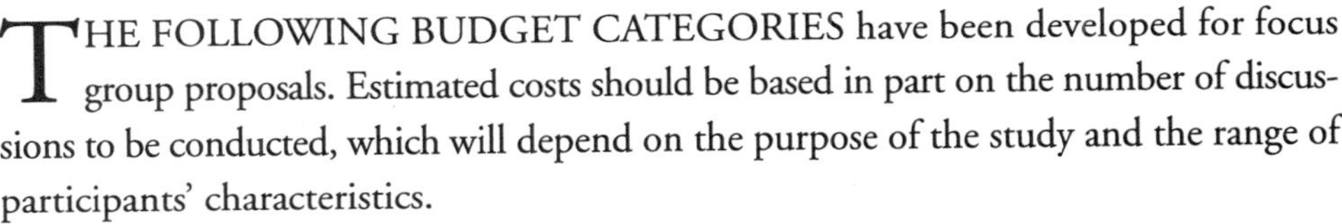

THE FOLLOWING BUDGET CATEGORIES have been developed for focus group proposals. Estimated costs should be based in part on the number of discussions to be conducted, which will depend on the purpose of the study and the range of participants' characteristics.

- Planning (possible extra sessions with representatives of implementing agencies or target groups, including transportation and meeting space)
- Recruitment of participants (recruitment questionnaire, transportation)
- Payment or gifts for participants (incentives)
- Refreshments
- Rental for space where discussions are held
- Child care
- Moderator and assistant moderator or note-taker fees
- Transportation for moderators and note takers
- Possible feedback sessions with moderators and note takers after the data collection
- Transportation for participants to and from the site
- Transcription of tapes (full day of secretarial service for each discussion held)

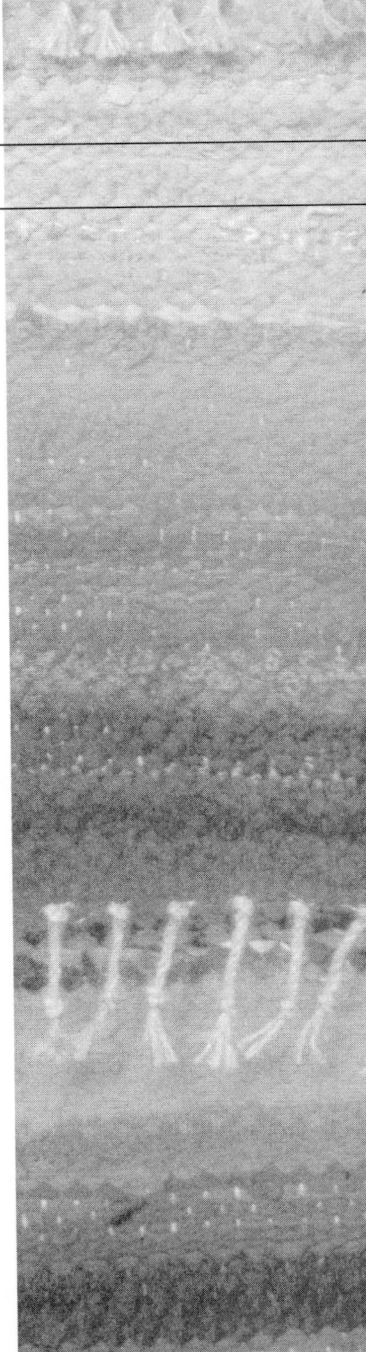

Adapted from Krueger 1994, pp. 235–237.

- Translation, if not included in transcription
- Data management (including computer software if used for coding and analysis, computer time, data entry personnel)
- Analysis, interpretation, and report preparation
- Typing and photocopying report
- Supplies and equipment (tape recorders, tapes, paper, overhead projector, and so on)
- Oral presentation of results (may involve meeting space, transportation, per diems, equipment rental, photocopying)
- Technical assistance (may involve multiple visits at several stages throughout the research)

APPENDIX SIX

Topic Guides for Focus Group Discussions on Reproductive Health

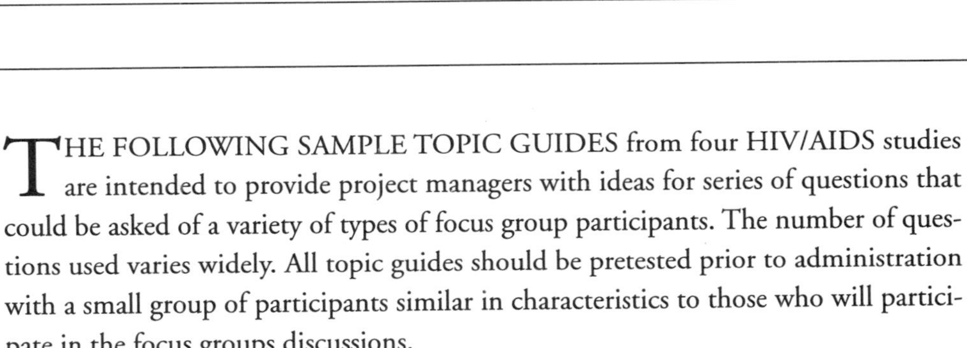

THE FOLLOWING SAMPLE TOPIC GUIDES from four HIV/AIDS studies are intended to provide project managers with ideas for series of questions that could be asked of a variety of types of focus group participants. The number of questions used varies widely. All topic guides should be pretested prior to administration with a small group of participants similar in characteristics to those who will participate in the focus groups discussions.

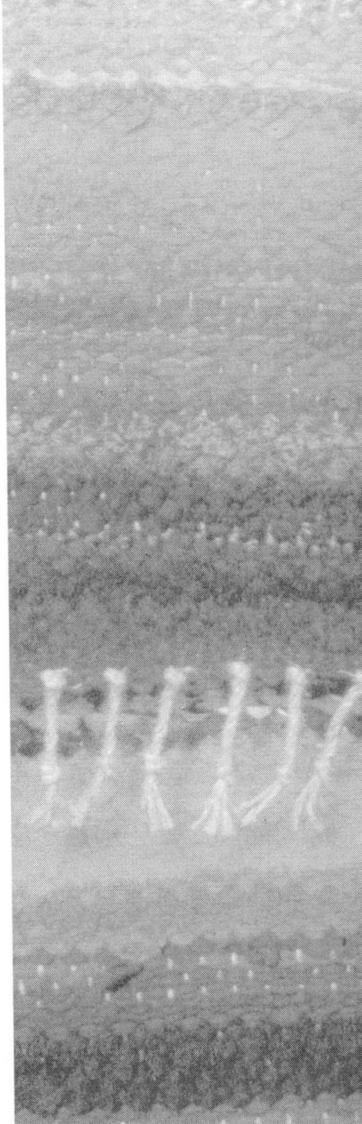

A. Sample Topic Guide for Research Examining the Features of Social Relationships among Homosexual and Bisexual Men at Risk for AIDS (O'Brien 1993)

The goals of the long-term program were to identify which features of social ties enhance the psychological health of men in this population as well as the ability to adhere to widely publicized behavioral guidelines for preventing transmission of HIV. Only four questions were used in a "funneling" sequence leading from a general topic to the specific interest—the influence of social relationships on psychological health and on safer sex practices.

1. How is your life different because of the HIV/AIDS epidemic? (This first question is the icebreaker, which allowed each participant to speak and helped the researchers to learn the language participants used for talking about their experiences.)

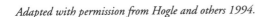

Adapted with permission from Hogle and others 1994.

2. When people get involved sexually, why is it that sometimes they have safer sex and sometimes they don't? (This question helped to focus the discussion on safer sex experiences and to allow the conversation to move toward a discussion of social interactions.)
3. What are some things other people have done that you have found supportive in dealing with the HIV/AIDS epidemic? (The researchers asked this question so that specific interventions, such as expressions of support for safer sex activities, could be identified.)
4. How can we best recruit men for the large-scale questionnaire phase of this study?

B. Sample Topic Guide for a Study to Explore Opinions on Sexual Practices (World Health Organization 1990)

1. Have you ever heard of people of the same sex having sex together in your society/community?
2. In general, do people in society accept that? Why or why not?
3. In general, which is more common: men having sex with men or women having sex with women? Why?
4. What do men do with each other when they have sex? (Try to elicit information on oral and anal sex.)
5. What do men and women do when they have sex? (Try to elicit information on oral and anal sex, differences between age groups, urban/rural differences.)
6. How common is it for men to go to prostitutes?

C. Sample Topic Guide to Explore Perceptions Concerning Norms Governing Sexual Decision Making and Behavior Associated with the Risk of HIV Transmission to Women in Haiti (Ulin and others 1995)

The format involves the use of a story to prompt discussion among the participants. This technique allows the participants to discuss the behavior of the story characters rather than their own behavior, thus revealing perceptions on social norms for sexual behavior.

STORY FOR DISCUSSION

Moderator: Joujou is living with a man by the name of René. René is working in a factory, but Joujou is not working. Joujou has four kids at home: the oldest one is seven years old, the youngest one and a half; and she is again pregnant. Before Joujou got pregnant with this last child, she wanted to start using family planning, but René did not want her to. René gives money for food in the house, but it is he who decides what to cook. When the children are sick, Joujou must ask René's permission before she takes them to the clinic.

QUESTIONS FOR DISCUSSION

1. What do you think about the way René and Joujou are living? (Kinds of decisions men and women make together, women's decisions, men's decisions)
2. Who makes the decision when a man and woman make love?
3. If a man feels like making love with his woman and the woman does not want to, what can she do? How does the man react? (Women's right to refuse sex, refusal strategies, partners' response)
4. What reasons might there be for a woman to refuse to make love with her man? (Women's rights under specific conditions, bargaining)

STORY FOR DISCUSSION

Moderator: There is another part to the story of Joujou and René. Let's continue it and see what happens.

Joujou is worried. She has learned that when René goes to town, he often goes to the houses of other women with whom he is having affairs. Joujou does not know what she should do. She does not want to leave René, but she is afraid he will give her AIDS.

QUESTIONS FOR DISCUSSION

5. What do you think this woman should do? (Expectations of behavior for women at risk of HIV)
6. If the woman does what you are saying, how do you think the man will react? (Expectations of male response to protective behavior)
7. Do you think that the woman should talk to the man about the fears she has of contracting AIDS? How can she bring up the subject? How will he react? (Male-female communication on AIDS and AIDS prevention)
8. If the man is having an affair with another woman, can he give the disease to his woman (at home)? How? (Knowledge of HIV transmission)
9. As far as you know, how do people (in general) get AIDS? (Knowledge of HIV transmission)
10. What kind of people get AIDS? Do you fear AIDS? (Transmission, belief in severity, sense of vulnerability, personal fear, appearance of HIV-infected people)
11. What are the consequences of this disease for the family? (Knowledge of the disease, belief in severity)
12. If a woman knows nothing about this disease, how can she get information? What do women want to know? (Formal and nonformal sources of information, desire for information)
13. (Women only) Do women talk to each other about AIDS? When? How do they feel in these discussions? (Nature and circumstances of informal discussion, emotional responses to discussion, level of interest)

STORY FOR DISCUSSION

Moderator: The woman in the story (Joujou) is afraid that her man may give her AIDS because she knows that he is having affairs with other women.

QUESTIONS FOR DISCUSSION

14. How can she protect herself? How will the man react? (Knowledge of prevention, spontaneous reference to condoms, right of women to protect themselves, initiating behavior change, barriers to prevention)
15. Does the woman have the right to ask the man to use condoms? How can she ask him? How will he respond?
16. If the man does not want to use condoms, can the woman convince him? How? (Empowerment, communication, male response, barriers)
17. In general, are women willing to use condoms? (Women's attitudes toward condoms, response of women to men who initiate condom use)
18. Where can a person get condoms?
19. Are women able to obtain (buy) condoms on their own? (Condom availability, barriers to obtaining condoms)
20. We have heard that not all women have the right to ask a man to use condoms. What can you tell us about that? (Types of women who have or do not have the right to demand condoms)
21. As far as you know, are young people in their teens in danger of contracting AIDS? Why? (Beliefs about adolescent sexual behavior and AIDS risk)
22. How do you think you might help young people avoid getting AIDS? (Responsibility of adults to counsel adolescents, appropriate advisers, nature of advice)
23. If you knew they were sexually active, would you advise young people to use condoms? (Belief in the appropriateness of condoms for adolescents)
24. Some parents say they would not talk to their children about sex. What do you think about that? (Responsibility of parents for sex education)
25. (Women only) You women know what AIDS is about. Do you believe you have a responsibility to protect yourselves? To protect your unborn babies? Please explain what you mean. (Responsibility for prevention, risk of perinatal transmission)
26. (Women only) How do you think women might help each other to be stronger in their relationships with men? (Mutual support for protection against AIDS, sense of collective responsibility)
27. (Men only) You men know what AIDS is about. Do you feel that you have a responsibility to protect your wives? Other women that you may be seeing? Yourselves? Please explain. (Responsibility for prevention, stable and casual partners)
28. As far as you know, would people benefit from talking about AIDS in small groups like this one? (Networking and support)

D. Sample FGD Topic Guide for Female Youth Exploring Knowledge about AIDS, Sexual Activity, and Condom Use to Guide Development of a Survey of Knowledge, Attitudes, Beliefs, and Practices (AIDSCAP/FHI 1993, unreferenced)

The following topic guide was designed for focus group discussions (FGDs) among female youth to assist in questionnaire development. In-country researchers collaborating with AIDSCAP adapt the guide to local situations, translate it into the language in which the guide will be used, and pretest it prior to use. The main objective is to investigate the dynamics of sexual behavior among young women in order to identify the vocabulary and phrasing they use to describe relationships and sexual activity, particularly condom negotiation and use. Using the FGD results, researchers then adapt core questionnaires for collecting data to establish the prevalence within target populations of various aspects of sexual behavior.

Following an introductory statement appropriate for the local context, the following questions could be used to elicit information about sexual beliefs and practices among young women.

SEXUAL ACTIVITY

1. Where do girls your age meet boys or men?
2. Is there an age difference between most of your female friends and their boyfriends/partners?
3. What kind of relationships are common among your female friends—for example, are many of your friends engaged, have regular boyfriends, have casual boyfriends, and so on?
4. Tell me about couples who are ______________ (regular, casual partners, and so on). How long do these arrangements usually last? Is it common for girls your age to have sexual relations with their boyfriends? About what age do girls your age have sexual intercourse for the first time? Why does it vary?
5. Before a girl reaches the age where she has sexual intercourse, are there other nonpenetrative sexual activities that are commonly practiced among girls and boys/men? Can you describe some of these activities? With whom might a girl practice these activities? (What is their relationship, partner's age?) At what age do girls your age begin these activities?
6. If a girl has a regular boyfriend, about how often might she see him during a week? About how many times might she have sexual intercourse with him during a one-week/one-month period?
7. Where might a couple your age go to have sex?
8. Is it common for girls your age to have sexual relations with more than one man, that is, to be with one man one night and another man on a different night?
9. Is it common for your female friends' boyfriends/partners to have sexual relationships with more than one girl/woman?

10. Have sexual practices among people your age changed over time? For example, are the common practices we have discussed today different from what your parents or grandparents might have experienced? How are they different? Which practices are the same?

CONDOM USE

1. Do girls your age who are having sex use anything to keep from getting pregnant? If so, what, which methods of birth control? Where do they obtain these methods?
2. Does anyone know what these are? (Show condom in and out of the package) What else are they called?
3. Who uses condoms, in your opinion? What kind of man/boy? What kind of woman/girl? Why?
4. Is it common among your female friends to use condoms? Why? Why not?
5. Among your friends who use condoms, who do you think initiates using a condom?
6. What would girls your age think if a man stated that he was going to use a condom?
7. What would a man/boy think if a girl asked him to use a condom? What would a man/boy think if a girl had a condom with her? Why? Can you explain that further?
8. Would you be insulted if a man said he wanted to use a condom? Do you think your partner would be insulted if you asked him to use a condom?
9. Have you ever used a condom before? Why? Why not?
10. Where could you go today to get a condom? How much do they cost?
11. Do you think using a condom is a good idea? Why? When? Why not?
12. Have you ever asked a partner to use a condom? Do you know if any of your friends have ever asked their partners to use a condom? What happened?
13. Can you imagine any circumstances under which you would ask a man to use a condom? Tell me about that.
14. If you were planning to have sex with a man, are there any circumstances under which you would change your mind and refuse to have sex with him? Under what circumstances?
15. How could you ask a man to use a condom, that is, what could you say?
16. If he refused, how might you respond to try and convince him?

LODGING

1. With whom are you living now?
2. Who pays for your
   Food
   Clothing
   Transportation
   Health care
   School fees
   Incidental expenses/pocket money

QUESTIONNAIRE REVIEW

One of this project's objectives is to do a survey of people your age to learn about the kinds of issues we have discussed today. What I would like to do now is to read you some questions from the questionnaire and see if you can suggest ways to improve the wording of the questions. I also want your opinion on whether you think young people will respond honestly to these questions.

1. If someone came to your home and asked you to participate in this survey, would you agree?
2. Please listen to the introduction of the questionnaire. What is this study about? How will the information be used?
3. After listening to this statement, are you confident that this information will not be shared with anyone? If yes, why? Which statements convinced you? If not, why? Which statements made you suspicious?
4. If you were doing the study and you knew that none of the information would ever be released to anyone outside of the staff, what would you say to convince respondents?

APPENDIX SEVEN

Sample Interviewer Training Program Agenda

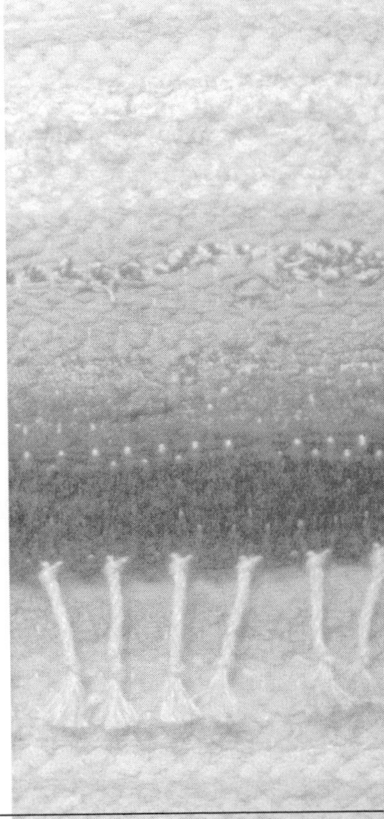

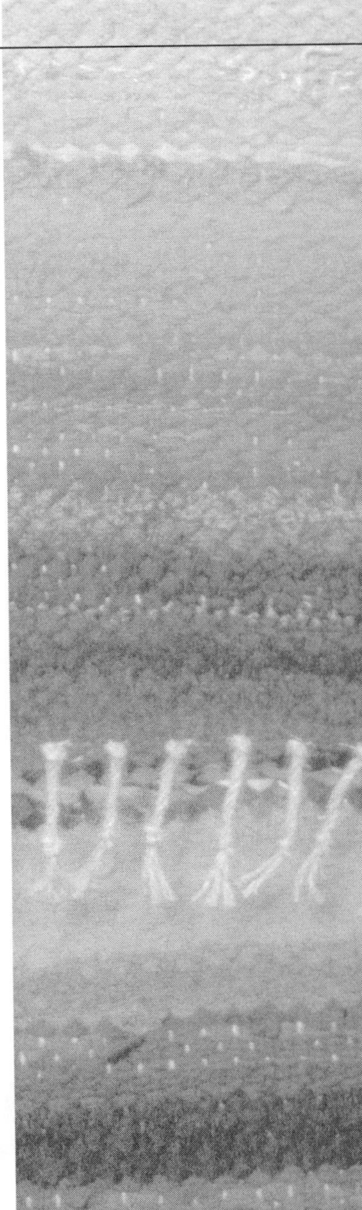

Norplant Study
Qualitative Methods Workshop
Dakar, Senegal
June 5–8, 1996
Eight Participants

WEDNESDAY, JUNE 5

Morning

Coffee and introductions

About Norplant

- Introduction to the method: what it is, how it works
- Findings of other studies: common concerns
- Norplant in Senegal

Handout: Fact sheet on Norplant

Break

Goals and objectives of the Norplant study

Study design

- Record review
- Focus groups discussion
- In-depth interviews
- How data will be analyzed

Discussion of ethical issues

Handout: Overview of the Norplant Study

Lunch

Afternoon
Techniques

- How to use a topic guide
- Asking questions in interviews and discussions
- Probes: verbal and nonverbal

Focus group discussion (FGD) demonstration

Break
Observations and discussion: managing interviews and focus groups

Handout: Steps in Leading a Focus Group Discussion

Assignment: Develop a topic guide for an in-depth interview or a focus group on Thursday morning

THURSDAY, JUNE 6

Morning
Role-playing: interviews and note taking

Handout: Tips for Interviewers

Break
Role-playing: FGD and note taking

Handout: Tips for Focus Group Moderators and Note Takers

Lunch

Afternoon
Preliminary analysis

- Group level
- Individual level
- Coding

Break
Review of study topic guides

Assignment: Review techniques and prepare to conduct an interview.

FRIDAY, JUNE 7

Morning
Field practice (by prearrangement at two clinics): Participants will observe and conduct one interview each and write up notes

Afternoon
Presentation of findings from morning interviews
Group discussion and critique

- Additional probing
- Revisions to guide
- Preliminary coding

Assignment: Each team prepares to conduct one focus group.

SATURDAY, JUNE 8

Morning
Field practice (by prearrangement at two clinics): Each team will pretest the continuing client FGD guide and transcribe tape for two FGDs. Each participant will observe one focus group and moderate or take notes in the other.

Lunch

Afternoon
Presentation of FGD findings
Group discussion and critique

- Additional probing
- Revisions to guide
- Preliminary coding

Summary and evaluation of training

APPENDIX EIGHT

Common Errors in Moderating Focus Groups

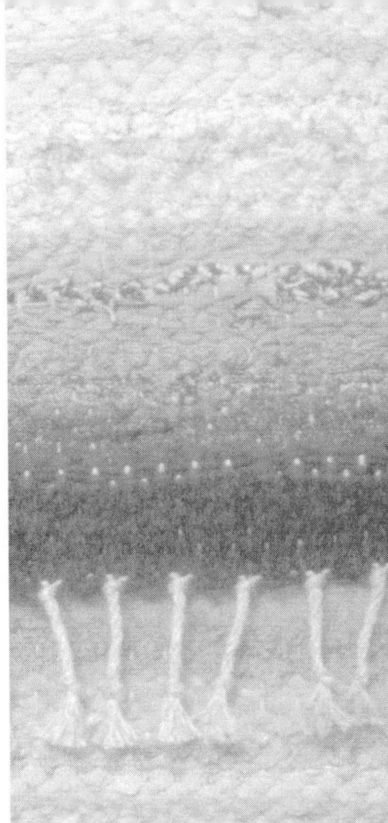

FACILITATING A FOCUS GROUP discussion on a sensitive topic is never easy, but moderators who are new to qualitative data collection can find that hearing all points of view and keeping the discussion on track can be especially challenging. It is not unusual for an interviewer to begin a qualitative project with a strong background in survey work. Many find it difficult at first to replace the structure of a quantitative interview with the flexibility that qualitative research demands—asking open-ended questions, probing answers, and following the participants' lead while keeping the discussion focused on the research problem.

Common errors that appear in focus group transcripts are the following:

- Allowing one or two participants to dominate the discussion or not enabling reticent participants to speak
- Remaining too long on a topic, continuing to repeat questions even after participants have nothing additional to say
- Using the same words to repeat a question instead of probing what has just been said or noticing new ideas and asking participants to elaborate
- Interrupting people who begin to express a different point of view by repeating the original question as if the speaker were not addressing it
- Accepting comments on what people should do without probing what they actually do and why there is a difference
- Not probing the logical conclusions of ideas ("If that, then what?" or simply, "Why?")
- Not probing assumptions to see where they come from ("Why do people say that?")
- Letting a good question drop if it is not answered immediately

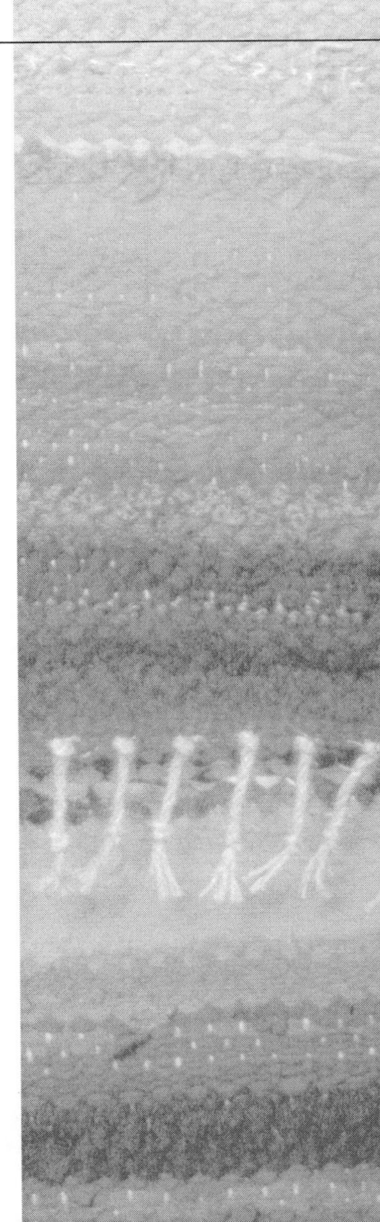

- Failing to explore vague or nonspecific terms or to clarify vernacular expression that may not be familiar to the researchers
- Allowing the group to talk only about married (more stable) relationships and to ignore casual (less stable) unions
- Asking leading questions that might bias the answers; for example, "Don't you think that . . . ?" or "Would you agree that . . . ?"

The examples we provide are taken from the transcripts of focus group discussions conducted in Haiti for the purpose of understanding women's perspectives on sexual decision making in relation to HIV/AIDS protection. Although they come from focus groups, most of these points apply equally to in-depth interviewing or any interactive technique in which the researcher must probe sensitive information.

Example 1

A group of women in casual relationships with male sexual partners are talking about protecting themselves if they suspect a partner is HIV-infected.

Moderator: Do you think you have a responsibility to protect yourself from getting AIDS?

Group (in unison): No.

Moderator: You don't feel you have any responsibility? Why do you think you don't have any responsibility?

Participant 1: Because we don't have husbands.

Moderator: You don't feel you have a responsibility to protect yourself from AIDS? Is that what you are saying?

Participant 2: I personally feel I should be using condoms. I have children, and I wouldn't like to have any more.

COMMENT

This moderator correctly probed the group's denial of responsibility, but she kept repeating the word when it may not have been clear what *responsibility* meant to participants. Her probe also seems like a leading question—as if the participants have given an unacceptable answer. She might have asked, "What do we mean by *responsibility for protection*?" Or she could have restated the question, probing the idea with different words: "Whose responsibility is it to protect the woman from AIDS? Is it up to the man? The woman? Someone else? What do you think that person should do to protect herself or himself?"

The answer "because we don't have husbands" offers another important clue that the moderator missed. She should have probed this response with such questions as "Why does having a husband or not having a husband make any difference?" "What is the responsibility of a woman with a husband?" "What about a woman without a husband?" "What about the responsibility of the husband, himself—or the man who is not her husband?" The moderator could also have clarified what the term *husband* meant to the participants, because in Haiti multiple relationships, both stable and non-stable, are common.

Participant 2 did not answer the question directly. The moderator could then have explored views on the uses of condoms and gradually brought the discussion back to the use of condoms as protection against sexually transmitted infection.

Example 2

A group of men are talking about the causes of AIDS.

Moderator: What are some of the ways that people can get AIDS?

Participant 1: If a man has sex with several women and the women have sex with several men, they will get AIDS.

Participant 2: If you go to the hospital and get an injection and the syringe has AIDS on it . . .

Participant 3: We know there is something called voodoo in our country. The [voodoo] priest prepares all kinds of diseases. He can prepare a powder. . . . he sends it to you. . . . you get a different kind of AIDS.

Moderator: What are some other ways you can get AIDS?

COMMENT

The moderator did not pursue this reference to a different form of AIDS. He should have asked in what way AIDS from powder is different from sexually transmitted AIDS, whether a person with voodoo AIDS can pass it to another person by sexual contact, whether it can be cured, and so forth. He then could have invited other participants to add to the discussion of this different kind of AIDS.

Example 3

A group of men are discussing a situation in which a man may have acquired the AIDS virus.

Participant: Superstitious people say that this infected person has supernatural AIDS.

Group laughs.

Moderator: Do you think he could give his AIDS to other people?

COMMENT

Again, the moderator let an important theme drop. The group's laughter suggests a strong reaction to the comment. Is it excitement, embarrassment, fear that the response might be socially unacceptable? The transcript did not say. The moderator might have asked the participants to talk more about what superstitious people and the transmission of supernatural AIDS mean to them and to others in the community.

How do the consequences of supernatural AIDS differ from the consequences of other kinds of AIDS?

Example 4

A group of women in married or stable sexual relationships have been discussing women's vulnerability to AIDS.

Moderator: Can a woman protect herself from AIDS?

Participant: We are afraid because now men do not want to stay with one woman; they want to live with them.

Moderator: When that happens, is there any way the woman can protect herself?

COMMENT

While keeping the discussion on the topic of protection, the moderator missed an opportunity to probe the implication that men are more promiscuous now than they used to be. She could have asked, "Why do men not stay with one woman?" "How has this changed?" "Why has it changed?" She might have been able to develop a new theme, namely, that women think men have more partners than they used to, and to identify factors that might contribute to the perceived change.

Example 5

A group of women in married or stable relationships have just agreed that many women do not use condoms.

Moderator: Why do women not use condoms?

Participant: I have other things I use.

Moderator: Are there others here who also will not use condoms?

COMMENT

The moderator missed the clue that (1) women may believe there are other ways to prevent HIV transmission; (2) women may be thinking of condoms only as contraception; or (3) women may have other ideas about condoms that were not expressed. She should have asked, "What other things?" and "In what ways do these protect the woman?" The question she did ask could be perceived as a leading question. The participant did not say she would not use condoms, but the moderator's next question reflects refusal and the possible implication that such behavior by others in the group would be unacceptable.

Example 6

A group of women in married or stable sexual relationships are talking about women's vulnerability in the AIDS epidemic.

Moderator: What can a woman do to protect herself from AIDS?

Participant: I can't imagine taking precautions myself, because I can't avoid making love. The only thing that could prevent me from making love would be if he would come on too strong; but as long as it isn't rape, there should be love and affection. If AIDS really exists, I will get it anyway from making love.

Moderator: Does anyone else have something to say?

COMMENT

This relatively complex comment contains at least two important clues that the moderator did not follow. First, she could have asked how a woman chooses between her duties as a wife or sexual partner and her need to protect herself from AIDS. And does the woman have any choice in the matter? The discussion might have taken a different turn at this point, expanding on the potential subordination of women in the sexual relationship and its effect on women's well-being.

A second clue was the participant's question as to the existence of AIDS. The moderator might have gently probed whether women in the group doubted its existence, whether other women they knew might suspect that it did not exist, and if so, what alternatives they would offer for the current widespread concern about this disease.

Example 7

A group of men are sharing what they know about HIV/AIDS transmission.

Moderator: What are some ways people get AIDS?

Participant: The person could have AIDS, and I can eat and drink with that person and never contract it—I am not susceptible. Another can just touch the person with AIDS and contract it.

Moderator: What do you mean by "not susceptible?"

COMMENT

The moderator did the right thing to probe perception of susceptibility, but the participant never answered his question. The moderator should have come back to it, asking why some people seem more susceptible than others, what made the speaker feel safe, whether this difference in susceptibility includes other kinds of sexual transmission, and so forth.

Example 8

A group of women in non-stable sexual relationships are talking about how women get AIDS.

Moderator: What are some ways that women can get AIDS?

Participant 1: If you're trying to survive by living on the streets and you're poor, you have no protection against it [AIDS]; it can happen to you more easily.

Participant 2: Women of ill repute [can get AIDS].

Moderator: Are those the only women who can catch the disease?

COMMENT

The moderator turned the discussion away from a very important theme: the ability of women with multiple partners to protect themselves and their partners. These participants were poor and in casual and other nonstable relationships. They were beginning to talk about the pressure on poor women to exchange sex for money or other support. The moderator should have probed the idea that poor women are more susceptible. She should have asked them to talk more about what it means to be a single woman and what poor and economically dependent women might do to protect themselves from AIDS. Probing responses in greater depth might have provided richer information on sexual decision making and barriers to protection in this highly vulnerable group.

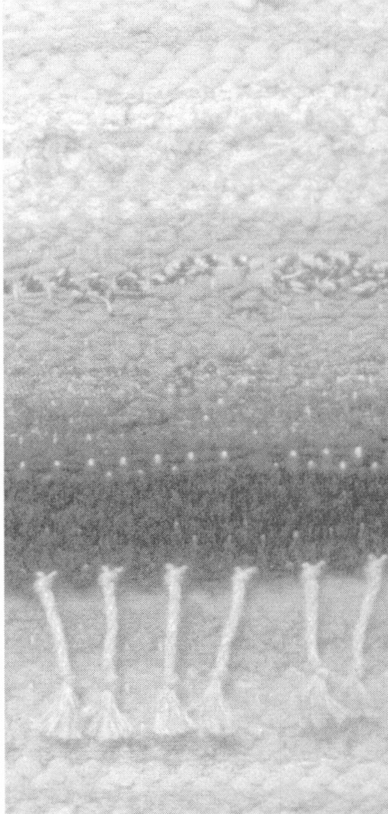

APPENDIX NINE

Critical Appraisal Skills Programme (CASP)

Ten Questions to Help You Make Sense of Qualitative Research

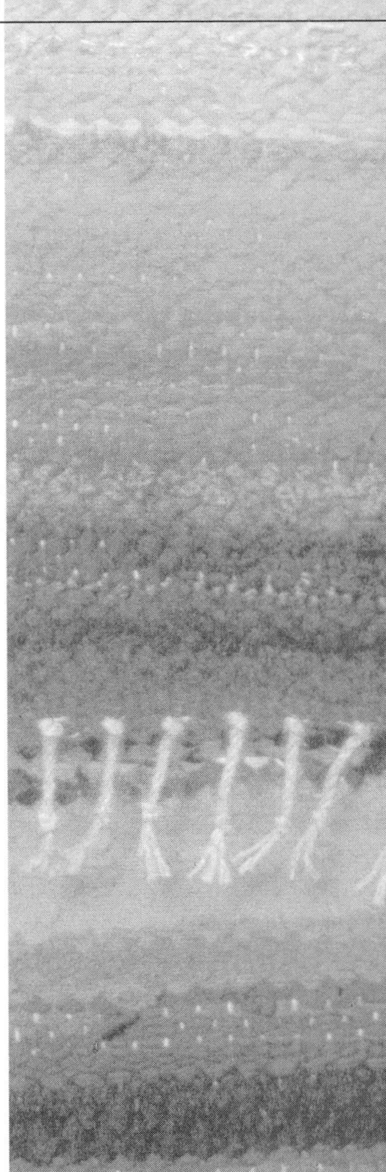

General Comments

The first two questions are screening questions and can be answered quickly. If the answer to both is "yes," it is worth proceeding with the remaining questions.

A number of italicized hints are given. These are designed to remind you why the question is important. It is important to emphasize that all of these prompts need not necessarily be met.

Several of the questions ask for a response on a scale ranging from "yes" to "no." Where there are subquestions, try to answer these first and then summarize the subquestions into one overall response by marking a cross on the scale.

The ten questions have been developed by the national CASP collaboration for qualitative methodologies.

Screening Questions

1. Was there a clear statement of the aims of the research? — Yes / No

   Hints: *What are/were they trying to find out?*
   Why is it important?
   What is its relevance?

2. Is a qualitative methodology appropriate? — Yes / No

   Hint: *Does the research seek to understand or illuminate the subjective experiences or views of those being researched?*

Detailed Questions

3. Sampling strategy
   Is it clear:
   a. From where the sample was selected and why?
   b. Who was selected and why?
   c. How were they selected and why?
   d. Was the sample size justified?
   e. Is it clear why some participants chose not to take part?

   Hint: *Consider saturation of data.*

   Was the sampling strategy appropriate to address the aims?

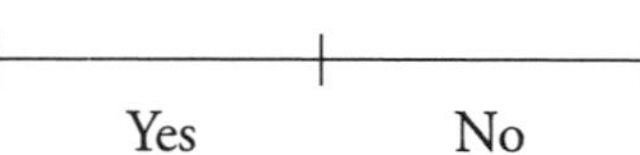

4. Data collection
   Is it clear:
   a. Where the setting of the data collection was, and why that setting was chosen?
   b. How was the data collected and why?
   Hints: Focus group, structured interview, and so on
   c. How the data were recorded and why?

   Hints: Recorded, made notes, and so on

   d. If the methods were modified during the process and why?

   Were the data collected in a way that addresses the research issue?

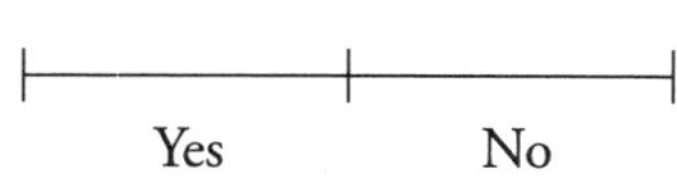

5. Data analysis
   Is it clear:
   a. How the analysis was done?
   b. How the categories/themes were derived from the data? Is there adequate description?
   c. If steps have been taken to test the credibility of the findings?

d. Are you confident that all the data were taken into account?

Hints: Is there adequate discussion of the evidence both for and against the researcher's arguments? Have attempts been made to feed results back to respondents, and/or using and comparing different sources of data about the same issue where that is appropriate (triangulation)? Was the analysis repeated by more than one researcher to ensure reliability?

Was the data analysis sufficiently rigorous?

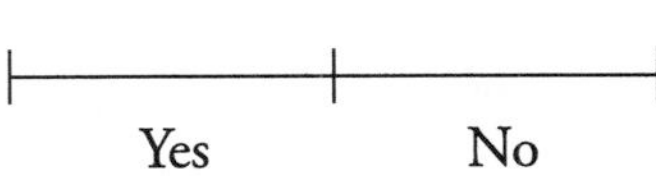

6. Research partnership relations

   Is it clear:

   a. If the researchers critically examined their own role, potential bias, and influence?
   b. Where the data were collected and why that setting was chosen?
   c. How the research was explained to the participants?

   Hint: Consider confidentiality, ethics, implications, and consequences for research findings for all of the above.

   *Has the relationship between researchers and participants been adequately considered?*Yes

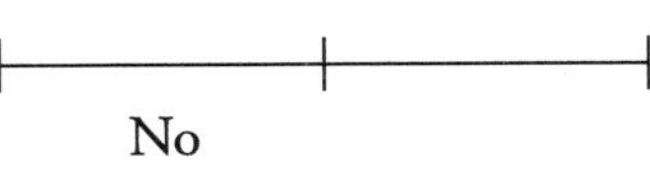

7. Findings

   Hints: What were the findings—are they explicit, easy to understand?

   Is there a clear statement of the findings?

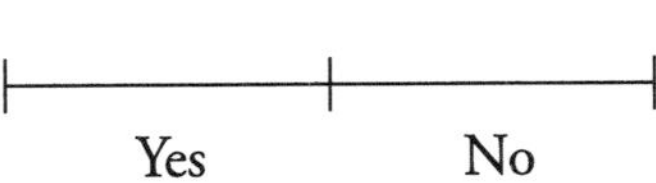

8. Justification of data interpretation

   a. Is there sufficient data presented to support the findings?
   b. Do the researchers explain how the data presented in the paper were selected from the original sample?

   Hints: Criteria for the selection of the quote, some details of the respondent, what is the role of the data—example, illustration, "nice" quote to share, and so on

   Do the researchers indicate links between data presented and their own findings on what the data contain?

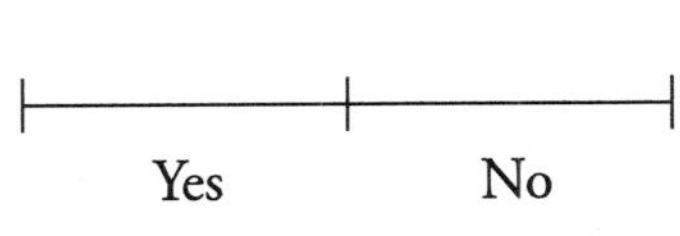

9. Transferability

   Hints: Consider:

   a. Whether the context and setting in which the study was performed is described in sufficient detail to determine similarities and differences to your own.
   b. If all the relevant clinically important outcomes were considered.

   Are the findings of this study transferable to a wider population?

   Yes No

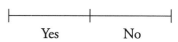

10. Relevance and usefulness
    a. In terms of addressing the research aim?
    b. In terms of contributing something new to understanding/new insight/different perspective?
    c. In terms of suggesting further research?
    d. In terms of impacting on policy/practice?

    How relevant is the research?

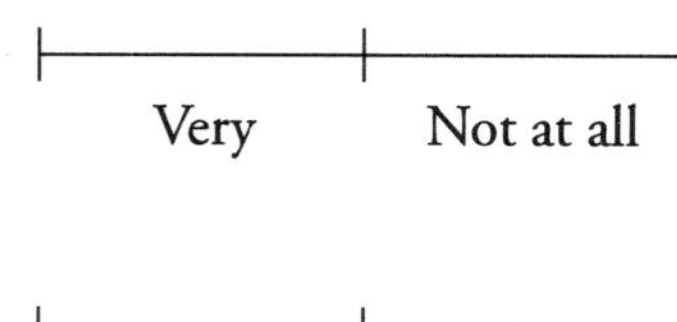

    a. To your patient/problem/scenario.
    b. To you personally.

    How important are these findings to your practice?

    Very Not at all

APPENDIX TEN

Where to Publish

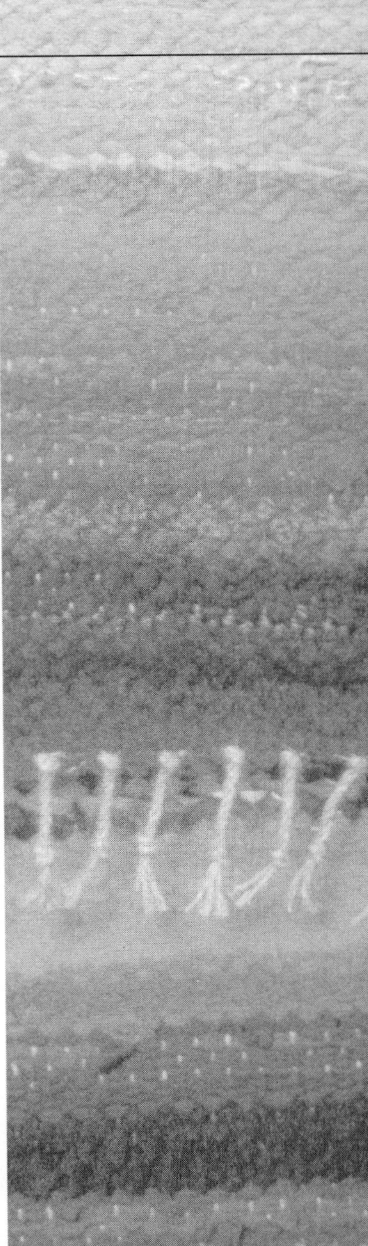

An INCREASING NUMBER of scientific journals that cover reproductive health issues are accepting articles that report on qualitative studies. The journals and presses listed here represent a selection of publishing venues for qualitative researchers to consider.

Journals

African Journal of Reproductive Health
Editor
Women's Health and Action Research Centre
4 Alofoje Avenue, off Uwasota Street
P.O. Box 10231, Ugbowo
Benin City, Edo State Nigeria
Tel: 234 52 602334/600151
Fax: 234 52 602091
E-mail: wharc@warri.rcl.nig.com
Web: http://www.wharc.freehosting.net

AIDS Education and Prevention
Francisco S. Sy, M.D., Dr.P.H., Editor
620 Peachtree St., NE, Suite 612
Atlanta, GA 30308 USA
Web: http://www.guilford.com/cgi-bin/cartscript.cgi?page=periodicals/jnai.htm&cart_id=170965.26683

American Anthropologist
New Manuscript Submissions
Fran Mascia-Lees and Susan Lees
Hunter College
695 Park Avenue, Room 715N
New York, NY 10021 USA
(212) 772-5428

American Ethnologist
Virginia R. Dominguez, Editor
University of Iowa
Department of Anthropology
114 Macbride Hall
Iowa City, IA 52242 USA
E-mail: aejournal@uiowa.edu
Web: http://www.nyu.edu/gsas/dept/anthro/aes/amereth.html

American Journal of Public Health
AJPH Submissions
800 I Street, N.W.
Washington, DC 20001-3710 USA
Tel: (202) 777-2742
E-mail: ajph.submissions@apha.org
Web: http://www.ajph.org/

American Journal of Sociology
Andrew Abbott, Editor
5835 S. Kimbark Avenue
Chicago, IL 60637-1684 USA
Tel: (773) 702-8580
Fax: (773) 702-6207
Web: http://www.journals.uchicago.edu/AJS/home.html

Cross Cultural Research (formerly *Behavior Science Research*)
Melvin Ember, Editor
Human Relations Area Files
755 Prospect Street
New Haven, CT 06511 USA
E-mail: hrafmem@minerva.cis.yale.edu
Web: http://www.sagepub.com/journal.aspx?pid=222

Culture, Medicine and Psychiatry
Byron J. Good, Editor-in-Chief, or Mary-Jo Delvecchio Good, Associate Editor
Department of Social Medicine
Harvard Medical School
641 Huntington Avenue
Boston, MA 02115 USA
Web: http://www.kluweronline.com/issn/0165–005X

Field Methods
Dr. H. Russell Bernard
Department of Anthropology
University of Florida
1112 Turlington Hall
Gainesville, FL 32606 USA
E-mail: ufruss@ufl.edu
Web: http://www.qualquant.net/FM/submit.htm

Health Education and Behavior
Marc A. Zimmerman, Ph.D., Editor
Department of Health Behavior and Health Education
University of Michigan
School of Public Health
1420 Washington Heights
Ann Arbor, MI 48109-2029 USA
Web: http://www.sph.umich.edu/hbhe/heb

Human Organization
Donald D. Stull, Editor
Department of Anthropology
University of Kansas
Lawrence, KS 66045 USA
Web: http://www.sfaa.net/ho/

International Quarterly of Community Health Education
Dr. George P. Cernada
P.O. Box 3585
Amherst, MA 01004-3585 USA
Web: http://www.baywood.com/journals/PreviewJournals.asp?Id=0272–684x

Journal of Contemporary Ethnography
Robert D. Benford, Editor
Southern Illinois University
Carbondale, IL 62901-4524 USA
Tel: (618) 453-7614
Fax: (618) 453-8926
E-mail: rbenford@siu.edu

Journal of Family Practice
Jeff Susman, M.D.
Room 141
Health Professions Building
Department of Family Medicine
University of Cincinnati
Eden and Bethesda Avenues
Cincinnati, OH 45267 USA
Tel: (513) 558-4021
Fax: (513) 558-3030
E-mail: jfp@fammed.uc.edu
Web: http://www.jfponline.com

Journal of Health and Population in Developing Countries
Editor
CB# 7411, 1107 McGavran-Greenberg
University of North Carolina at Chapel Hill
Chapel Hill, NC 27599-7411 USA
Tel: (919) 966-1938
Fax: (919) 966-6961
E-mail: HPJournal@unc.edu
Web: www.jhupdc.unc.edu

Journal of Immigrant Health
Kluwer Academic Plenum Publishers
Mr. Bill Tucker
233 Spring Street, 7th Floor
New York, NY 10013-1578 USA
Phone: (212) 620-8035
Fax: (212) 647-1898
E-mail: bill.tucker@wkap.com
Web: http://www.kluweronline.com/issn/1096–4045

Journal of Interpersonal Violence
Jon R. Conte, Editor
School of Social Work JH-30
University of Washington
4101 15th Avenue, N.E.
Seattle, WA 98195 USA

Journal of Women's Health and Gender-based Medicine
Andrew P. Marvel, Assistant Editor
University of Pennsylvania
3508 Market St., Suite 251
Philadelphia, PA 19104 USA
Tel: (215) 662-3348
Fax: (215) 662-4690
E-mail: j.womens.health@uphs.upenn.edu

Lancet (England)
Editor
32 Jamestown Road
London, NW1 7BY UK
Tel: 44 (0) 20 7424 4910
Fax: 44 (0) 20 7424 4911
E-mail (inquiries only): editorial@lancet.com

Lancet (United States)
360 Park Avenue South
New York, NY 10010-1710 USA
Tel: (212) 633-3810
Fax: (212) 633-3850
E-mail (inquiries only): editorial@lancet.com

Medical Anthropology: Cross-Cultural Studies in Health and Illness
Stacy Leigh Pigg, Editor
Department of Sociology and Anthropology
Simon Fraser University
8888 University Drive
Burnaby, BC V5A1S6 Canada

Medical Anthropology Quarterly
Dr. Pamela I. Erickson, Editor
Department of Anthropology
354 Mansfield Rd, U-2176
University of Connecticut
Storrs, CT 06269-2176 USA

Psychology and Health
Paul Norman, Editor
Department of Psychology
University of Sheffield
Sheffield, UK S10 2TP
Tel: (44-114) 2226505
Fax: (44-114) 2766515
E-mail: P.Norman@sheffield.ac.uk

Qualitative Health Research
Dr. Janice Morse, Editor
International Institute for Qualitative Methodology
6–10 University Extension Centre
Edmonton, Alberta T6G 2T4 Canada
E-mail: Judy-norris@ualberta.ca

Qualitative Inquiry
Norman K. Denzin, Editor
Department of Sociology
326 Lincoln Hall
University of Illinois
Urbana, IL 61801 USA
Tel: (217) 333-1950
Fax: (217) 333-5225
E-mail: n-denzin@uiuc.edu
Web: http://www.sagepub.com/journals/10778004.htm

Qualitative Sociology
Robert Zussman, Editor
University of Massachusetts
Sociology Department, Thompson Hall
200 Hicks Way
Amherst, MA 01002-9277 USA
Tel: (413) 545-2729; (413) 545-0072
Fax: (413) 545-3204
E-mail: qsoc@soc.umass.edu
Web: http://www.kluweronline.com/issn/0162–0436

Reproductive Health Matters
Marge Berer, Editor
444 Highgate Studios
53–79 Highgate Road
London, NW5 1 TL UK
Tel: 44 20 7267 6567
Fax: 44 20 7267 2551
E-mail: RHMjournal@compuserve.com
Web: http://authors.elsevier.com/JournalDetail.html?PubID=622668&Precis=&popup=

Social Science and Medicine
Dr. Ryan Mowat
MRC Social and Public Health Sciences Unit
4 Lilybank Gardens
Glasgow, G12 8RZ UK
Tel: 0141 357 7571
Fax: 0141 357 0219
E-mail: ryan@msoc.mrc.gla.ac.uk
Web: http://www.elsevier.com/wps/find/journaldescription.cws_home/315/description#description

Sociological Quarterly
Kevin T. Leicht, Editor
Department of Sociology
505 Seashore Hall
University of Iowa
Iowa City, IA 52242-1401 USA
E-mail: tsq@uiowa.edu
Web: http://www.ucpress.edu/journals/tsq/

Studies in Family Planning
Julie Reich, Managing Editor
Population Council
One Dag Hammarskjold Plaza
New York, NY 10017 USA
E-mail: sfp@popcouncil.org
Web: http://www.popcouncil.org/sfp

Symbolic Interaction
Simon Gottschalk, Editor
Department of Sociology
University of Nevada, Las Vegas
4505 Maryland Parkway
Las Vegas, NV 89154-5033 USA
Web: http://www.ucpress.edu/journals/si/edsub.htm

Books and Monographs

Alta Mira Press
Ethnographic Alternatives
Rosalie M. Robertson, Senior Editor
Anthropology, Ethnic Studies
1630 North Main Street, #367
Walnut Creek, CA 94596 USA
Tel: (925) 938-7243
Fax: (925) 933-9720
E-mail: rrobertson@altamirapress.com

Duke University Press
Ken Wissoker, Editor-in-Chief
905 West Main Street, Suite 18B
Durham, NC 27701 USA
Tel: (919) 687-3600
Fax: (919) 688-4574
E-mail: kwissoker@duke.edu

Indiana University Press
Janet Rabinowitch, Editorial Director
601 North Morton Street
Bloomington, IN 47404 USA
Tel: (812) 855-5063
Fax: (812) 855-8507
E-mail: jrabinow@indiana.edu

Jossey-Bass/Pfeiffer
989 Market Street
San Francisco, CA 94103-1741 USA
Web: http://www.jossey-bass.com

New York University Press
Qualitative Studies in Psychology Series
Eric Zinner, Editor-in-Chief
838 Broadway, 3rd Floor
New York, NY 10003-4812 USA
Tel: (212) 998-2575
Fax: (212) 995-3833
E-mail: eric.zinner@nyu.edu
Web: http://www.nyupress.nyu.edu/

Oxford University Press
Executive and Editorial Offices
198 Madison Avenue
New York, NY 10016 USA
Tel: (212) 726-6000
Web: http://www.oup-usa.org/

Routledge (England)
11 New Fetter Lane
London, EC4P 4EE UK
Tel: 44 020 7583 9855
Fax: 44 020 7842 2298
Web: http://www.routledge.com

Routledge (United States)
29 West 35th Street
New York, NY 10001 USA
Tel: (212) 216-7800
Fax: (212) 564-7854
Web: http://www.routledge-ny.com

Rutgers University Press
Adi Hovac, Editorial Assistant, Sciences and Social Sciences
100 Joyce Kilmer Avenue
Piscataway, NJ 08854-8099 USA
Tel: (732) 445-7762
Fax: (732) 445-7039
E-mail: adih@rci.rutgers.edu

Sage Publications, Ltd. (England)
1 Oliver's Yard 55 City Road
London, EC1Y 1SP UK
Tel: 44 020 7374 0645
Fax: 44 020 7374 8741
E-mail: info@sagepub.co.uk

Sage Publications (United States)
Lisa Cuevas Shaw, Research Methodology, Evaluation, Statistics and Qualitative Research
2455 Teller Road
Thousand Oaks, CA 91320 USA
Tel: (805) 499-0721
Fax: (805) 499-0871
E-mail: lisa.cuevas@sagepub.com
Web: www.sagepub.com

Sage Publications (India)
M-32 Market
Greater Kailash-Part-1
Post Box 4215
New Delhi, 110048 India
Tel: 91 11 6419884/6444958
Fax: 91 11 6472426
E-mail: sageind@giasdl01.vsnl.net.in
Web: http://indiasage.com/

Temple University Press
Janet M. Francendese, Editor-in-Chief
1601 North Broad Street, USB 306
Philadelphia, PA 19122-6099 USA
Tel: (215) 204-8787
Fax: (215) 204-4719
Web: http://www.temple.edu

University of Chicago Press
Editorial Department
1427 East 60th Street
Chicago, IL 60637 USA
Tel: (773) 702-7700
Fax: (773) 702-9756
Web: http://www.press.uchicago.edu

University of Michigan Press
P.O. Box 1104
839 Greene Street
Ann Arbor, MI 48106-1104 USA
Tel: (734) 764-4388
Fax: (734) 936-0456
E-mail: umpress-www@umich.edu
Web: http://www.press.umich.edu

University of North Carolina Press
P.O. Box 2288
Chapel Hill, NC 27515-2288 USA
Tel: (800) 848-6224
Fax: (919) 966-3829
Web: http://uncpress.unc.edu

University of Pennsylvania Press
Peter A. Agree or Walda Metcalf, Social Science Editors
4200 Pine Street
Philadelphia, PA 19104-4011 USA
Tel: (215) 898-6261
Fax: (215) 898-0404
Web: http://www.upenn.edu/pennpress

Zed Books
7 Cynthia Street
London, N1 9JF UK
Tel: 44 020 7837 0384
Web: http://www.zedbooks.co.uk

APPENDIX ELEVEN

Sample Research Brief on the Female Condom

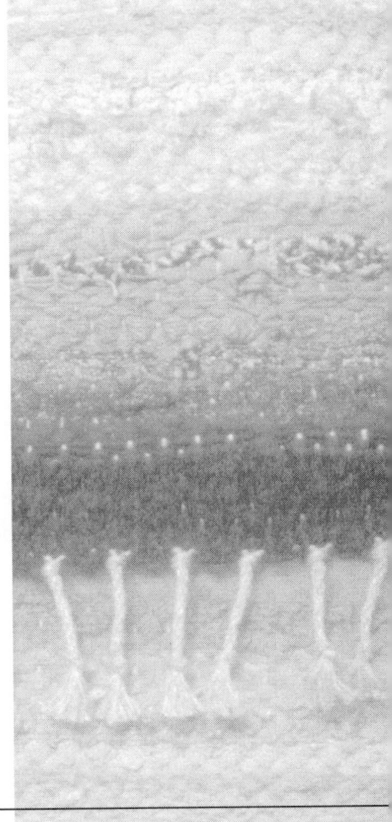

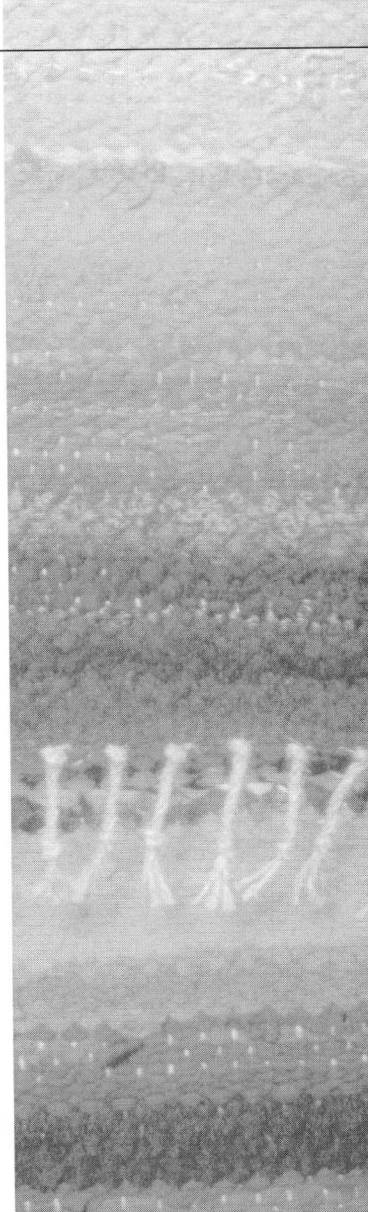

Lessons from a Female Condom Community Intervention Trial in Rural Kenya

What impact will a general distribution of the female condom have on sexually transmitted infection (STI) rates in a rural area? To address this question, FHI conducted a community intervention trial and follow-up service delivery assessment in rural Kenya, collaborating with the University of Nairobi, Department of Medical Microbiology, and the Family Planning Association of Kenya. The researchers concluded:

- The availability of the female condom did not reduce STI rates, relative to the reductions achieved by distribution of the male condom alone.
- Female condom users generally liked the device, recognized its dual protection properties and appreciated its advantages over the male condom.
- Provider preconceptions may have limited opportunities for women to use the device.

The community intervention trial was conducted in six matched pairs of tea, coffee and flower plantations, each served by at least one primary health care clinic. Each matched pair comprised an intervention and a control site. In the intervention areas, providers and outreach workers received training in providing male and female

---

Reprinted with permission of Family Health International. FHI produced these research briefs as part of an information dissemination effort supported by the Bureau for Africa/Office of Sustainable Development, U.S. Agency for International Development. For more information, please visit FHI's Web site at http://www.fhi.org.

condoms, STI risk reduction and treatment, and were supplied with free male and female condoms. The control areas received training, supplies and training only on the male condom. A thorough educational campaign reached residents throughout all sites with activities in control sites covering only the male condom.

The study followed about 1,600 women, testing and treating them at baseline, six months and 12 months for three infections—gonorrhea, chlamydia, and trichomoniasis. At both control and intervention plantations, about 24 percent of the women tested and treated had one or more of the three STIs at the beginning of the study. After 12 months, STI rates had declined to about 18 percent at both the intervention and control sites.[1] These results indicate that adding the female condom to the male condom distribution system did not contribute to any additional reductions in disease prevalence. At the same time, the intensive promotional campaign in the male-condom-only distribution system was not sufficient to have an important impact on disease rates either.

Reported female condom use was not sufficiently frequent to make a substantial difference in the overall number of protected sex acts in the intervention sites. Also, providing female condoms did not result in more overall condoms distributed in intervention sites. At the end of the study, 58 percent of study participants in intervention sites reported that they had not used the female condom at all in the previous six months.[2]

SERVICE DELIVERY IMPACT

To assess why so few women used the female condom, researchers visited 16 of the 23 sites participating in the community trial, including a balance of high- and low-performing intervention and control sites. At each site, surveys were conducted with all available clinicians, outreach workers, recent family planning clients, and community key informants. Also, researchers observed all family planning service delivery encounters in the clinic on the day of the visit.[3]

A gap existed between clinicians' reported condom promotion activities and their observed behaviors. In 42 observed family planning visits, the woman in every case chose a hormonal method, but only once did a provider suggest a condom as a supplemental method for STI protection. Moreover, 91 percent of providers interviewed said they had a major influence on whether clients used condoms. Many clinicians viewed the female condom as a feasible method only for single women and sex workers, not for women in stable unions. This provider opinion regarding appropriate female condom users may have contributed to inadequate interest on the part of clients. Only one of 10 intervention site clinics distributed female condoms all 12 months of the trial as called for by the protocol.

Despite the provider behaviors, outreach workers reported that the female condom was viewed by clients as an acceptable method, credited for being warmer, roomier, and stronger than the male condom. Some women felt safer with the female condom because it was perceived as being less prone than the male condom to break. Further, women appreciated being able to insert the female condom themselves, avoiding the risk of men tampering with the device, as was suspected with the male condom.

At the same time, social norms and personal preferences appeared to limit true acceptability of the female condom and impede its introduction into sexual relationships. Community members expressed concern that the female condom may allow women too much freedom, enabling them to "move around" on their husbands. Some feared that intensified distribution of condoms might lead to increased prostitution.

With limited understanding of female anatomy, some users expressed fears that it could "slip into the stomach," get "lost inside the womb," or get "stuck in the vagina." Others rumored it was laced with HIV or that the lubricant could cause infertility or produce infections. Some men worried that a woman can take semen captured in the female condom to a witch doctor and put a hex on the partner.

When considering the introduction of the female condom in rural areas, program planners need to take into consideration the local culture and address the negative influence that traditional gender roles can have on female condom use.

NOTES

1. Feldblum PJ, Kuyoh MA, Bwayo JJ, et al. Female condom introduction and sexually transmitted infection prevalence: results of a community intervention trial in Kenya. AIDS 2001 May 25;15(8):1037–1044.

2. Welsh MJ, Feldblum PJ, Kuyoh MA, et al. Condom use during a community intervention trial in Kenya. Int J AIDS STDs 2001 July;12(7):469–474.

3. Toroitich-Ruto C. Assessment of the Intervention: Was It Implemented as Intended? Presented at Conference on Female Condom and STDs: A Community Intervention Trial, May 9, 2000, Nairobi, Kenya.

APPENDIX TWELVE

Who Is an Author?

IN QUALITATIVE RESEARCH the data collection and analysis phases tend to be less temporally distinct than in quantitative research, and team members who collect study data are called on to conduct iterative analysis as they go. Such active participation by all study team members in refining questions, coding data, and generating insights has implications for authorship roles on study papers. Although different journals have different rules for authorship, this one, by the International Committee of Medical Journal Editors (2003), is most widely accepted:

> Authorship credit should be based on 1) substantial contributions to conception and design, or acquisition of data, or analysis and interpretation of data; 2) drafting the article or revising it critically for important intellectual content; and 3) final approval of the version to be published. Authors should meet conditions 1, 2, and 3.
>
> When a large, multi-center group has conducted the work, the group should identify the individuals who accept direct responsibility for the manuscript. These individuals should fully meet the criteria for authorship defined above, and editors will ask these individuals to complete journal-specific author and conflict of interest disclosure forms. When submitting a group author manuscript, the corresponding author should clearly indicate the preferred citation and should clearly identify all individual authors as well as the group name. Journals will generally list other members of the group in the acknowledgements. The National Library of Medicine indexes the group name and the names of individuals the group has identified as being directly responsible for the manuscript.
>
> Acquisition of funding, collection of data, or general supervision of the research group, alone, does not justify authorship.

All persons designated as authors should qualify for authorship, and all those who qualify should be listed.

Each author should have participated sufficiently in the work to take public responsibility for appropriate portions of the content.

Some journals now also request that one or more authors, referred to as "guarantors," be identified as the persons who take responsibility for the integrity of the work as a whole, from inception to published article, and publish that information.

Increasingly, authorship of multi-center trials is attributed to a group. All members of the group who are named as authors should fully meet the above criteria for authorship.

The order of authorship on the byline should be a joint decision of the co-authors. Authors should be prepared to explain the order in which authors are listed.

APPENDIX THIRTEEN

Sample Brochure to Share Qualitative Study Findings with Participating Communities

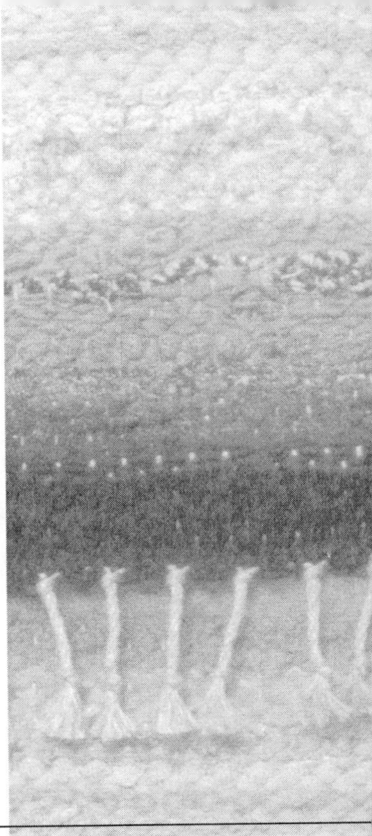

THIS BROCHURE was developed by Susan Settergren and the staff of the POLICY Project to share findings with members of the communities in Zimbabwe where a qualitative study on unsafe abortion and postabortion care was conducted. It is reprinted with permission from the POLICY Project, an international effort funded by the U.S. Agency for International Development and undertaken by the Futures Group International, Research Triangle Institute, and the Centre for Development and Population Activities in 1999. For more information, see http://www.policyproject.com/pubs/policymatters/pm-01.pdf.

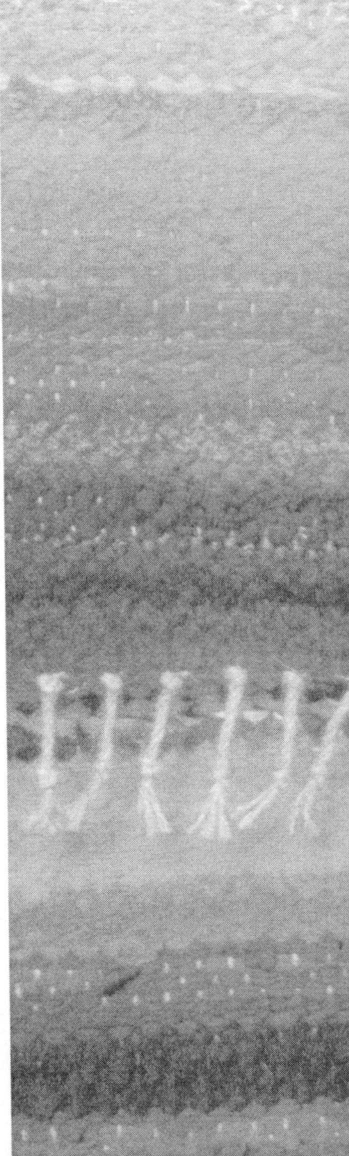

Actions That You Recommended

- Sensitise and educate community members (parents, teachers, youth, leaders) on the dangers and the issues.
- Discuss unwanted pregnancy, unsafe abortion, and postabortion care at church, residents' association and burial society meetings, and sports clubs. Talk with family members and neighbors.
- Network with other organisations and develop community action plans.
- Broadcast information on the radio and in newspapers.
- Host drama performances and workshops.
- Sensitise izinyanga about the dangers of performing abortions.
- Seek prompt medical treatment when abortion complications occur.
- Establish youth centers for counseling and employment development.
- Expand and improve postabortion care services by offering confidentiality, counseling, and support.
- Continue dialogue on policy issues related to unsafe abortion and postabortion care.
- Be better parents: Spend time with children, teach them about sex and reproductive health, exercise discipline, be good role models.
- Teach sex education in schools.

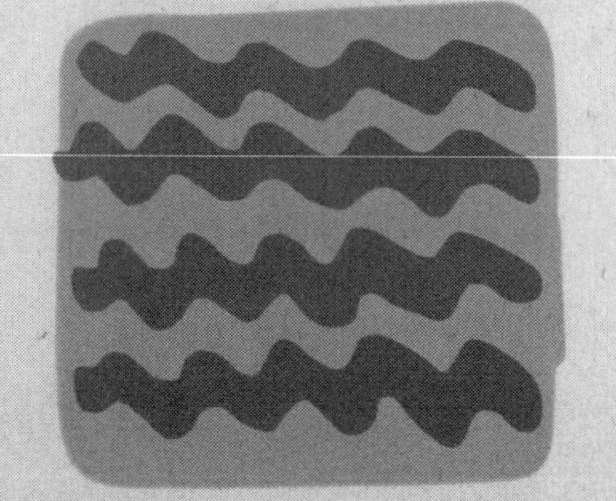

"Don't - Ungaqali"

Community Perspectives on Unsafe Abortion and Postabortion Care

"There is no point in blaming this or that. Abortion is a community problem."
- *Woman at a performance discussion*

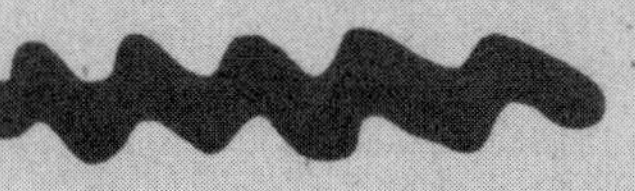

Amakhosi Theatre Group

P.O. Box 7030, Mzilikazi, Bulawayo, Zimbabwe
Phone: 79379, Fax: 77412, Email: amakhosi@telconet.co.zw

Performances, Discussions, and Interviews

In November and December 1998, Amakhosi Theatre Group performed the play, *Don't - Ungaqali,* in communities throughout Bulawayo and Hwange. The play tells the story of a teenage couple who engages in sex and the girl becomes pregnant. The girl has an illegal abortion and suffers complications. Her life is saved because she gets medical attention in time, but she can bear no more children.

Over 2,500 people saw the play and nearly 500 of them participated in discussions on unsafe abortion following the performances. We took notes on those discussions and also interviewed 60 community members to learn more about your views on unsafe abortion and postabortion care.

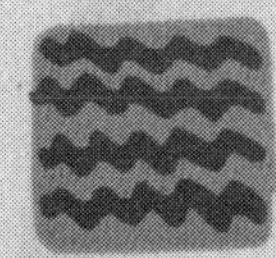

What We Heard From You

- Unsafe abortion is a well-known problem, although most abortions are done secretly. It's often only when someone dies or gets sick that the problem becomes known.
- Young girls are at highest risk of unwanted pregnancy and unsafe abortion. However, women of all ages induce abortions.
- Causes of unwanted pregnancy are many. They include economic hardship that leads to sex for income, poor parenting, ignorance about sex and reproductive health, early physical maturity and experimentation with sex, promiscuity, unprotected sex, peer pressure to have sex, shift from traditional to modern societal values, inaccessibility of contraceptives, women's lack of control of their sexuality, inadequate family accommodation, boys and men cheating girls into having sex by promising marriage, and lack of respect between a man and a woman.
- Men's denial of responsibility for the pregnancy and fear of family members finding out about the pregnancy are major causes for abortion.
- Abortions are obtained from a variety of sources, including izinyanga, community elders, and medical doctors. They also are self-induced, sometimes with assistance from friends and other community members. Most abortionists are unskilled, although some are more qualified than others.
- The law requires health care facilities to report abortion cases to the police. However, the practice of reporting appears to vary among service delivery sites and individuals. Parents and community members also report cases to authorities. Frequently, they file these reports because they want the abortionist to be arrested.
- Those who experience complications of induced abortion often delay, or do not seek, medical treatment. Fear of being reported to the police by clinic or hospital staff; fear of harsh treatment and exposure by nurses, and fear of reactions from parents, friends, and community members are the primary reasons for avoiding medical attention. People reported that nurses gossip and treat clients, especially youth, harshly. On the other hand, nurses expressed frustration with a client's failure to explain the reason for her condition and her delay in seeking treatment until complications were severe.

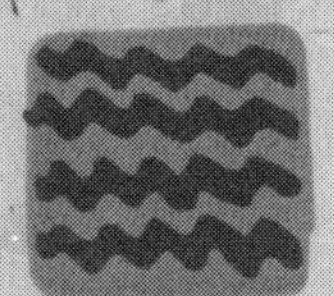

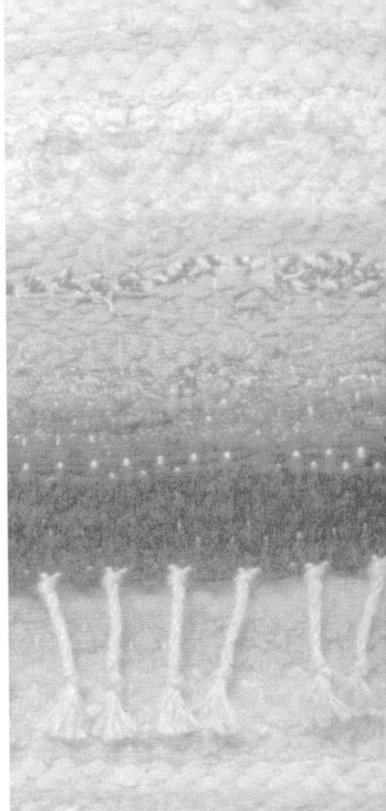

APPENDIX FOURTEEN

Making Study Findings Accessible to Other Researchers

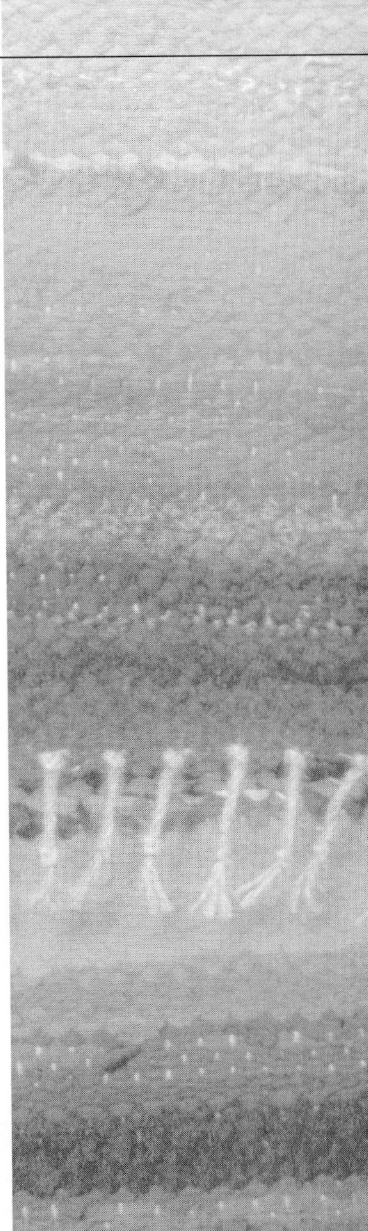

YOU CAN MAKE your study findings more accessible to other researchers nationally, regionally, and internationally in four important ways:

- Add standardized cataloging information to the title page or inside cover of your report.
- Submit your report or article to bibliographic indexing databases and information clearinghouses.
- Make your study report or data set available to other researchers through physical and electronic libraries.
- Ask a health organization or research partner organization to post your report on its Web site.

Following are some general guidelines based on advice from qualitative researchers and librarians. Where you submit your materials may depend on your study topic and region.

Cataloging Information

INTERNATIONAL STANDARD BOOK NUMBER (ISBN)

If your institution is registered as a publisher with the ISBN system, assign an ISBN number and print the number with other title page or cover information in your document.

U.S. LIBRARY OF CONGRESS (LC)

People throughout the world searching for information on publications use the LC database. There are two options for getting your book into the LC database. Both require providing information to LC before publication:

1. Register the book electronically by completing the LC Preassigned Control Number Program form before publication. You will receive an LC Control Number (LCCN) that should be printed in the book, usually on the back of the title page. You are required to send a copy of the book to the LC when it is published. When the LC receives the book, it will catalog the book and add it to its database. The LCCN and the database make it much easier for libraries and dealers to find your book and the catalog information. For more information and electronic registration forms, go to http://pcn.loc.gov/pcn.
2. Register with the LC Cataloging In Publication (CIP) program. Before printing, generally at the final draft stage, you send the complete text of the book in electronic form to the LC for cataloging. The LC will send you the complete bibliographic record of your book, including classification numbers and subject headings. This information should be printed in the book when it is published. Having the catalog record in the book makes it much easier for libraries to process the book and for anyone to select, locate, and order it. You must send a copy of the book to the LC once it is published. For more information on the CIP, contact

   Mr. John Celli, Chief
   Cataloging in Publication Division (CIP)
   Library of Congress
   101 Independence Avenue, S.E.
   Washington, DC 20540-4320 USA
   E-mail: jcel@loc.gov

For general information or to view the forms and register, go to http://cip.loc.gov/cip.

Bibliographic Indexing Databases and Information Clearinghouses

Consider submitting your report or article to bibliographic indexing databases and information clearinghouses, such as the following.

POPULATION INFORMATION ONLINE (POPLINE)

POPLINE at http://db.jhuccp.org/popinform/basic.html is the world's largest bibliographic database on population, family planning, and related health issues. POPLINE provides citations with abstracts for over 275,000 records representing published and unpublished literature in the field.

POPLINE Digital Services (PDS) provides authoritative, accurate, and up-to-date reproductive health information in electronic formats for developing-country health professionals and policymakers. Full-text copies of most of the documents cited in POPLINE are available to individuals or institutions in developing countries free of charge, upon request. PDS also provides full-text documents on the Internet. For more information, contact

POPLINE Digital Services (PDS)
111 Market Place, Suite 310
Baltimore, MD 21202 USA
Tel: (410) 659-6300
Fax: (410) 659-6266
E-mail: popline@jhuccp.org

SOCIAL SCIENCE INFORMATION GATEWAY (SOSIG)

SOSIG at http://www.sosig.ac.uk is a fully searchable subject-based catalog of international Internet resources on social science. This service, funded by the Economic and Social Research Council of the United Kingdom, offers access to a catalog of thousands of high-quality social science resources from around the world including

- Research reports and papers
- Electronic journals and texts
- Statistics and software
- Databases and data
- Learning and teaching resources
- Internet links to university social science departments

If you would like to recommend that SOSIG post your study citation or data sets or publicize information related to your work, you must complete registration information at the SOSIG Internet address at www.sosig.ac.uk/about_us/contacts.html or write to

The Social Science Information Gateway
Institute for Learning and Research Technology
University of Bristol
8–10 Berkeley Square
Bristol, BS8 1HH UK
Tel: 44 0 117 928 7117
Fax: 44 0 117 928 7112

DEVELOPMENT EXPERIENCE CLEARINGHOUSE (DEC)

If your research is done with support from the U.S. Agency for International Development (USAID), you may submit your study reports or documents for inclusion in the DEC Development Experience System (DEXS). This database at www.dec.org was developed to ensure that valuable USAID experience is preserved and gains wider exposure. Once processed into the DEXS system, your documents will be searchable and accessible online over the Internet, and the public can order paper copies at any time. For instructions on how to submit your material, see http://www.dec.org/submit.cfm or contact

Document Acquisitions
USAID Development Experience Clearinghouse
8403 Colesville Road, Suite 210
Silver Spring, MD 20910-6344 USA
Tel: (301) 562-0641
E-mail: docsubmit@dec.cdie.org

ASIA-PACIFIC POPIN

Asia-Pacific POPIN is a decentralized network involving regional, subregional, national, and nongovernmental population information centers in the Economic and Social Commission for Asia and the Pacific (ESCAP) region. To submit studies conducted in Asia or the Pacific to the ESCAP directory of current population research, contact

Director, Population and Rural and Urban Development Division
ESCAP, United Nations Building
Rajdamnern Avenue
Bangkok, 10200 Thailand
Tel: 66-2 288-1536
Fax: 66-2 288-1009
E-mail: ertuna.unescap@un.org

For more information visit the ESCAP Web site at http://www.un.org/popin/regions/escap.html or the main POPIN Web site at http://www.un.org/popin.

U.S. LIBRARY OF CONGRESS (LC)

The size and variety of its collections make the LC the largest library in the world. Collections include research materials in more than 450 languages. By sending a copy of your research report to the LC, you contribute to the preservation of knowledge and public access to your materials—whether available in hard copy or in a full-text electronic version. To submit your report, send a copy to

Mr. Michael Albin, Chief
Anglo/American Acquisitions Division (LS/ACQ/ANAD)
Library of Congress
101 Independence Avenue, S.E.
Washington, DC 20540-4170 USA
Tel: (202) 707-5361
Fax: (202) 707-9440
E-mail: malb@loc.gov

For more information, see http://www.loc.gov/rr/collects.html.

U.S. NATIONAL LIBRARY OF MEDICINE (NLM)

The NLM provides online access to MEDLINE, PubMed, and other specialized databases on HIV/AIDS, bioethics, public health, and health services research at http://www.nlm.nih.gov/hinfo.html. To request that your publication or document be cataloged and made accessible through the NLM, contact

The National Library of Medicine
Cataloging Section
8600 Rockville Pike
Bethesda, MD 20894 USA
Tel: (301) 496-5497
Fax: (301) 402-1211
E-mail: custserv@nlm.nih.gov

WORLDCAT

Submit your publication to the WorldCat database, the most consulted database in higher education. WorldCat is managed by the Online Computer Library Center, Inc. (OCLC), a global library cooperative. It holds over forty-six million cataloging records created by libraries around the world, with four hundred languages represented. Request that your publisher send your document to a participating library to catalog. Libraries that participate in the OCLC may submit the record to the WorldCat database and may be willing to undertake the cataloging work in exchange for a free copy of your material. To locate a member library, visit http://www.oclc.org/contacts/libraries/default.htm. For more information, contact

OCLC Online Computer Library Center, Inc.
6565 Frantz Road
Dublin, OH 43017-3395 USA
Tel: (614) 764-6000/(800) 848-5878 (USA/Canada)
Fax: (614) 764-6096
E-mail: oclc@oclc.org

BIREME'S SCIENTIFIC ELECTRONIC LIBRARY ONLINE (SCIELO)

BIREME is a project of the Centro Latino-Americano e do Caribe de Informação em Ciências da Saúde (Latin American and the Caribbean Center on Health Sciences Information) and the Fundação de Amparo à Pesquisa do Estado de São Paulo (FAPESP)—a governmental foundation in Brazil aimed at supporting scientific research. The BIREME project promotes a common methodology for the preparation, storage, retrieval, and evaluation of electronic publications through the use of information and communication technologies. One of the applications of the methodology is SciELO at www.scielo.org, a virtual library comprising scientific publications produced in Latin America and the Caribbean. For more information on how to submit your study report to SciELO, contact

FAPESP/BIREME Project for Electronic Scientific Publications
Centro Latino-Americano e do Caribe de Informação em Ciências da Saúde
Rua Botucatu, 862-04023-901
Vila Clementino 04023-901
São Paulo SP, Brazil
Tel: 55 11 576 9863
Fax: 55 11 5575 8868
E-mail: scielo@bireme.br

Depositing Data Sets

To make your research permanently available to the international community, seek opportunities to deposit your data set at a national or regional university library or faculty of social sciences.

INTER-UNIVERSITY CONSORTIUM FOR POLITICAL AND SOCIAL RESEARCH (ICPSR)

ICPSR, established in 1962, is the main repository for social science research in the United States. ICPSR maintains and provides access to a vast archive of social science data for research and instruction, and it offers training in quantitative methods to facilitate effective data use. ICPSR preserves data to ensure that data resources are available to future generations of scholars, migrating the data to new storage media as changes in technology warrant. In addition, ICPSR provides user support to assist researchers in identifying relevant data for analysis and in conducting their research projects.

ICPSR, a unit within the Institute for Social Research at the University of Michigan, encourages researchers to deposit their own computer-readable data in the archive for long-term preservation and for use in secondary analysis by other social science researchers.

For instructions on how to prepare a data set for deposit, visit the ICPSR Web site at http://www.icpsr.umich.edu/ACCESS/deposit. For more information, contact

The Inter-University Consortium for Political and Social Research
P.O. Box 1248
Ann Arbor, MI 48106-1248 USA
Tel: (734) 647-5000
Fax: (734) 647-8200
E-mail: netmail@icpsr.umich.edu

THE SOCIAL SCIENCE DATA ARCHIVES (SSDA)

Located in the Research School of Social Sciences at the Australian National University, the SSDA was established in 1981 to collect and preserve computer-readable data and make the data available for further analysis. SSDA actively seeks deposit of data sets from research by academic, government, and private organizations in order to preserve them for future use. For information on how to deposit data, visit http://assda.anu.edu.au/depositing.html or contact

Australian Social Science Data Archive
18 Balmain Crescent
The Australian National University
ACTON ACT 0200
Tel: +61 2 6125 4400
Fax: +61 2 6125 0627
E-mail: assda@anu.edu.au

DUBLIN CORE METADATA INITIATIVE

The Dublin Core is a directory of directories. One way to help other researchers find your report or locate your data sets—if these materials are available on the Internet—is to make sure the final HTML Web pages are annotated with Dublin Core metatags or indexing information. Dublin Core metadata supplement existing methods for searching and indexing Web-based metadata, regardless of whether the corresponding resource is an electronic or physical document. Adding Dublin Core metatags promotes greater access to your information by anyone searching the World Wide Web. Even if your study report will not immediately be posted on the Internet, you can add bibliographic descriptors to your data set or report using the Dublin Core metadata element set. Some people also use Dublin Core elements for cataloging.

To download the Dublin Core metadata, see http://dublincore.org/documents/2000/07/16/usageguide. For a copy of this guide in other languages, see http://dublincore.org/resources/translations.

Web Sites

IBIBLIO

If your organization—or a research partner's organization—has posted your material on a Web site, explore the group's interest in permitting a major Web hub such as ibiblio.org to replicate the material in the social or applied sciences sections of its collections. Ibiblio, a collaboration of the Center for the Public Domain and the University of North Carolina at Chapel Hill, is home to one of the largest collections of freely available full-text online information used for teaching, research, and public service. For more information, visit http://ibiblio.org/collection.html.

AMEDEO

If you own the copyright to your research report, do not plan to submit your data to a peer-review journal, and would like to see your findings made freely available to the public, consider submitting your text electronically to AMEDEO.com, the Medical Literature Guide, at http://www.amedeo.com. The editors will post your report on the following Web sites, which archive scientific research and ideas: http://publiclibraryofscience.com or http://www.FreeMedicalJournals.com.

Suggested Readings and Selected Internet Resources

I. General Texts on Qualitative Research Methods

Bernard HR. 1995. Research methods in anthropology: qualitative and quantitative approaches. 2nd ed. Walnut Creek, CA: Altamira Press.

Campbell O, Cleland JG, Collumbien M, Southwick K. 1999. Social science methods for research on reproductive health. Geneva: World Health Organization.

Denzin NK, Lincoln YS, editors. 1994. Handbook of qualitative research. Thousand Oaks, CA: Sage.

Hudelson PM. 1996. Qualitative research for health programmes. Geneva: World Health Organization.

Patton MQ. 1990. Qualitative evaluation and research methods. 2nd ed. Newbury Park, CA: Sage.

Rossman GB, Rallis FR. 1998. Learning in the field: an introduction to qualitative research. Thousand Oaks, CA: Sage.

Schensul JJ, LeCompte MD, editors. 1999. Ethnographer's toolkit. Vols. 1–9. Walnut Creek, CA: Altamira Press.

Yoddumnern-Attig B, Allen-Attig G, Boonchalaksi W, Richter K, Soonthorndhada A, editors. 1993. Qualitative methods for population and health research. Nakhon Pathom, Thailand: Mahidol University, Institute for Population and Social Research.

II. Theoretical Basis of Qualitative Research

Kelle U. 1997. Theory-building in qualitative research and computer programs for the management of textual data. Sociological Research Online 2(2). Available at: http://www.socresonline.org.uk/socresonline/2/2/1.html.

Patton MQ. 1990. In: Patton MQ. Qualitative evaluation and research methods. 2nd ed. Newbury Park, CA: Sage. Chap. 3, Variety in qualitative inquiry: theoretical orientations.

Strauss A, Corbin J. 1990. Basics of qualitative research: grounded theory procedures and techniques. Newbury Park, CA: Sage.

Trotter RT II. 1997. Anthropological midrange theories in mental health research: selected theory, methods and systematic approaches to at-risk populations. Ethos 25(2):259–74.

III. Participant Observation

Bernard HR. 1995. Research methods in anthropology: qualitative and quantitative approaches. 2nd ed. Walnut Creek, CA: Altamira Press. Chap. 9, Participation observation.

DeWalt KM. 2001. Participant observation: a guide for fieldworkers. Walnut Creek, CA: Altamira Press.

Schensul JJ, LeCompte MD, Nastasi BK, Borgatti SP. 1999. Enhanced ethnographic methods. In: Schensul SL, Schensul JJ, LeCompte MD, editors. Ethnographer's toolkit. Vol. 3, Enhanced ethnographic methods. Walnut Creek, CA: Altamira Press.

Schensul SL, Schensul JJ, LeCompte MD. 1999. Chap. 5, Exploratory or open-ended observation. In: Schensul SL, Schensul JJ, LeCompte MD, editors. Ethnographer's toolkit. Vol. 2, Essential ethnographic methods: observations, interviews, and questionnaires. Walnut Creek, CA: Altamira Press.

Spradley JP. 1980. Participant observation. New York: Holt, Rinehart and Winston.

IV. In-Depth Interviewing

Patton MQ. 1990. Qualitative evaluation and research methods. 2nd ed. Newbury Park, CA: Sage. Chap. 7, Qualitative interviewing.

Rubin HJ, Rubin IS. 1995. Qualitative interviewing: the art of hearing data. Thousand Oaks, CA: Sage.

V. Focus Group Research

Debus M. 1986. Handbook for excellence in focus group research. Washington, DC: Academy for Educational Development.

Morgan DL, Krueger RA, editors. 1998. The Focus Group Kit. Thousand Oaks, CA: Sage.

VI. Social Network Analysis

Scott J. 1991. Social network analysis: a handbook. Newbury Park, CA: Sage.

Trotter RT II. 1999. Chap. 1, Friends, relatives, and relevant others: conducting ethnographic network studies. In: Schensul JJ, LeCompte MD, editors. Ethnographer's toolkit. Vol. 4, Mapping social networks, spatial data, and hidden populations. Walnut Creek, CA: Altamira Press.

VII. Data Management and Analysis

Huberman AM, Miles MB. 1994. Data management and analysis methods. In: Denzin NK, Lincoln YS, editors. Handbook of qualitative research. Part 4, Methods of collecting and analyzing empirical materials. Thousand Oaks, CA: Sage.

Krueger, RA. 1998. Analyzing and reporting focus group results. In: Morgan DL, Krueger RA, editors. The Focus Group Kit. Vol. 6. Thousand Oaks, CA: Sage.

Miles MB, Huberman AM. 1994. Qualitative data analysis: an expanded sourcebook. 2nd ed. Thousand Oaks, CA: Sage.

Patton, MQ. 1999. Enhancing the quality and credibility of qualitative analysis. Health Serv Res 34(5):1189–1208.

Silverman D. 1998. The quality of qualitative health research: the open-ended interview and its alternatives. Soc Sci Health 4(2):104–17.

VIII. Combining Qualitative and Quantitative Methods

Caracelli V, Greene J. 1993. Data analysis strategies for mixed-method evaluation designs. Policy Anal 15(2):195–207.

Dixon-Woods M, Agarwal S, Jones D, Sutton A, Young B. 2004. Integrative approaches to qualitative and quantitative evidence. A review of the literature by UK Health Development Agency. Available online as PDF file at: http://www.hda.nhs.uk/documents/integrative_approaches.pdf.

Morgan DL. 1998. Practical strategies for combining qualitative and quantitative methods. Qualitative Health Res May;8(3):362–76.

Pedersen D. Qualitative and quantitative: two styles of viewing the world or two categories of reality? 1992. In: Scrimshaw NS, Gleason GR, editors. Rapid assessment procedures: qualitative methodologies for planning and evaluation of health-related programmes. Boston: International Nutrition Foundation for Developing Countries.

Sandelowski M. 2000. Combining qualitative and quantitative sampling, data collection, and analysis techniques in mixed method studies. Res Nurs Health Jun;23(3):246–55.

Tashakkori A, Teddlie C. 1998. Mixed methodology: combining qualitative and quantitative approaches. Thousand Oaks, CA: Sage.

IX. Ethical Issues

Alty A, Rodham K. 1998. The ouch! factor: problems in conducting sensitive research. Qualitative Health Res 8(2):275–82.

Association of Social Anthropologists of the UK and Commonwealth. 1999. Ethical guidelines for good research practice. Available at: http://www.theasa.org/ethics.htm.

Ringheim K. 1995. Ethical issues in social science research with special reference to sexual behavior research. Soc Sci Med 40:1691–97.

Rivera R, Borasky D, Rice R, Carayon F. 2001. Research Ethics Training Curriculum. Research Triangle Park, NC: Family Health International.

Seal DW, Bloom FR, Somlai AM. 2000. Dilemmas in conducting qualitative sex research in applied field settings. Health Educ Behav Feb;27(1):10–23.

World Health Organization. 1999. Putting women's safety first: ethical and safety recommendations for research on domestic violence against women. Geneva: World Health Organization.

X. Writing Qualitative Reports

Richardson L. 1990. Writing strategies: reaching diverse audiences. Newbury Park, CA: Sage.

Wolcott HF. 1990. Writing up qualitative research: qualitative research methods. No. 20. Newbury Park, CA: Sage.

XI. Special Issues and Applications

Chambers R. 1985. Shortcut methods of gathering information for rural development projects. In: Cernea M, editor. Putting people first: sociological variables in rural development. New York: Oxford University Press.

Knodel J. 1997. A case for nonanthropological qualitative methods for demographers. Popul Dev Rev Dec;23(4):847–53.

Petchesky RP, Judd K, editors. 1998. Negotiating reproductive rights: women's perspectives across countries and cultures. London: Zed Books.

Scrimshaw S, Hurtado E. 1987. Rapid assessment procedures for nutrition and primary health care. Tokyo: UN University.

University of British Columbia, Institute of Health Promotion Research, B.C. Consortium for Health Promotion Research. 1995. Study of participatory action in health promotion: review and recommendations for the development of participatory research in health promotion in Canada. Ottawa: Royal Society of Canada.

XII. E-mail lists

PSYCH-NARRATIVE: Discussion of narrative in everyday life
To subscribe, send the following message to majordomo@massey.ac.nz:

subscribe psych-narrative

QUALRS-L: Qualitative research for the human sciences
To subscribe, send the following message to listserv@listserv.uga.edu:

subscribe QUALRS-L<your name>

or go to http://www.listserv.uga.edu/cgi-bin/wa?SUBED1=qualrs-l&A=1.

Qual-software: Qualitative analysis computer programs
To subscribe send the following message to jiscmail@jiscmail.ac.uk:

join qual-software<your name>

or go to http://www.jiscmail.ac.uk/cgi-bin/wa.exe?SUBED1=qual-software&A=1.

XIII. Web Sites

Council for the Development of Social Science Research in Africa (CODESRIA)
http://www.codesria.org

National Centre for Social Research, Qualitative Research Unit
http://www.scpr.ac.uk/natcen/pages/hw_qualitative.htm

Qualitative Methods Workbook
http://www.ship.edu/~cgboeree/qualmeth.html

Qualitative Research Resources
http://www.vanguard.edu/faculty/dratcliff/qual

QualPage: Resources for Qualitative Research
http://www.qualitativeresearch.uga.edu/QualPage/

XIV. Online Journals

The Qualitative Report
http://www.nova.edu/ssss/QR

Forum: Qualitative Social Research
http://www.qualitative-research.net/fqs/fqs-eng.htm

References

Adioetomo SM, Eggleston E. 1998. Helping the husband, maintaining harmony: family planning, women's work and women's household autonomy in Indonesia. J Popul 4(2 Special edition):7–31.

Adrien A, Cayemittes M. 1991. Le Sida en Haïti: connaissances, attitudes, croyances, et comportements de la population. Bureau du Coordination du Programme National de Lutte contre le SIDA. Port-au-Prince: Institut Haïtien de l'Enfance.

Alty A, Rodham K. 1998. The ouch! factor: problems in conducting sensitive research. Qualitative Health Res 8(2):275–282.

Association of Social Anthropologists of the Commonwealth. 1999. Ethical guidelines for good research practice. Available at: http://www.asa.anthropology.ac.uk/ethics2.html. Accessed 1999.

Babbie E. 1998. The practice of social research. 8th ed. Belmont, CA: Wadsworth.

Bandura A. 1977. Self-efficacy: toward a unifying theory of behavior change. Psych Rev 84:191–215.

Bandura A. 1986. Social foundations of thought and action: a social cognitive theory. Englewood Cliffs, NJ: Prentice Hall.

Bandura A. 1989. Perceived self-efficacy in the exercise of control over AIDS infection. In: Mayes VM, Albee GW, Schneider SF, editors. Primary prevention of AIDS: psychological approaches. London: Sage. p 128–41.

Barnett B, Eggleston E, Jackson J, Hardee K. 1996. Case study of the Women's Center of Jamaica Foundation Program for Adolescent Mothers (WP96–03). Research Triangle Park, NC: Family Health International.

Barnett B, Stein J. 1998. Women's voices, women's lives: the impact of family planning. Research Triangle Park, NC: Family Health International.

Basch CE. 1987. Focus group interview: an underutilized research technique for improving theory and practice in health education [review]. Health Educ Q Win;14(4):411–48.

Beck T, Stelcner M. 1996a. Guide to gender-sensitive indicators. Quebec: Canadian International Development Agency.

Beck T, Stelcner M. 1996b. The why and how of gender-sensitive indicators: a project level handbook. Quebec: Canadian International Development Agency.

Bender DE, Baker R, Dusch E, McCann MF. 1990. Integrated use of qualitative and quantitative methods to elicit women's differential knowledge of breastfeeding and lactational amenorrhea in periurban Peru. J Health Popul Developing Countries 1(1):68–84.

Bender DE, Castro D. 2000. Explaining the birthweight paradox: Latina immigrants' perceptions of resilience and risk. J Immigrant Health Jul;2(3):155–173.

Bender DE, Harbour C. 2001. Tell me what you mean by "si": perceptions of quality of prenatal care among immigrant Latina women. Qualitative Health Res Nov;11(6):780–94.

Bentley M, Fullem A, Srirak N, Jogelkar N, Khumalo-Sakutukwa G, Mwafulira L, Celentano D, Kelley C, Rosenberg Z, Nelson K. 2000. Acceptability of novel, microbicide BufferGel during a phase I safety trial in Thailand, Zimbabwe, and Malawi. Presentation at the Microbicides 2000 conference, Washington, DC, 2000 Mar 13–16. Abstract in: AIDS 2001 Feb;15(Suppl 1):S30.

Bentley ME, Fullem AM, Tolley EE, Kelly C, Jogelkar N, Srirak N, Mwafulirwa L, Khumalo-Sakutukwa G, Celentano DD. 2004. Acceptability of a microbicide, BufferGel, among women and their partners in a four-country phase I trial. Am J Publ Health 94(7): 1159–64.

Berer M, Ravindron TKS, eds. Safe motherhood initiatives: critical issues. London: Reproductive Health Matters, 2000.

Bernard HR. 1995. Research methods in anthropology: qualitative and quantitative approaches. 2nd ed. Walnut Creek, CA: Altamira Press.

Bertrand J, Brown L, Kinzonzi M, Mansilu M, Djunghu B. 1992. AIDS knowledge in three sites in Bas-Zaire. AIDS Educ Prev 4:251–66.

Blumer H. 1969. Symbolic interactionism: perspective and method. Englewood Cliffs, NJ: Prentice Hall.

Bogdewic SP. 1992. Participant observation. In: Crabtree BF, Miller WL, editors. Doing qualitative research. Vol. 3, Research methods for primary care. Newbury Park, CA: Sage.

Bond KC, Valente TW, Kendall C. 1999. Social network influences on reproductive health behaviors in urban northern Thailand. Soc Sci Med Dec; 49(12):1599–614.

Borgatti SP, Everett MG, Freeman LC. 2001. UCINET V Network analysis software manual. Harvard, MA: Analytic Technologies. Available at: http://lrs.ed.uiuc.edu/tse-portal/analysis/social-network-analysis.

Brown LK, DiClemente RJ, Reynold LA. 1991. HIV prevention for adolescents: utility of the health belief model. AIDS Educ Prev 3(1):50–9.

Bruce J. 1990. Fundamental elements of the quality of care. Stud Fam Plann 21(2):61–91.

Bryman A, Burgess RG. 1999. Qualitative research. 4 Vols. London: Sage.

Buckner BC, Tsui, AO, Hermalin AI, McKaig C. 1995. A guide to methods of family planning program evaluation: 1965–1990: with selected bibliography. Chapel Hill, NC: Evaluation Project.

Burgess RG. 1984. In the field: an introduction to field research. London: Allen and Unwin.

Burrell G, Morgan G. 1979. Sociological paradigms and organizational analysis. London: Heinemann.

Buston K. 1999. NUD*IST in action: its use and its usefulness in a study of chronic illness in young people. In: Bryman A, Burgess RG, editors. Qualitative research. Vol. 3, Analysis and interpretation of qualitative date. London: Sage. p 183–202.

Cabaraban M, Morales B. 1998. Social and economic consequences of family planning use in the southern Philippines. Research Triangle Park, NC: Family Health International.

Cáceres CF. 1999. La (re)configuracion del universo sexual. Lima, Peru: REDESS Jóvenes.

Campbell O, Cleland JG, Collumbien M, Southwick K. 1999. Social science methods for research on reproductive health. Geneva: World Health Organization.

Carey JW. 1993. Linking qualitative and quantitative methods: integrating cultural factors into public health. Qualitative Health Res Aug;3(3):298–318.

Carey JW, Wenzel PH, Reilly C, Sheridan J, Steinberg JM, Harbison K. 1998. CDC-EZ-Text: Software for collection, management, and analysis of semi-structured qualitative databases. Version 3.0. Atlanta: Conwal Incorporated for the Centers for Disease Control and Prevention. Available at: http://www.cdc.gov/hiv/software/ez-text.htm.

Caro DA. 1995. What you count is not what I am: notions of gender in quantitative analysis [unpublished manuscript]. GENESYS Project, U.S. Agency for International Development.

Carr D. 2004. Improving the health of the world's poorest people. Health Bulletin 1. Washington, DC: Population Reference Bureau.

Castle S, Konaté MK, Ulin PR, Martin S. 1999. A qualitative study of clandestine use in urban Mali. Stud Fam Plann 30(3):231–48.

Catania JA, Kegeles SM, Coates TJ. 1990. Towards an understanding of risk behavior: an AIDS risk reduction model (ARRM). Health Educ Q 17(1):53–72.

Cernada GP. 1982. Knowledge into action: a guide to research utilization. Vol. 1, Community health education monographs. Farmingdale, NY: Baywood.

[CERPOD] Centre d'Études et de Recherche sur la Population pour le Développement. 1999. Lorsque l'entourage hésite . . .: résultats d'une étude réalisée dans le district de Bamako. Bamako, Mali: CERPOD.

Cicourel AV. 1973. Cognitive sociology. Language and meaning in social interaction. London: Penguin Education.

Cobas JA, Balcazar H, Benin MB, Keith VM, Chong Y. 1996. Acculturation and low-birth-weight infants among Latino women: a reanalysis of the HHANES data with structural equation models. Am J Publ Health 86(3):394–96.

Coffey A, Holbrook B, Atkinson P. 1999. Qualitative data analysis: technologies and representations. In: Bryman A, Burgess RG, editors. Qualitative research. Vol. 3, Analysis and interpretation of qualitative data. London: Sage. p 165–81.

Cohen, C and Wills TA. 1995. Stress, social support, and the buffering hypothesis. Psychological Bulletin 98(2):310–57.

Communications Initiative Partners Meeting. 2000. Transcript of meeting at the Rockefeller Foundation, New York, 2000 May 15–17. Tapes 9–10.

Cornwall A, Jewkes R. 1995. What is participatory research? Soc Sci Med 41(12):1667–76.

Cortes LM, Gittelsohn J, Alfred J, Palafox NA. 2001. Formative research to inform intervention development for diabetes prevention in the Republic of the Marshall Islands. Health Education and Behavior 28(6):696–715.

Crabtree BF, Miller WL, editors. 1992. Doing qualitative research. Vol. 3, Research methods for primary care. Newbury Park, CA: Sage.

Critical Appraisal Skills Programme. 1998. Critical Appraisal Skills Programme (CASP): Ten Questions to Help You Make Sense of Qualitative Research. Oxford: Critical Appraisal Skills Programme.

Dagron AG. 2001. Making waves: stories of participatory communication for social change. New York: Rockefeller Foundation.

Debus M. 1986. Handbook for excellence in focus group research. Washington, DC: Academy for Educational Development.

Denison J. 1996. Behavior change: a summary of four major theories. Arlington, VA: Family Health International.

Denzin NK. 2000. The practices and politics of interpretation. In: Denzin NK, Lincoln YS, editors. Handbook of qualitative research. 2nd ed. Part 5, The art and practices of interpretation, evaluation, and representation. Thousand Oaks, CA: Sage. p 897–922.

Denzin NK, Lincoln YS, editors. 2000. Handbook of qualitative research. 2nd ed. Thousand Oaks, CA: Sage.

DeVellis BM, DeVellis RF. 2000. Self-efficacy and health. In: Baum A. and Revenson T., editors. Handbook of health psychology. New York: Erlbaum.

Devers, KJ. 1999. How will we know "good" qualitative research when we see it? Beginning the dialogue in health services research. Health Serv Res 34(5):1153–88.

Díaz M, Simmons R. 1999. When is research participatory? Reflections on a reproductive health project in Brazil. J Women's Health 8(2):175–84.

Dickin K, Griffiths M, Piwoz E. 1997. Designing by dialogue: a program planner's guide to consultative research for improving young child feeding. Washington, DC: Academy for Educational Development, Health and Human Resources Analysis Project.

Emmons KM, Thompson B, McLerran D, Sorensen G, Linnan L, Basen-Enquist K, Biener L. 2000. The relationship between organizational characteristics and the adoption of workplace smoking policies. Health Education & Behavior 27(4)483–501.

Eng E, Blanchard L. 1991. Action-oriented community diagnosis: A health education tool. International Quarterly of Community Health Education 11(2):93–110.

Eng E, Parker E. 1994. Measuring community competence in the Mississippi Delta: The interface between evaluation and empowerment. Health Educ Q 21(2):201–20.

Fetterman DM. 1992. A walk through the wilderness: learning to find your way. In: Shaffir WB, Stebbins RA, editors. Experiencing fieldwork: an inside view of qualitative research. Newbury Park, CA: Sage.

Fishbein M, Triandis HC, Kanfer FH, Becker M, Middlestadt SE, Eichler A. 1997 [Original publication 1991]. Factors influencing behavior and behavior change: final report—theorist's workshop. Washington, DC: American Cancer Society. In: Glanz K, Lewis FM, Rimer BK, editors. Health behavior and health education: theory, practice and research. 2nd ed. San Francisco: Jossey-Bass.

Flick U. 1998. An introduction to qualitative research. Thousand Oaks, CA: Sage.

Francis DP, Heyward WL, Popovic V, and others. 2003. Candidate HIV/AIDS vaccines: Lessons learned from the world's first phase III efficacy trials. AIDS 17(2):147–56.

Freudenberg N, Eng E, Flay B, Parcel G, Rogers T, Wallerstein N. 1995. Strengthening individual and community capacity to prevent disease and promote health: in search of relevant theories and principles. Health Educ Q 22(3):290–306.

Gans H. 1968. The participant observer as a human being: observations on the personal aspects of fieldwork. In: Becker HS, Greer B, Reisman D, and others, editors. Institutions and the person. Chicago: Aldine. p 300–17.

Gergen MM, Gergen KJ, editors. 2000. Qualitative inquiry: tensions and transformations. In: Denzin NK, Lincoln YS, editors. Handbook of qualitative research. Part 6, The future of qualitative research. Thousand Oaks, CA: Sage. p 1025–46.

Gilchrist VJ. 1992. Key informant interviews. In: Crabtree BF, Miller WL, editors. Doing qualitative research. Vol. 3, Research methods for primary care. Newbury Park: Sage.

Gittelsohn J, Toporoff EG, Evans M, Anliker J, Davis S, Sharma A, White J. 2000. Food perceptions and dietary behavior of American-Indian children, their caregivers, and educators: formative assessment findings from Pathways. Journal of Nutrition Education 32(1):2–13.

Glanz K, Lewis FM, Rimer BK, editors. 2002. Health behavior and health education: theory, practice and research. 3rd ed. San Francisco: Jossey-Bass.

Glanz NM, Halperin DC, Hunt LM. 1998. Studying domestic violence in Chiapas, Mexico. Qualitative Health Res May;8(3):377–92.

Glaser B, Strauss A. 1967. The discovery of grounded theory. Chicago: Aldine.

Golden-Biddle K, Locke L. 1999. Appealing work: an investigation of how ethnographic texts convince. In: Bryman A, Burgess RG, editors. Qualitative Research. Vol. 3, Analysis and interpretation of qualitative data. London: Sage. p 369–96.

Goldstein E, Wrubel J, Faigles B, DeCarlo P. 1998. Sources of information for HIV prevention program managers: a national survey. AIDS Educ Prev 10(1):63–74.

Greenhalgh S. 1997. Methods and meanings: reflections on disciplinary difference. Popul Dev Rev 23(4):819–24.

Grimes DA. 1999. Communicating research. In: O'Brien PM, Pipkin FB, editors. Introduction to research methodology for specialists and trainees. London: FCOG Press. p 210–7.

Guba EG, Lincoln YS. 1994. Competing paradigms in qualitative research. In: Denzin NK, Lincoln YS, editors. Handbook of qualitative research. Part 2, Major paradigms and perspectives. Thousand Oaks, CA: Sage. p 105–17.

Guest G, McLellan E, Matia D, Pickard R, Fuchs J, McKirnan D, Neidig J. 2004. HIV vaccine efficacy trial participation: men-who-have-sex-with-men's experience of risk reduction counseling and perceptions of behavior change. AIDS Care. Forthcoming.

Harris E, Tanner M. 2000. Health technology transfer. Br Med J Sep 30;321(7264):818.

Havelock RG. 1969. Planning for innovation through dissemination and utilization of knowledge. Ann Arbor, MI: Center for Research on Utilization of Scientific Knowledge, Institute for Social Research.

Heise L, McGrory CE, Wood SY. 1998. Practical and ethical dilemmas in the clinical testing of microbicides. New York: International Women's Health Coalition.

Helitzer-Allen D, Makhambera M, Wangel AM. 1994. Obtaining sensitive information: the need for more than focus groups. Reprod Health Matters May;3:75–82.

Hess DJ. 1989. Teaching ethnographic writing: a review essay. Anthropol Educ Q 20;163–76.

Hogle J, Stalker M, Hassig S, Henry K, Young L. 1994. Conducting effective focus group discussions. Arlington, VA: Family Health International.

Holstein JA, Gubrium JF. 1999. Active interviewing. In: Bryman A, Burgess RG. Qualitative research. Vol. 2, Methods of qualitative research. London: Sage. p 105–21.

Huberman AM, Miles MB. 1994. Data management and analysis methods. In: Denzin NK, Lincoln YS, editors. Handbook of qualitative research. Part 4, Methods of collecting and analyzing empirical materials. Thousand Oaks, CA: Sage. p 428–44.

Hudelson PM. 1996. Qualitative research for health programmes. Geneva: World Health Organization.

Human Interaction Research Institute. 1976. Putting knowledge to use: a distillation of the literature regarding knowledge transfer and change. Los Angeles: Human Interaction Research Institute.

International Committee of Medical Journal Editors. 2003. Uniform requirements for manuscripts submitted to biomedical journals. Available at: http://www.icmje.org.

Janesick VJ. 2000. The choreography of QR design: minuets, improvisations and crystallization. In: Denzin NK, Lincoln YS, editors. Handbook of qualitative research. Part 3, Strategies of inquiry. Thousand Oaks, CA: Sage. p 379–99.

Janowitz B, Holtman M, Hubacher D, Jamil K. 1997. Can the Bangladeshi family planning program meet rising needs without raising costs? Int Fam Plann Perspect Sep;23(3):116–21.

Janowitz B, Jamil K, Chowdhury J, Rahman B, Holtman M. 1996. Productivity and costs for family planning service delivery in Bangladesh: the NGO program. Research Triangle Park, NC: Family Health International.

Kaler A. 2001. "It's some kind of women's empowerment": the ambiguity of the female condom as a marker of female empowerment. Soc Sci Med 52(5):783–96.

Kelle U. 1997. Theory-building in qualitative research and computer programs for the management of textual data. Sociological Research Online 2(2). Available at: http://www.socresonline.org.uk/socresonline/2/2/1.html.

Kelly JA, Somlai AM, DiFranceisco WJ, Otto-Salaj LL, McAuliffe TL, Hackl KL, Heckman TG, Holtgrave DR, Rompa D. 2000. Bridging the gap between the science and service of HIV prevention: transferring effective research-based HIV prevention interventions to community AIDS service providers. Am J Public Health Jul;90(7):1082–8.

Kidder LH. 1981. Qualitative research and quasi-experimental frameworks. In: Brewer MB, Collins BE, editors. Scientific inquiry and the social sciences. San Francisco: Jossey-Bass.

King G, Keohane RO, Verba S. 1994. Designing social inquiry. Princeton, NJ: Princeton University Press. p 26–7.

Kirk J, Miller ML. 1986. Reliability and validity in qualitative research. Newbury Park, CA: Sage.

Kitua AY, Mashalla YJS, Shija JK. 2000. Coordinating health research to promote action: the Tanzanian experience. Br Med J Sep 30;321(7264):821–3.

Knodel J. 1994. Conducting comparative focus group research: cautionary comments from a coordinator. Health Transition Rev 4(1):99–104.

Knodel J. 1997. A case for nonanthropological qualitative methods for demographers. Popul Dev Rev Dec;23(4):847–53.

Koo HP, Woodsong C. 1997. Conceptual model for study of the dynamics and meaning of unintended pregnancy [Unpublished manuscript]. Research Triangle Institute.

Krueger RA. 1994. Focus groups: a practical guide for applied research. Newbury Park, CA: Sage.

Krueger RA. 1998. Analyzing and reporting focus group results. In: Morgan DL, Krueger RA, editors. The Focus Group Kit. Vol. 6. Thousand Oaks, CA: Sage.

Lau RR. 1982. Origins of health locus of control beliefs. J Personality Soc Psych 42(2):322–34.

Lincoln YS, Guba EG. 1985. Naturalistic inquiry. Beverly Hills, CA: Sage.

Lincoln YS, Guba EG. 1999. Establishing trustworthiness. In: Naturalistic inquiry. Chap. 62. Beverly Hills, CA: Sage.

Lofland J. 1974. Styles of reporting qualitative field research. American Sociologist 9(3):101–111.

Machado A. 1997. Proverbios y cantares, verse XXIX. In: Poesias completas. Northford, CT: Elliot's Books.

Mason J. 1996. Qualitative researching. London: Sage.

McLellan E, Strotman R, MacGregor J, Dolan D. 2004. AnSWR users guide. Atlanta, GA: Centers for Disease Control and Prevention. Available at: http://www.cdc.gov/hiv/software/answr.htm.

McLeroy KR, Bibeau D, Steckler A, Glanz K. 1988. An ecological perspective on health promotion programs. Health Educ Q 15:351–78.

Meetoo D, Temple B. 2003. Issues in multi-method research: Constructing self-care. International Journal of Qualitative Methods 2(3):1–8.

Menou MJ. 1993. Measuring the impact of information on development. Ottawa: International Development Research Centre.

Menou MJ. 1999. Impact of the Internet: some conceptual and methodological issues, or how to hit a moving target behind a smoke screen. In: Nicholas D, Rowlands I, editors. The Internet: its impact and evaluation. London: ASLIB.

Merton RK, Fiske M, Kendall PL. 1956. The focused interview: a manual of problems and procedures. 2nd ed. New York: Free Press.

Miles MB, Huberman AM. 1994. Qualitative data analysis: an expanded sourcebook. 2nd ed. Thousand Oaks: Sage.

Miller WL, Crabtree BF. 2000. Clinical research. In: Denzin NK, Lincoln YS, editors. Handbook of qualitative research. Part 3, Strategies of inquiry. Thousand Oaks, CA: Sage. p 607–31.

Mokdad AH, Marks JS, Stroup DF, Gerberding JL. 2004. Actual causes of death in the United States. Journal of the American Medical Association 291(10):1238–45.

Morgan DL. 1988. Focus groups as qualitative research. Newbury Park, CA: Sage.

Morgan DL. 1998. Practical strategies for combining qualitative and quantitative methods. Qualitative Health Res May;8(3):362–76.

Morris LL, Fitz-Gibbon CT, Freeman ME. 1987. How to communicate evaluation findings. Newbury Park, CA: Sage.

Morse JM. 1994. Designing funded qualitative research. In: Denzin N, Lincoln Y, editors. Handbook of qualitative research. Thousand Oaks, CA: Sage.

N6 (Non-numerical unstructured data indexing searching and theorizing) qualitative data analysis program. 2002. Version 6.0. Melbourne, Australia: QSR International Pty Ltd.

Nachbar N, Baume C, Parekh A. 1998. Assessing safe motherhood in the community: A guide to formative research. Arlington, VA: MotherCare/John Snow.

National Bioethics Advisory Committee. 2001. Ethical and policy issues in international research. Bethesda, MD: National Bioethics Advisory Committee.

Nichter M. 1990. Eight stages of formative research: Model developed for the International Network of Clinical Epidemiology. Available as PDF file (3 p) at: http://www.medanthro.net/academic/tools/nichter_formative_research.pdf.

[NVivo] NVivo qualitative data analysis program. 2002. Version 2.0. Melbourne, Australia: QSR International Pty Ltd.

Obermeyer CM. 1997. Qualitative methods: a key to better understanding of demographic behavior? Popul Dev Rev 23(4):813–18.

O'Brien K. 1993. Improving survey questionnaires through focus groups. In: Morgan DL, editor. Successful focus groups. Newbury Park, CA: Sage.

Olesen VL. 2000. Feminisms and qualitative research at and into the millennium. In: Denzin NK, Lincoln YS, editors. Handbook of qualitative research. Part II, Paradigms and perspectives in transition. Thousand Oaks, CA: Sage.

Pan American Health Organization. 1997. Workshop on gender, health, and development: facilitator's guide. Washington, DC: Regional Program on Women, Health, and Development, Pan American Health Organization.

Patton MQ. 1990. Qualitative evaluation and research methods. 2nd ed. Newbury Park, CA: Sage.

Patton, MQ. 1999. Enhancing the quality and credibility of qualitative analysis. Health Serv Res 34(5):1189–208.

Paulson S, Gisbert ME, Quiton M. 1996. Case studies of two women's health projects in Bolivia. Research Triangle Park, NC: Family Health International.

Pedersen D. 1992. Qualitative and quantitative: two styles of viewing the world or two categories of reality? In: Scrimshaw NS, Gleason GR, editors. Rapid assessment procedures: qualitative methodologies for planning and evaluation of health-related programmes. Boston: International Nutrition Foundation for Developing Countries.

Petchesky RP, Judd K, editors. 1998. Negotiating reproductive rights: women's perspectives across countries and cultures. London: Zed Books.

Pino R, Schensul J, Romero M. 1999. The roles of cousins in the social networks of drug-using youth in Hartford. Presentation at the American Anthropological Association annual meeting; 1999 November 17–21; Chicago, Illinois.

Piotrow PT, Kincaid DL, Rimon JG, Rinehart W. 1997. Health communication: lessons from family planning and reproductive health. Westport, CT: Praeger.

Pool IS. 1957. A critique of the twentieth anniversary issue. Public Opinion Quarterly 21:190–198.

Population Council. 1994. Communication strategy: the Africa operations research and technical assistance project II [unpublished manuscript]. Population Council.

Porter RW, Hicks I. 1995. Knowledge utilization and the process of policy formation: toward a framework for Africa. Washington, DC: Academy for Educational Development.

Porter RW, Prysor-Jones S. 1997. Making a difference to policies and programs: a guide for researchers. Washington, DC: Academy for Educational Development.

Potter J, Wetherell M. 1987. Discourse and social psychology: beyond attitudes and behaviour. London: Sage.

Prochaska JO, DiClemente CC, Norcross JC. 1992. In search of how people change: applications to addictive behaviors. Am Psychologist 47(9):1102–14.

Prochaska JO, Redding CA, Evers KE. 2002. The transtheoretical model and stages of change. In: Glanz K, Lewis FM, Rimer BK, editors. Health behavior and health education: theory, practice and research. San Francisco: Jossey-Bass. p 99–120.

Qualitative Research & Publishing (QUARC). 2004. QDA overview. Qualitative Research & Consulting. Available at: http://www.quarc.de/body_overview.html.

Richardson L. 1990. Writing strategies: reaching diverse audiences. Newbury Park, CA: Sage.

Rist RC. 2000. Influencing the policy process with qualitative research. In: Denzin NK, Lincoln YS, editors. Handbook of qualitative research. 2nd ed. Part V, The art and practices of interpretation, evaluation, and representation. Thousand Oaks, CA: Sage.

Rogers EM. 1983. Diffusion of innovations. 3rd edition. New York: Free Press.

Rogers EM, Storey JD. 1987. Communication campaigns. In: Berger CR, Chafee SH. Handbook of communication science. Beverly Hills, CA: Sage.

Ronai CR. 1995. Multiple reflections of child sex abuse: an argument for a layered account. J Contemp Ethnography Jan;23(4):395–426.

Rosenstock I, Strecher V, Becker M. 1994. The health belief model and HIV risk behavior change. In: Clemente RJ, Peterson JL, editors. Preventing AIDS: theories and methods of behavioral interventions. New York: Plenum Press. p 5–24.

Rosenstock IM. 1974. Historical origins of the Health Belief Model. Health Education Monographs 2:328–335.

Rossman GB, Rallis FR. 1998. Learning in the field: an introduction to qualitative research. Thousand Oaks, CA: Sage.

Rothman J. 1980. Using research in organizations. Beverly Hills, CA: Sage.

Rubin HJ, Rubin IS. 1995. Qualitative interviewing: the art of hearing data. Thousand Oaks, CA: Sage.

Rutter M. 1993. Resilience: some conceptual considerations. J Adol Health 14(8):626–31.

Ryan GW, Bernard HR. 2000. Data management and analysis methods. In: Denzin NK, Lincoln YS, editors. Handbook of qualitative research. 2nd ed. Part 5, The art and practices of interpretation, evaluation, and representation. Thousand Oaks, CA: Sage. p 769–802.

Sallis JF, Owen N. 2002. Ecological models of health behavior. In: Glanz K, Rimer BK, Lewis FM, editors. Health behavior and health education. San Francisco: Jossey-Bass.

Schensul JJ, LeCompte MD, Nastasi BK, Borgatti SP. 1999. Ethnographic toolkit. In: Schensul JJ, LeCompte MD, editors. Volume 3, Enhanced ethnographic methods. Walnut Creek, CA: Altamira Press.

Schuler SR, McIntosh EN, Goldstein MC, Pande BR. 1985. Barriers to effective family planning in Nepal. Stud Fam Plann Sep/Oct;16(5):260–70.

Scribner R, Dwyer JH. 1989. Acculturation and low birthweight among Latinos in the Hispanic HANES. Am J Publ Health 79(9):1263–67.

Seidel J. 1998. The ethnograph v5.0: a user's guide. Thousand Oaks, CA: Sage.

Seidel R. 1993. Notes from the field in communication for child survival. Washington, DC: Academy for Educational Development.

Selltiz C, Wrightsman LS, Cook SW. 1976. Research methods in social relations. New York: Holt, Rinehart and Winston.

Shah MK. 1999. Listening to young voices: facilitating participatory appraisals of reproductive health with adolescents. Washington, DC: FOCUS on Young Adults.

Sharma RR. 1996. An introduction to advocacy: training guide. Washington, DC: Academy for Educational Development.

Smith PH, Earp JAL, DeVellis R. 1995. Measuring battering: development of the Women's Experience with Battering (WEB) scale. Women's Health: Research on Gender, Behavior, and Policy 1(4):273–88.

Smith PH, Tessaro J, Earp JAL. 1995. Women's experiences with battering: a conceptualization from quantitative research. Women's Health Issues 5(4):173–95.

Smith WA. 1995. Mass communication for health: a behavioral perspective. Presentation at the National Academy of Sciences Expert Meeting on Reproductive Health, 1995 Jan 25, Washington, DC.

Spencer L, Ritchie J, Lewis J, Dillon L. 2003. Quality in qualitative evaluation: A framework for assessing research evidence. Government Chief Social Researcher's Office, UK National Center for Social Research. Available as PDF file [170 p] at: http://policyhub.gov.uk/docs/qqe_rep.pdf.

Spradley JP. 1979. The ethnographic interview. New York: Holt, Rinehart and Winston.

Steckler A, Ethelbah B, Martin CJ, Stewart D, Pardilla M, Gittelsohn J, Stone E, Fenn D, Smyth M, Vu M. 2003. Pathways process evaluation results: a school-based prevention trial to promote healthful diet and physical activity in American Indian third, fourth, and fifth grade students. Preventive Medicine 37:S80–S90.

Steckler A, McLeroy KR, Goodman RM, Bird ST, McCormick L. 1992. Toward integrating qualitative and quantitative methods: an introduction. Health Educ Q 19(1):1–8.

Stevens WF, Tornatzky LG. 1980. The dissemination of evaluation: an experiment. Eval Rev Jun;4(3):339–54.

Stokols D, Allen J, Bellingham R L. 1996. The social ecology of health promotion: Implications for research and practice. American Journal of Health Promotion 10:247–51.

Strauss A. 1987. Qualitative analysis for social scientists. New York: Cambridge University Press.

Strauss A, Corbin J. 1990. Basics of qualitative research: grounded theory procedures and techniques. Newbury Park, CA: Sage.

Tashakkori A, Teddlie C. 1998. Mixed methodology: combining qualitative and quantitative approaches. Thousand Oaks, CA: Sage.

Tesch R. 1990. Qualitative research: analysis types and software tools. New York: Falmer.

Thomas WI, Thomas DS. 1929. The child in America. New York: Knopf.

Thorngate W. 1995. Measuring the effect of information on development. In: McConnell P, editor. Making a difference: measuring the impact of information on development. Ottawa: International Research Centre.

Timyan J. 1991. Guidelines for gathering qualitative data for HAPA PVO grants project evaluation. Baltimore, MD: Johns Hopkins University, Institute for International Programs, School of Hygiene and Public Health.

Tolley E, Dev A, Hyjazi Y, and others. 1998. Context of abortion among adolescents in Guinea and Côte d'Ivoire. Research Triangle Park, NC: Family Health International.

Tolley E, Nare C. 2001. Access to Norplant removals: an issue of informed consent. African Journal of Reproductive Health 5(1):90–99.

Tolman DL, Szalacha LA. 1999. Dimensions of desire: bridging qualitative and quantitative methods in a study of adolescent sexuality. Psych Women Q Mar;23(1):7–39.

Toroitich-Ruto C. 2000. Assessment of the intervention: was it implemented as intended? Presentation at Conference on Female Condom and STDs: A Community Intervention Trial, May 9, 2000, Nairobi, Kenya.

Tourigny SC. 1998. Some new dying trick: African American youths "choosing" HIV/AIDS. Qualitative Health Res Mar;8(2):149–67.

Trotter RT II. 1997. Anthropological midrange theories in mental health research: selected theory, methods and systematic approaches to at-risk populations. Ethos 25(2):259–74.

Trow M. 1957. Comment on participant observation and interviewing: a comparison. Human Org 16:33–5.

Ulin PR. 1992. African women and AIDS: Negotiating behavioral change. Social Science and Medicine 34(1):62–73.

Ulin, PR, Cayemittes M, Metellus E. 1995. Haitian women's role in sexual decision-making: the gap between AIDS knowledge and behavior change. Research Triangle Park, NC: Family Health International.

Ulin PR, Robinson ET, Tolley EE, McNeill ET. 2002. Qualitative methods: A field guide to applied research in sexual and reproductive health. Research Triangle Park, NC: Family Health International.

[UNAIDS] Joint United Nations Programme on HIV/AIDS. 2000a. Ethical considerations in HIV preventive vaccine research. Geneva: UNAIDS.

[UNAIDS] Joint United Nations Programme on HIV/AIDS. 2000b. Report on the global HIV/AIDS epidemic. Geneva: World Health Organization.

United Nations. 1994. Programme of action for the International Conference on Population and Development. New York: United Nations.

United Nations. 1995. Platform for action of the Fourth World Conference on Women. New York: United Nations.

VanLandringham MJ, Suprasert S, Grandjean N, and others. 1995. Two risky views of sexual practices among northern Thai males: the health belief model and the theory of reasoned action. J Health Soc Behavior 36(2);195–212.

Varga, CA. 1997. The condom conundrum: barriers to condom use among commercial sex workers in Durban, South Africa. Afr J Reprod Health Mar;1(1):74–88.

Wallston KA, Wallston BS, DeVellis R. 1978. Development of the multidimensional health locus of control (MHLC) scales. Health Educ Monographs 6:160–70.

Wang CC. 1999. Photovoice: a participatory action strategy applied to women's health. J Women's Health 8(2):185–92.

Wang CC, Burris M. 1997. Photovoice: concept, methodology, and use for participatory needs assessment. Health Educ Behavior 24(3):369–87.

Webb EJ, Campbell DT, Schwartz RD, Sechrest L. 1966. Unobtrusive measures: nonreactive research in the social sciences. Chicago: Rand McNally.

Weitzman PF, Levkoff SE. 2000. Combining qualitative and quantitative methods in health research with minority elders: lessons from a study of dementia caregiving. Field Methods 12(3)195–208.

Welsh MJ, Feldblum PJ, Kuyoh MA, Mwarogo P, Kungu D. 2001. Condom use during a community intervention trial in Kenya. Int J AIDS STDs 12(7):469–74.

Werner EE. 1993. Risk, resilience and recovery: perspectives from the Kauai Longitudinal Study. Dev Psychopathology 5:303–15.

Williams WC. 1984. The doctor stories. Coles R, compiler. New York: New Directions Books.

Williamson N. 1995. Protecting study participants in social science research versus biomedical research [unpublished manuscript]. Research Triangle Park, NC: Family Health International.

Winch PJ, Wagman JA, Malouin RA, Mehl GL. 2000. Qualitative research for improved health programs: guide to manuals for qualitative and participatory research on child health, nutrition, and reproductive health. Washington, DC: Academy for Educational Development.

Wolcott HF. 1990. Writing up qualitative research: qualitative research methods, No. 20. Newbury Park, CA: Sage.

Wolff B, Knodel J, Sittitrai W. 1991. Focus groups and surveys as complementary methods: examples from a study of the consequences of family size in Thailand. Research report no. 91–213. Ann Arbor: University of Michigan, Population Studies Center.

World Health Organization. 1990. A guide to the use of focus group discussions in sexual behavior and AIDS research. Geneva: World Health Organization/GPA.

World Health Organization. 1996. Revised 1990 estimates of maternal mortality: a new approach by WHO and UNICEF. Geneva: World Health Organization.

World Health Organization. 2000. Preparing a research project proposal: guidelines and forms. 3rd ed. Geneva: World Health Organization.

Xie Z, Gu B, Hardee K. Family planning and women's lives in three provinces of the People's Republic of China. 2000. Final report. Research Triangle Park, NC: China Population Information and Research Center, Family Health International, and the Futures Group.

Yin RK. 1994. Case study research: design and methods. Thousand Oaks, CA: Sage.

Yoddumnern-Attig B, Allen-Attig G, Boonchalaksi W, and others, editors. 1993. Qualitative methods for population and health research. Nakhon Pathom, Thailand: Mahidol University, Institute for Population and Social Research.

The Authors

Priscilla R. Ulin, M.N., Ph.D., is a senior research scientist in the behavioral and social sciences division at Family Health International. She first discovered the power of qualitative methods while conducting survey research in Botswana in 1970. Since then she has combined qualitative and quantitative techniques in research, teaching, and technical assistance in sexual, reproductive, and maternal and child health in the United States and developing countries. A medical sociologist, her focus is primarily on social change and health decision making, especially in relation to the influence of family and community in reproductive health decisions and protection against HIV/AIDS and other sexually transmitted infections and in community participation in research. Dr. Ulin worked in Haiti under the auspices of the Family Health International (FHI) AIDSTECH project, where she used qualitative methods to explore women's sense of vulnerability in the AIDS epidemic. She was the deputy director of FHI's Women's Studies Project, a multinational program of social and behavioral science research, both qualitative and quantitative, on the consequences of family planning for women's lives. In this capacity she also directed research in sub-Saharan Africa on women's strategies to adopt modern family planning in the face of community opposition, on the impact of family planning on women's participation in economic development, and on the influence of family on contraceptive decisions. Dr. Ulin received a master's degree in nursing from Yale University and a doctorate in sociology from the University of Massachusetts at Amherst.

Elizabeth T. Robinson, M.S., is director for information programs at FHI. She manages FHI publications, information dissemination activities, and technical assistance in communications. Since joining FHI in 1985, she has served in various capacities, including as managing editor for FHI's scientific periodicals *Network, Network en français,* and *Network en español;* editor of numerous reports, books, and articles; member of FHI's Gender Advisory Committee; team leader and Web architect for FHI's multilingual Web site; and manager of FHI's international health journalism training and scientific paper-writing programs. She worked on FHI's Women's Studies Project, codeveloping a process evaluation to determine the inclusion of women's advocates in the research process, and has served on interagency working groups on female genital cutting, emergency contraception, and gender. Ms. Robinson has held consultancies with the World Health Organization, the American Social Health Association, and the International Monetary Fund. Prior to coming to FHI, she worked as a journalist in metropolitan New York; Washington, DC; North Africa; and francophone West Africa—experience that provided rich comparisons with qualitative approaches used to study reproductive health. Ms. Robinson received an M.S. in journalism from the Columbia University Graduate School of Journalism in New York and held a fellowship in the Columbia University School of International and Public Affairs Fellows Program.

Elizabeth E. Tolley, M.A., is a senior research associate at FHI and a full-time doctoral student at the School of Public Health, University of North Carolina at Chapel Hill. She was first introduced to the use of qualitative methods for research in health in 1991 while living in Mumbai, India, where she became involved in a project funded by the Ford Foundation and administered by Johns Hopkins University School of Public Health to train Indian researchers in the use of qualitative methods. The project enabled her to learn side-by-side with her Indian counterparts from an internationally recognized team of experts including Dr. Margaret Bentley, Dr. Perti Pelto, Dr. Joel Gittelsohn, and Dr. Moni Nag. Since joining FHI in 1995, she has used qualitative research methods to examine a range of topics, including access to early removal of Norplant, the context of adolescent abortion in West Africa, women's experiences with menstrual changes related to contraceptive use, and most recently the acceptability and long-term use of HIV risk-reduction behaviors, like the use of vaginal microbicide gels. She is especially interested in exploring ways to make qualitative analysis more systematic and rigorous and ways to make qualitative and quantitative approaches more compatible. Ms. Tolley received her M.A. in Social Change and Development from Johns Hopkins University Nitze School of Advanced International Studies.

The Contributors

Sri Moertiningsih Adioetomo, Ph.D., is senior researcher of the Demographic Institute, Faculty of Economics, University of Indonesia. She received her doctorate in demography from Australian National University, Canberra, in 1994. She has conducted research and analysis in demography, population, and related issues; was principal investigator of a study in Indonesia on women's work and women's household autonomy for the Family Health International (FHI) Women's Studies Project; and has published numerous articles on family planning and fertility. From 1998 to 2002 she was the director of the Demographic Institute Faculty of Economics, University of Indonesia. From 2002 to 2003 she served as the deputy coordinating minister for people's welfare in charge of women's empowerment.

Patricia Bailey, Ph.D., has been a researcher with FHI for twenty years, focusing largely on programmatic evaluation in the areas of maternal health, adolescents, and HIV prevention. She is experienced in both quantitative and qualitative research methods and has provided technical assistance to colleagues in the field on study design, sampling, questionnaire development, and data management systems and analysis, using both complex statistical techniques and text analysis. Since 1996 she has focused on safe motherhood efforts, working in Mozambique, Nicaragua, and Peru on Columbia University's Averting Maternal Death and Disability Program, as well as in Guatemala and Honduras with MotherCare and the Maternal and Neonatal Project. As a senior researcher with FHI's Women's Studies Project, she collaborated on a manual for reproductive health providers in Bolivia to incorporate a gender perspective into services and conducted a study of adolescents in Brazil to determine the impact of abortion or motherhood on educational status, self-esteem, and family relationships.

David Bell, M.A., Ed.D., is an educator and psychologist who, since 1992, has worked in community development projects throughout southern Africa. His particular interests focus on empowerment and the role of education in social transformation in developing countries. He is currently assistant professor in international development and social change in the International Development, Community, and Environment Program at Clark University in Worcester, Massachusetts.

Deborah E. Bender, Ph.D., M.P.H., is a professor in the School of Public Health at the University of North Carolina at Chapel Hill. Her research interests focus on reproductive health issues for Latina women in the Americas. She has worked extensively in the Andean region and with immigrant Latina populations in North Carolina. Her methodological strength lies in the integration of quantitative and qualitative methods of data collection. Through this linkage her findings have enriched the validity of women's explanations and strengthened the generalizability of findings related to specific reproductive issues.

Marge Berer, M.A., cofounded and has been the editor of the journal *Reproductive Health Matters* since 1993. She is currently cochairperson of the International Consortium for Medical Abortion. From 1996 through 2001, she served as chairwoman of the Gender Advisory Panel of the Department of Reproductive Health and Research, World Health Organization (WHO). She is also the co-editor of *Safe Motherhood Initiatives: Critical Issues* (Reproductive Health Matters, 2000) and the author of numerous articles about making abortion safe and legal, women, HIV, reproductive and sexual health, and other aspects of reproductive health and rights policies. For the past twenty-five years, she has been a feminist and international advocate for women's reproductive rights.

Lorie Broomhall, Ph.D., is an anthropologist in the Behavioral and Social Sciences Division of Family Health International. She has over twelve years of experience in community-based research related to HIV/AIDS, youth, reproductive health, drug abuse, and gender and sexuality. Dr. Broomhall has designed and participated in ethnographic and formative research studies used to develop programs for prevention of HIV transmission and sexually transmitted infection, family planning, and drug abuse. In addition, she developed and directed behavioral components for microbicide clinical trials and has worked among underserved and culturally diverse populations in sub-Saharan Africa, Latin America, and the United States. Her current work combines qualitative and quantitative methods in reproductive health in Kenya, Uganda, South Africa, and Mexico. She also conducts training in qualitative methods and capacity building for ethnographic research.

Sarah Castle, Ph.D., is a lecturer in the Centre for Population Studies at the London School of Hygiene and Tropical Medicine. She has conducted research for more than fifteen years in Mali, where she first started doing fieldwork on infant feeding and illness management. More recently, her research interests have focused on reproductive health. She is currently involved in setting up and evaluating a peer education program to improve sexual health among the young people of the Mopti region in Mali.

Dina C. Castro, M.P.H., Ph.D., is a researcher at the FPG Child Development Institute at the University of North Carolina at Chapel Hill. She has worked for twenty years in public health and education research and has conducted interventions to improve the quality of life of low-income children and families in her native Peru and in the United States. Her current work focuses on program policies and practices that affect Latino children's and families' access to and use of health and early childhood education services.

Edmond Bagdé Dingamhoudou, a journalist and social worker with the Population Council in Senegal, formerly served at the Centre d'Etudes et de Recherche sur la Population pour le Développement in Bamako, Mali, where he was responsible for communicating and disseminating findings from the institute's regional research.

Baochang Gu, Ph.D., currently serves as deputy executive director and director for international cooperation, China Family Planning Association, Beijing. He is a member of numerous advisory boards and panels on population and reproductive health. Dr. Gu served as principal investigator of a study in China on the effect of family planning on women's lives for FHI's Women's Studies Project. The main topics of his work are population dynamics and fertility trends, family planning and reproductive health, sex ratio at birth and women's status, quality of care and informed choice, and urbanization and migration. He has served as deputy chair and associate professor of the department of sociology, Peking University, Beijing; United Nations Population Fund adviser on population and development to the Democratic People's Republic of Korea; and senior program associate, the Population Council, New York. He received his doctorate in sociology and demography from the University of Texas at Austin.

Theresa Hatzell, M.P.H., Ph.D., is a senior associate in FHI's Health Services Research group. Dr. Hatzell's recent research supports programming and policy formulation regarding the interface between family planning and STI/HIV prevention. Dr. Hatzell has worked in Niger, Ethiopia, Senegal, Democratic Republic of Congo (formerly Zaire), the Philippines, Sri Lanka, South Africa, Kenya, Tanzania, and Madagascar. She earned her doctorate from the department of health policy and administration at the University of North Carolina at Chapel Hill, where she had previously received a master's degree in public health, specializing in maternal and child health.

Barbara Janowitz, Ph.D., is director of Health Services Research at FHI, where she has worked since 1977. In recent years she has concentrated her research on cost analysis and cost effectiveness analysis. Her published work in economics includes a paper exploring the impact of introducing contraceptive implants into the Thailand family planning program, on the costs and outputs of community-based distribution programs in Tanzania, and on the costs of family planning services in Bangladesh. Her work in both Bangladesh and Tanzania included analyses of the costs of programs that provided family planning services to women in their homes. She has worked on studies through FRONTIERS, an operations research program for developing countries, to determine the costs of adding reproductive health services to family planning clinics in Zimbabwe; of improving quality of care in Egypt and

Uganda; of providing reproductive health services to youths in Kenya; of involving men in the maternity care of their partners in South Africa, and through HORIZONS to determine the costs of preventing vertical transmission of HIV. Dr. Janowitz served on the faculty of Kent State University for several years and received her doctorate in political economy from Johns Hopkins University.

Shireen J. Jejeebhoy, Ph.D. is senior programme associate at the Population Council in New Delhi, where she is involved in social science and operations research on various aspects of sexual and reproductive health. Her particular areas of focus have been gender issues and adolescent sexual and reproductive health and development. Her previous work includes *Towards Adulthood: Exploring the Sexual and Reproductive Health of Adolescents in South Asia* (coedited with Sarah Bott, Iqbal Shah, and Chander Puri), *Research Approaches to the Study of Reproductive Tract Infections and Other Gynaecological Morbidities* (coedited with Michael Koenig and Christopher Elias), *Women's Reproductive Health in India* (coedited with Radhika Ramasubban), and *Women's Education, Autonomy, and Reproductive Behaviour: Experiences from Developing Countries.* She holds a doctorate in demography from the University of Pennsylvania.

Naveeda Khawaja, M.Sc., M.P.H., currently works as UNFPA's regional adviser for Behavior Change Communication, Advocacy and Adolescent and Sexual Reproductive Health (ASRH) for the agency's Country Support Services Team for South and Western Asia. Previously, Ms. Khawaja worked as the coordinator of the Technical Alliance for Social Change, Pakistan, a technical resource unit that focused on building nongovernmental and private-sector capacity to use community-based information, education, and communications strategies to improve reproductive health and early child care. Ms. Khawaja has varied experience working with government, nongovernmental organizations, the private sector, and donors. She has held leadership positions on projects and for organizations such as UNICEF; the British Council; MotherCare/John Snow, Inc.; and USAID and has served as a consultant to the Asia Foundation, the World Bank, the World Food Program, and the Marie Stopes Society. She is a graduate of Punjab University with a master's degree in nutrition, was awarded a USAID Jefferson Fellowship, and studied international health and behavioral sciences at Emory University's Rollins School of Public Health.

Kathleen M. MacQueen, M.P.H., Ph.D., is a senior scientist with the Behavioral and Social Sciences Division at Family Health International. A biocultural anthropologist by training, much of her work has been in the area of applied research ethics and HIV prevention trials. Both domestically and internationally, she has collaborated in preparations for HIV vaccine trials, microbicide trials, and most recently the prophylactic use of an antiretroviral to prevent acquisition of HIV. Before coming to FHI in 2001, she spent ten years at the Centers for Disease Control (CDC), where she worked as a researcher and science director in the National Center for HIV, STD, and TB Prevention. She is one of the developers of AnSWR, a CDC-based qualitative data management and analysis software program, and is a strong proponent of research that integrates qualitative and quantitative approaches. She has a doctorate in anthropology from Binghamton University/State University of New York and a master's in public health degree from the Rollins School of Public Health at Emory University.

Susanna Rance, Ph.D., is a researcher and activist affiliated with the organization La Paz in Bolivia. She teaches courses on gender, health, and qualitative research methods. She received her doctoral degree from the department of sociology, Trinity College, Dublin, with a thesis on medical discourse concerning abortion. She teaches courses on gender, health, issues of human rights and citizenship, qualitative research methods, and research ethics. Her publications include books on the family planning debate in Bolivia and on humane treatment in medical education.

Suzanne Smith Saulniers, Ph.D., is a rural sociologist and specialist in gender and development planning. She has worked as a development project and program designer for more than twenty-eight years in Pakistan, Asia, and Africa. She has worked directly in reproductive health projects and in program design, implementation and evaluation in Haiti, Kenya, and the Democratic Republic of Congo (formerly Zaire). At the time of the study described in this book, she served as assistant representative of the Asia Foundation's office in Pakistan. Dr. Smith Saulniers holds a doctorate from the University of Wisconsin in sociology. She taught social research methodology for seven years at Huston-Tillotson College in Texas. She is currently senior gender analyst for the Asia and Near East Technical Support Project for USAID/Asia Near East Bureau at the Academy for Educational Development.

Iqbal Shah, M.A., M.Sc., Ph.D., is a social scientist working with the Department of Reproductive Health and Research at WHO in Geneva. He has worked at WHO since 1985 and is primarily responsible for the implementation of activities on social science and operations research in reproductive health. His recent publications include articles on dynamics of contraceptive use, infant mortality, abortion, condom use, and indicators for reproductive health. His academic training is in sociology, public health, and demography. Prior to joining WHO, Dr. Shah worked for the World Fertility Survey, International Statistical Institute.

Michele G. Shedlin, Ph.D., is principal investigator and deputy director of International and Immigrant Health Research, Center for Drug Use and HIV Research at the National Development and Research Institutes. Dr. Shedlin is a medical anthropologist with U.S. and international experience in qualitative health research. She has consulted for community-based organizations, policy institutions, governmental agencies, and the private sector in program design, evaluation, teaching, and training in qualitative research methodology. Her experience in Latin America and with Latino populations in the United States and her work in maternal and child health, substance abuse, and HIV/AIDS have resulted in numerous reports and publications. Currently, she is the principal investigator of two NIH-funded research projects on Hispanic immigrants and HIV risk (New York) and drug use and HIV risk (Nicaragua) as well as co-investigator of two NIH-funded studies of men who have sex with men and HIV risk behavior.

Nancy Stark, R.N., Ph.D., is a medical anthropologist with experience in international health, particularly maternal and child health and reproductive and family planning decision making. Dr. Stark is currently a research associate and Cancer Control Fellow at Wake Forest University School of Medicine. Her research interests include breast and other reproductive cancers, symptom management, tobacco use in India, and complementary and alternative medicines. Recent publications by Dr. Stark include articles on the effects of lymphedema on the quality of life of breast cancer survivors and issues related to minority accrual to clinical trials.

Allan Steckler, Dr.P.H., is professor of health behavior and health education and associate dean of global health at the School of Public Health, University of North Carolina at Chapel Hill. He teaches graduate courses in qualitative evaluation methods, models of health education practice, organizational change, and diffusion of innovation. Since 1980, Dr. Steckler has been involved in research and evaluation of school and community health programs. Funded projects have included evaluation of school and medical self-care programs in Appalachian West Virginia; a rural health initiative; an evaluation of drug and pregnancy prevention curricula in North Carolina; and smoking prevention curricula in middle schools, funded by the National Cancer Institute. Currently he is a co-investigator of the National Heart, Lung, and Blood Institute project Pathways, which is studying obesity prevention through schools among Native American youth. Dr. Steckler has published widely on public health policy and evaluation, including the book *Process Evaluation for Public Health Interventions and Research,* edited with Dr. Laura Linnan (Jossey-Bass, 2002).

Cynthia Woodsong, Ph.D., a medical anthropologist, is a senior scientist at FHI, where her work focuses on vaginal microbicides; reproductive health, including STIs/HIV; and the provision of comprehensive support to the informed consent process in clinical trials research. She provides assistance to staff at FHI and elsewhere on the use of qualitative methodologies, including integrated and mixed-method designs.

Index

A

B

C

G

H

I

R

S

T